Constitutional Facial
Acupuncture

Content Strategist: Claire Wilson

Content Development Specialist: Catherine Jackson

Project Manager: Julie Taylor

Designer/Design Direction: Miles Hitchen

Illustration Manager: Jennifer Rose

Illustrator: Kinesis Illustration

Cover and author photograph: Neale Albert

Photographs: Janneke Vermeulen

Constitutional Facial Acupuncture

Mary Elizabeth Wakefield

Licensed Acupuncturist, Masters of Science,
Diplomate in Acupuncture, certified by the National Certification
Commission for Acupuncture and Oriental Medicine (USA).
Educator of the Year, American Association of
Acupuncture and Oriental Medicine (USA).

Creator/Instructor of the 2-year International GOLD STANDARD FACIAL
ACUPUNCTURE® Certification Program at Northwestern Health Sciences
University, Bloomington, MN, USA, Creator of the facial acupuncture
elective at Pacific College of Oriental Medicine, New York, NY (2007-2011).
Creator, Diamond Acupuncture Facial™ for 2005 Academy Awards,
Los Angeles, CA, President, Chi-Akra Center and Muse L' Herbal,
New York, NY, USA

Foreword by
Lillian Bridges

President, Lotus Institute, Inc., Issaquah, Washington, USA
Author of Face Reading in Chinese Medicine, Second Edition,
pub. Elsevier ©2012

EDINBURGH   LONDON   NEW YORK   OXFORD   PHILADELPHIA   ST LOUIS   SYDNEY   TORONTO   2014

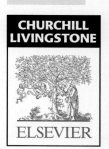

CHURCHILL LIVINGSTONE

ELSEVIER

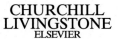

ISBN 978 0 7020 4947 7

British Library Cataloguing in Publication Data
A catalogue record for this book is available from the British Library

Library of Congress Cataloging in Publication Data
A catalog record for this book is available from the Library of Congress

Notices
Knowledge and best practice in this field are constantly changing. As new research and experience broaden our understanding, changes in research methods, professional practices, or medical treatment may become necessary.

Practitioners and researchers must always rely on their own experience and knowledge in evaluating and using any information, methods, compounds, or experiments described herein. In using such information or methods they should be mindful of their own safety and the safety of others, including parties for whom they have a professional responsibility.

With respect to any drug or pharmaceutical products identified, readers are advised to check the most current information provided (i) on procedures featured or (ii) by the manufacturer of each product to be administered, to verify the recommended dose or formula, the method and duration of administration, and contraindications. It is the responsibility of practitioners, relying on their own experience and knowledge of their patients, to make diagnoses, to determine dosages and the best treatment for each individual patient, and to take all appropriate safety precautions.

To the fullest extent of the law, neither the Publisher nor the authors, contributors, or editors, assume any liability for any injury and/or damage to persons or property as a matter of products liability, negligence or otherwise, or from any use or operation of any methods, products, instructions, or ideas contained in the material herein.

ELSEVIER your source for books, journals and multimedia in the health sciences
www.elsevierhealth.com

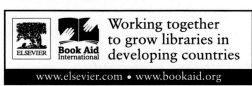

Working together to grow libraries in developing countries

www.elsevier.com • www.bookaid.org

The publisher's policy is to use paper manufactured from sustainable forests

Printed in China
Last digit is the print number: 10 9 8 7 6 5 4 3 2

Contents

Foreword

The face is an incredibly important aspect of identity. We are recognized, evaluated, and scrutinized by the signs on our faces and the expressions that we make. There are simply so many clues about personality and health that can be seen from the face, particularly if you know how to read the lines caused by previous expressions and assess the colors and markings that correspond to organ function. Faces clearly mirror what is going on inside the body and the mind, emotionally, psychologically, and physically.

As a professional Face Reader, coming from the ancient tradition of physiognomy in Classical Chinese Medicine, it is heartening to see my teachings applied by Mary Elizabeth Wakefield in a holistic way. While there are many Acupuncturists successfully treating patients cosmetically, a constitutional acupuncture treatment is more profound and the rejuvenating results are longer-lasting when the constitution is supported and enhanced. She also recognizes and treats the deeper issues underlying the aging face and compassionately guides her patients through the individual transformations that result in changes to their faces. She is now gifting her students with the wisdom of her methods in this book, which is rich with pointers, tips, and advice on how to treat and what to expect, along with detailed treatment protocols.

The modern focus on the face tends to emphasize ideals of perfection – celebrities are judged to have the best features, and magazines and the cosmetic industry create a dread and fear of any signs of aging on the face. This has led to a huge beauty industry that persuades millions of people to change their faces with plastic surgery, injectable fillers, laser resurfacing, and botox. However, these treatments create the illusion of beauty, when real beauty resides in the emanation of the individual spirit, which the ancient Chinese called Shen. The face and the eyes show this spirit through a glow, and removal of the emotional blockages that lodge in the body allows the Shen to manifest.

Mary Elizabeth Wakefield's method allows the patient's Shen to show, which is more important than focusing solely on the specific signs of aging, such as wrinkles. Wrinkles can certainly be lessened with facial acupuncture, but these lines will come back when the patient keeps on using the same expressions until the cycle is altered. Helping patients to understand why they have the lines is critical to the process and I am delighted that Mary Elizabeth's method encompasses this aspect of treatment.

As the Baby Boomer generation now enters its fifties and sixties, there will be ever larger numbers of aging adults seeking to look younger, stay healthier and maintain their attractiveness. Therefore, this will be a growing field and it is the perfect time for Acupuncturists around the world to learn and apply the techniques in *Constitutional Facial Acupuncture* in their clinical practices.

Lillian Bridges

Acknowledgements

"A friend is someone who knows the song in your heart and can sing it to you when you forget the words."
—Unknown

I had no idea what a massive undertaking this book would be, or how long it would take me to complete it! I have been writing this book all over the world, in between my international teaching engagements – from Sydney to London, Zurich, Amsterdam, New York, Minneapolis, Los Angeles, and Vancouver.

There are many friends, colleagues and loved ones that I would like to thank for all of their support, love, knowledge, and generosity, and for their willingness to offer assistance in whatever way they could.

I would not have been able to accomplish this task without the support and expert help from my husband, Michael, who is both a dear friend and collaborator in my seminars, a teacher in his own right, an author, composer, and an exquisite opera singer!

He is my precious companion, love and colleague, who knows and understands the song in my heart. When I have forgotten the words and the melody, been discouraged, doubted myself, or couldn't remember the tune out of sheer exhaustion, due to the accumulated demands of traveling, teaching and writing, he has been there, quite literally, to sing it to me.

He has read, re-typed all my chapters, pre-edited and formatted the text and the photos and e-mailed the final product to Elsevier. I dedicate this book to you, Michael … I am deeply grateful, and feel simultaneously blessed and joyful to have you in my life, both professionally and personally.

I would also like to thank Janneke Vermeulen, acupuncturist, gifted photographer and friend, for the wonderful facial acupuncture photographs. We shot them in Holland under less than ideal circumstances; Janneke, being a perfectionist, with a finely tuned eye, took some gorgeous, clear pictures, which beautifully illustrate the facial needling and the other tools used in the treatment protocols.

Many thanks to my gorgeous model and friend, Ineke van der Ham, Lic. Acup., from Amsterdam, who, with her high cheekbones and gift of natural beauty, made an exquisite model. I am grateful to both of my Dutch colleagues for their humor, patience and willingness to spend the long hours necessary to produce these wonderful photographs for my book.

Neale Albert also deserves thanks for my professional photograph and the excellent photo of the Diamond Acupuncture Facial™ I created for the Academy Awards that grace the book's cover.

Thank you, Deborah Malone, such a beautiful model, for your willingness to take time out from your busy schedule to have these photos taken. It would not have been possible to use these particular photographs without the assistance of Michael Taylor, a fine photojournalist from Australia, who kindly converted them into the CMYK format necessary for inclusion in the book. Tanya Sydney of Illumine Arts deserves a 'Brava' for her beautiful original print of Kuan Yin, which appears in Chapter 1.

My Content Strategist, Claire Wilson, deserves special praise and my gratitude for her patience with me in negotiating my contract, for immediately answering my every question, and for her willingness to mentor me with kindness, reassurance, compassion, clarity and humor. Without you, Claire, I might not have written his book. You are a light and a blessing.

I also wish to acknowledge my Content Development Specialist, Catherine Jackson, who always kept me on track, gently nudged and reminded me to submit all the requisite documents and permissions, as well as the other materials necessary to the publication process. Many thanks to Julie Taylor, my Project Manager, for her positive support during the editing, proofing and printing process, and for placing my manuscript with a wonderful and knowledgeable Copyeditor, Marcela Holmes.

I would like to thank the Elsevier staff who worked on this project for the time and energy that has been contributed to the creation of this book.

Two wonderful colleagues actually encouraged me in the very beginning, when I first conceived the idea of writing a book on my system of facial acupuncture:

Many thanks to my friend and colleague, Lillian Bridges, author of *Face Reading in Chinese Medicine,* who facilitated my connection to the proper channels at Elsevier, and has always championed and supported me. Thank you, Lillian, for your generosity of spirit.

Grazie mille to Giovannia Maciocia for answering my questions, and kindly advising me about the challenges of authoring my first book. It was greatly helpful, Giovanni, and I thank you for sharing your expertise.

Praise and thank yous are very important for my knowledgeable colleagues who looked over various chapters, provided feedback, corrected mistakes and made suggestions regarding edits.

I would first like to acknowledge and thank my fellow acupuncturist and journalist, Abba Anderson, M.S.O.M., L.Ac., who edited the Introduction, Chapter 1, Chapter 3 and the Constitutional Facial Acupuncture protocols in Chapter 7. Thank you for providing practical insights, advice and excellent suggestions for organizing the material.

Special thanks are due to my friend, Anne Harris, L.Ac., M.S.T.C.M., who, many years ago, arranged my very first seminar in northern California, for her detailed, knowledgeable and grounded advice, and special eye to organizing information in a precise and clear format.

Much appreciation to another colleague, Alexis Bennett, L.Ac., M.S., for her creative vision, sense of symmetry, and her understanding of the nature of beauty in words.

Many thanks to Virginia Bell, author and friend, who provided valuable assistance with the initial, more conceptual chapters, and emphasized clarity and communication with the general public, as well as acupuncturists.

I would like to acknowledge Carolyn Bengston, D.A.O.M., L.Ac., who taught me my first intradermal facial protocol at Tri-State College of Acupuncture in New York City, and my colleague, Peggy McMeekin, D.A.O.M., L.Ac., my personal acupuncturist, who ensured that I could escape from the 'human chair' position my body had acquired through sitting and writing for many hours at a time. Also thanks to Peggy for confirming that I have correctly remembered certain protocols in Chapter 4.

Many thanks are owing to Matt Callison, M.S., L.Ac., author and colleague, for encouraging me to set a standard for facial acupuncture, to raise the bar of excellence in this field, and to write a definitive book on this topic. Well, Matt, here it is. I also created a 2-year International GOLD STANDARD FACIAL ACUPUNCTURE® Certification Program, premiering it at Northwestern Health Sciences University (NWHSU) in Bloomington, Minnesota.

I would also like to thank NWHSU for their fantastic facilities and willingness to take a chance on this program. In particular, many 'bravas' to Diana Berg, Director, and Jenny Bell, Conference/Marketing Coordinator, and the rest of the Continuing Education Department, for their confidence in me, and their capacity to move heaven and earth to make the GOLD STANDARD a reality.

I especially wish to thank the students and colleagues who have committed themselves to this GOLD STANDARD FACIAL ACUPUNCTURE® Program.

They have arranged their schedules in order to attend, journeyed to Minnesota from all parts of the globe, and further inspired me with their excitement and enthusiasm for this burgeoning field in Chinese medicine. Thank you for your courage and willingness to undergo this transformational process.

I wish to thank Lin Sister Herb Shop in Chinatown, New York – in particular, the late Susan Lin, Master Herbalist, and beautiful friend, who advised me on my *Muse L' Herbal* topical herbal formulations. Her brother, Frank, my present herbalist, keeps me healthy, generously shares his herbal expertise, and reminds me to be mindful about preserving my vital energies. Thank you for your caring, Frank. I am so appreciative of my Lin Sister extended Chinese family, every one of you.

I would be remiss if I did not thank all my students worldwide, who have faith in me, and the courage to approach facial acupuncture at a more profound level. I continually learn from all of you, and respect your individual wisdom and abilities. I am always happy to see that you are abundant, flourishing and performing Constitutional Facial Acupuncture with skill and a sense of accomplishment.

I have created all these facial acupuncture protocols for my patients, and am honored that they have chosen me to be their practitioner, trusting me to help them. I appreciate your loyalty.

A big thanks to all of the universities, colleges, herbal companies, schools, centers and businesses, conferences and symposiums, which have allowed me to reach out to a wide range of people and practitioners through my teaching. I enjoy collaborating with you, and appreciate your professional support.

I am blessed with a family that has always encouraged my communication skills and creative endeavors. They are writers, artists, musicians, professors, teachers and other professionals, who also have a practical business sense. I am grateful to my late mother, the gorgeous Kathryn Wakefield Bovard, who was a fine writer, artist and a passionate English teacher. Thank you for correcting my grammar and spelling on a regular basis, reading my stories and poems, and encouraging me to write.

Much love and appreciation is due to my late father, Ray B. Wakefield, who was a scientist, musician and teacher. Thank you for supporting my artistic side, and ensuring that I received both voice and flute lessons during my childhood. I still miss your joie de vivre, melodious laughter and passion for life.

Here's to my brother, Ray, a professor of medieval German with unique, innovative communication and teaching skills. Thank you for encouraging me to discover new ways to inspire my students.

I am grateful to my beautiful sister, Barbara, another teacher, who is funny and brave, and who has always encouraged and supported me unconditionally, both in the writing of this book and my other creative ventures.

'Bravos' go to my brother, Bill, who always had a joke to tell me when I was tired or stressed. Thank you for making me laugh and uplifting my spirits.

Much love and thanks to my grandparents, aunts and uncles, all my cousins, nieces and nephews, and extended family, for all of your life force, resilience, and love of laughter and celebration.

Of course, a book might be regarded as an exercise in futility without readers, and I am grateful to all of you who are reading these acknowledgements at this moment. I wish you a pleasurable journey into the world of Constitutional Facial Acupuncture. Perhaps a story in the following pages will touch you; or you will be inspired to try a different way of needling a patient, or incorporate some new facial protocols into your practice.

I do hope that this book motivates you to become an advocate of ageless aging, that it fosters the recognition of a beauty that lies deep within – one of joy, vitality and humility, imbued with a sense of grace.

Mary Elizabeth Wakefield
New York, NY
www.chiakra.com
2013

Constitutional Facial Acupuncture: Changing The Face Of Aging

"Man cannot discover new oceans until he has courage to lose sight of the shore."
—Unknown

There is a growing demand for an organic, natural process of aging that involves not only the treatment of the body, but also the recognition of the mind/spirit connection in the healing process. Constitutional Facial Acupuncture, both an ancient and a revolutionary system, fills this demand, because it links inner beauty and radiance with outer physical balance.

This unique modality empowers and encourages people to reassess how they think about beauty and aging. It also offers a preventative alternative to cosmetic surgery and other invasive procedures, takes an integrative approach to health, and addresses the totality of the individual patient to enhance both beauty and longevity, while simultaneously promoting quality of life and youthful vigor.

We are presently experiencing a quantum evolution in our perceptions of the aging process, which involves the elimination of outmoded ideas about what it means to be elderly. This paradigm shift has been facilitated by half a billion Baby Boomers[1] worldwide, who have provided a powerful stimulus for a collective change to the "face of aging." This is not the previous silent generation, but an outspoken, entitled demographic, which, by force of their sheer numbers, is amending existing conscious and unconscious social contracts.

Why is this dramatic realignment of attitudes occurring at this particular moment in time? Perhaps it is simply a question of critical mass, for example, the "100th monkey" effect, originally formulated by biologist Lyall Watson in his 1979 book, *Lifetide*. In a thought-provoking study, Watson describes the proliferation of an adapted behavior among a tribe of monkeys on the Japanese island of Koshima. Certain members of this group had begun washing sweet potatoes, given to them by Japanese researchers, prior to eating them. However, after reaching a certain threshold, which Watson referred to as the "100th monkey," the entire group began to participate in this ritual.

Even more remarkably, an identical pattern suddenly became apparent on a nearby island, and later on the mainland. These later manifestations occurred without direct contact between the simian collectives.[2] This occurrence lends credence to the idea that innovative ideas possess an archetypal thrust that influences collective behavior on a subconscious level. More recently, biologist Rupert Sheldrake has offered his theory of morphic resonance, in which what he calls morphogenetic fields "work by imposing patterns on otherwise random or indeterminate patterns of activity."[3]

A parallel notion was advanced by author Malcolm Gladwell in his book, *The Tipping Point;* he describes how certain types of fashion trends go from being confined to a small group of innovators to establishing a significant presence in the greater culture. He cites the notable example of Hush Puppies, a style of 1960s shoes that was all but extinct. These antediluvian fashion accessories experienced a hipster revival in the mid-1990s, thanks to the unwitting influence of a small coterie of cool kids in the trendy East Village of New York City. Their sporting of this unconventional and "retro" footwear attracted the attention of famous fashion designers, who later featured the symbolically transformed Hush Puppies in their runway shows. It was only a matter of time before everyone wanted a pair!

However, I would argue that we are dealing with more than just the arrival of either the 101st middle-aged monkey who refuses to go with the program or a coterie of sexagenarians, 60+ year olds, who are following the latest fashion trends. This development is far-reaching in its implications, and seeks to redress a profound imbalance within the societal framework. It reminds us that, prior to the emergence of our global youth-obsessed popular culture, individual merit was assigned based upon contributions to society accrued over several decades of living. Only recently have we have re-configured adulthood as a protracted adolescence, and worshiped at the twin altars of physical attractiveness and youthful perfection.

Moreover, there is a new twist to this reconfiguration of the landscape of aging; 65, once considered retirement age, and the threshold of a period of physical and mental decline, is now being regarded as the beginning of a new, active and creative phase of life.

Around the globe, there are unprecedented numbers of people who regard themselves as middle-aged; in fact, the population of individuals over 50 years of age is the largest in recorded history. With dramatic advances in Western medical technology and a parallel expansion of consciousness about the effectiveness of alternative strategies to promote and maintain optimum health, these prosperous and high-functioning people expect to live longer than their parents, with a level of vitality and enjoyment that would have been considered unrealistic by previous generations.

The impact of this revolution is also beneficial to younger generations, who are observing the Boomers as they actively reject pre-existing beliefs about health, beauty, creativity and vitality being the exclusive property of the young. These trailblazers are pursuing natural, holistic, and less invasive approaches to maintain a youthful appearance without sacrificing their wisdom and integrity. They adhere to a concept of beauty that embraces the totality of their experience, keeps them productive, and authentically transforms body and spirit.

In alignment with these changing attitudes, scientific evidence is emerging to suggest that aging itself may not merely be a function of the biological clock set by our DNA or ancestral Qi. One's self-image, as a product of societal conditioning, may also contribute decisively. According to Dr. Ellen J. Langer, Harvard Professor of Psychology, and author of the international bestseller, *Mindfulness*,[4] unconscious cues involving aging shape how individuals think, dress, act, behave and live.

Dr. Langer's earliest research in this area involved an experimental group of elderly people at a nursing home, who were given decision-making tasks and definite responsibilities. They chose when to water houseplants, how and where to meet guests, whether in their rooms, in the lounge, or outside. In contrast, the members of the control group were given no choices about the arrangement of their daily activities.

The research project lasted only three weeks, however, when Dr. Langer and her researchers returned to the facility over 18 months later, they found that their test patients had remained autonomous, vigorous and sociable, while the control group had lapsed into characteristic apathy and passivity.

More importantly, the changed attitudes and increased responsibility encouraged by the experiment had a beneficial effect upon the target group. They had subsequently demonstrated longer life spans compared to the control group. By providing these nursing home residents with choices and some semblance of self-determination, the experiment compelled them to remain active, which stimulated their mental and physical self-expression. It decisively contributed to both greater quality of life and enhanced longevity.

Dr. Langer cites another innovative study in her most recent book,[5] one which we might call figurative time travel. On this occasion, a group of elderly men, ranging in age from 75–80, was transported to a country retreat, where they remained in isolation and surroundings that evoked a period 20 years earlier. All of the furnishings, books, and movies available to them reminded them of that time in their lives when they were in their physical prime. If individuals from the experimental group chose to reminisce, they were required to frame those recollections in the present tense, as if the events they were "recalling" were, in fact, happening in the moment. The intent of the experiment was to cultivate a less aged mindset, and observe what other effects might result. The test subjects were instructed to immerse themselves completely in the alternative reality.

Conversely, the control group was told to regard their altered living arrangements as rather more anomalous, and not to yield to the illusion of a return to the past. If they decided to share any memories with others, *their* recollections of these experiences were to remain just that, anecdotes of events that had occurred at the time, rather than in an imaginary "now."

After just a week, the experimental group looked 3 years younger; their gait and posture were improved. Joint flexibility and finger length increased. They had gained weight. Their short-term memory had improved, and they were uniformly more positive and energetic in their outlook on life.

The control group also demonstrated an improvement in their appearance, due in part to healthy sleep and some weight gain, but they were not as spry and youthful as their time traveling counterparts. Langer concluded that the impact of turning the clock back was not merely psychological, but also physiological.

The success of Dr. Langer's unorthodox experiment demonstrates for us that it is possible to trick the biological clock by releasing ingrained belief systems about aging, and negative conditioning that may affect us on a subliminal level. Armed with this knowledge, we are empowered to say "no" to limits placed upon our well-being, and to assume greater responsibility for our health.

These studies send a powerful message to us as Chinese Medicine practitioners, because they challenge the complacency of a system that consigns the elderly to a marginal existence of limited productivity and vitality. Not only does this scientific evidence support our innate understanding that every stage of life is one of intrinsic meaning and potential richness, it also calls into question our own choices regarding health and well-being as we contemplate that transition for ourselves.

As acupuncturists, we stand poised to address the concerns of all our patients, both the elder ones *and* the young, who, already primed by popular consensus, fear old age as a time of decline and illness. Metaphorically, we can function as a bridge, straddling the separate worlds of Western medicine and other complementary disciplines.

We are representatives of a medical tradition that has endured for thousands of years, that makes use of both logic and intuitive insight. Oriental medicine is both an art and a science; it respects individual differences and the significance of specific patterns or archetypal imbalances that may arise during the course of treatment. We embrace the inherent paradox of Yin and Yang, the diametrically polar opposites that are also one and the same. Our philosophy emphasizes the Five Phases that arise and flow throughout the entire course of our lives, from our first breath to our final gasp, a transformation from spirit to matter to spirit that mirrors the perennial cycle of Earth's seasons and the evolution of the Universe itself.

Philosophically, we are students of the Mystery and followers of the Way of the Tao as documented in the opening words of the *Tao Te Ching*:

> *"The way that can be mapped is not the Way.*
> *The name that can be named is not the eternal Name."*[6]

As students of the Tao, we know that the healing process is not a linear journey. Our position is unique. We have the capacity, while remaining true to the spirit of our medicine, to facilitate an active and mutually respectful dialogue between a wide range of modalities, and at the same time, to educate potential patients about the possibility of change, which empowers them to make mindful decisions about their own health.

Throughout my many years of instructing practitioners and treating patients, I have found that my system of Constitutional Facial Acupuncture is a wonderful way to support the individual transformational process. The face functions as a natural barometer of the health and well-being of the entire body; with a constitutionally based treatment strategy, we can guide our patients along a path of increased health, and help them to experience greater harmony, inside and out.

Renewal vs. Rejuvenation

> *"I intend to live forever; so far, so good."*
> —Unknown

The cornerstone of my philosophy is the belief that beauty can be achieved at any age. As practitioners, we are not facilitators of a narcissistic quest for the Fountain of Youth. We are, rather, guides that support our patients' processes of change, while simultaneously cultivating renewal and increased longevity in every season of their lives.

While *rejuvenation* is commonly used to describe the results of facial acupuncture treatments, I choose instead, to employ the word *renewal*, because it suggests more than a mere re-attainment of youth as the desired goal.

The noun *rejuvenation* derives from the Latin adjective *juvenis,* meaning *young.*[7] The usage of this particular term in the context of facial acupuncture treatments implies that the sole purpose of rejuvenating the face is to restore youthful features and appearance. In contrast, *renewal* refers to an ability to regenerate, to transform oneself while freshly resuming life after an interval of trauma or change. Therefore, the purpose of *renewal* is to support the evolutionary development of the patient on a spiritual level, not just to make them look younger.

The subtle energetic distinctions between these two concepts affect how we, as practitioners, approach facial acupuncture treatments, and in turn, how our patients view their own transformational journeys.

In my facial acupuncture practice, I have found that patients often seek me out when they have experienced some profound upheaval in their lives. They may have suffered a loss, such as the death of a child, parent, spouse or friend; they may be experiencing empty nest syndrome, as their children leave the home environment for the first time. They may have undergone a break-up of a relationship with a boyfriend, girlfriend, spouse, or significant other. Often, they have received a wake-up call in the form of a genuine health crisis, to which allopathic medicine has no answer.

These situations require them to step outside their normal routines, and can open them to an alternative way of being that holds the potential of authentic transformation.

I treat people of all ages; some of them may not be searching for a way to look younger. However, whatever their expectations may be of facial acupuncture, the outcome is usually more than they anticipated. Each tends to manifest what they need in their lives, as long as they can release outmoded belief systems that no longer serve them, and are willing to surrender to the possibility of change.

I believe that every season of life is rich with significance and the promise of rebirth. Wisdom, the authentic fruit of our having endured the vicissitudes of living, is a blessing, and stunningly beautiful. The freedom and self-understanding that result from this transformative journey allows my patients to exhibit qualities of individual beauty that belie their age or outward appearance. These attributes are manifestations of the most profound depths of soul.

Renewal is a revolution that originates from within. The combustion of Shen spirit, the purest emanation of our heart's compassion, sparks a refiner's fire that blazes outward, illuminating the entire spectrum of our existence.

Therefore, by learning and employing the treatment protocols of Constitutional Facial Acupuncture, you will be able to offer your patients a comprehensive constitutional treatment which is anything but cosmetic, one which views the face as a mirror of the overall health and well-being of the body. It is necessary for us to achieve more than a pretty face as a result of our efforts; my approach seeks to *transform and renew* the original essence and beauty of life.

In the following chapters, I have progressively outlined my philosophy and protocols for Constitutional Facial Acupuncture treatments. There are also learning tools, such as diagrams, charts, drawings, and photographs of the protocol, to aid you in understanding, and later utilizing and integrating this unique system.

Chapter 1 examines the myths around beauty and explores how the conventions and definitions of beauty change in each era, especially for women. Two archetypes of timeless beauty, Kuan Yin and Venus, representative of Eastern and Western perspectives, are introduced, compared and contrasted. We also examine how these powerful archetypes of the divine feminine continue to inform our unconscious notions about beauty.

Chapter 2 discusses and explains "Bodyscapes," the three levels of constitutional treatment – the Jing, Ying and Wei. This is an important component of my Constitutional Facial Acupuncture protocols, and distinguishes it from a "cosmetic-only" approach.

Chapter 3 addresses the Jing level and the Eight Extraordinary Meridians, how they are applied to enhance longevity, and specifically how they are used in my Constitutional Facial Acupuncture treatment protocols.

Chapter 4 focuses on the Twelve Regular Meridians, and provides useful and practical information, including a constitutional treatment protocol, recommended acupuncture points and a consideration of pathology from both a Traditional Chinese Medicine (TCM) and Five Element perspective.

Chapter 5 outlines the Wei level and tendinomuscular meridians. In addressing protective Qi, suggestions are given for various syndromes, like "Coat Hanger syndrome," as well as definitions and usage of "Ashi" and motor points.

Chapter 6 provides all the practical information required for the treatment protocols: contraindications, benefits, required supplies, operational information, treatment length and timeline, managing realistic expectations, maintenance treatments, and the long-term effects of Constitutional Facial Acupuncture.

Chapter 7 introduces the face as the most emotive part of the body, the principle of "the Shen leading the Qi," and the facial landscape, which includes the twelve areas of the face, their muscle function, emotional expression, associated lines and wrinkles, and origin and insertion techniques of the Constitutional Facial Acupuncture treatment protocols. Muscle diagrams and photos highlight each stage of the treatment protocol.

Chapter 8 expands upon the face's expressive role, and how the simple act of needling the face can release hidden, frozen emotions. Because emotions may arise during treatment, Kidney Spirit and the Three Shen points, accompanied by essential oil application, are introduced to support and address psychospiritual issues.

Chapter 9 details strategies for achieving more effective results, including Chinese herbal modular recipes for dermatological issues, that can be customized for each patient, essential oils, hydrosols, jade rollers, and a step-by-step treatment protocol that integrates constitutional and facial needling with these topical herbal preparations.

Chapter 10 provides guidelines and personal recommendations drawn from my 30 years of professional experience, not only to expedite your patients' personal transformation, but also to encourage you on your own journey of renewal and ageless aging.

REFERENCES

1. Current estimate for the worldwide Baby Boomer population is 450 million. Source: http://trendwatching.com/trends/boomingbusiness.htm, quoting MIT Agelab.

2. Watson L. Lifetide. New York, NY: Bantam Books; 1980. p. 147–48.

3. URL: http://www.sheldrake.org/Articles&Papers/papers/morphic/morphic_intro.html; Accessed 07/08/13.

4. Langer EJ. Mindfulness. Cambridge, MA: Da Capo Books; 1989.

5. Langer EJ. Counterclockwise: Mindful Health and the Power of Possibility. New York, NY: Ballantine Books; 2009.

6. Lao-Tzu. (Blakney RB, translator), The Way of Life. New York, NY: New American Library, Inc.; 1955.

7. *Webster's 7th New Collegiate Dictionary*. Springfield, MA: G. & C. Merriam Company; 1972. p. 723.

CHAPTER 1

The Mythic Quest for Beauty

From Venus to Kuan Yin

"The snow goose need not bathe to make itself white. Neither need you do anything to be yourself."
— Lao Tzu

What is beauty, and what does it mean to be called beautiful? The word beauty comes from the Latin *bellus* which means 'pretty,' and is related to the Latin *bonus*, which translates as 'good,' implying that there is goodness in beauty, which can be defined as "the aggregate of qualities in a person or thing that gives pleasure to the senses or pleasurably exalts the mind or spirit."[1]

Therefore, what we regard as beautiful must be cherished; it must please us both esthetically and viscerally, and it must manifest those perfections of harmony that we associate with the divine, a source of ultimate good.

This notion of beauty as embodying goodness implies that naturalness and unselfconsciousness is sufficient to itself. Alex Kuczynski, author of the book *Beauty Junkies*, cites the 16th century *Book of the Courtier*, written by Baldassare Castiglione, in which he opines that for a beautiful woman to seek approval for her beauty renders her less beautiful:

> *"Her manners need to be simple, with natural gestures and an unawareness of others watching her."[2]*

To what degree did the demure deportment of those noble ladies diverge from the narcissism of the icons of today's celebrity culture, with its emphasis on vanity and perfection at all cost, facilitated by today's beautification rituals of cosmetic surgery, Botox and cosmetic fillers?

> *"At age fifty, every man has the face he deserves …"[3]*
> *— George Orwell*

These surgical and pharmaceutical treatments, in addressing the symptoms of aging, casually eliminate individual character in favor of an idealized template of commercialized beauty. This secularization of beauty takes no account of its spiritual dimension, an aspect that embraces both physical aging and the soul's journey through life.

In other words, to erase the lines and change the contour of our faces is a way of obliterating our personal history. But, if we acquiesce to arbitrary standards of physical desirability, we are forced to disconnect from our genetic ancestry and withhold our accumulated wisdom from future generations whom it could benefit.

Antecedents: Beauty in Ancient Greece and Elsewhere

Throughout history, different cultures have adhered to their own particular ideas about the qualities that separate what is beautiful from what is not. In ancient Greece, the chorus of Muses chanted, "Only that which is beautiful is loved." When a question about the nature of beauty was proposed to Apollo's oracle at Delphi, the Pythian priestess responded, "The Most Beautiful is the Most Just."[4] Beauty was not merely associated with physical appeal.

In book 3 of the *Iliad,* the tale of the war between the Trojans and the Mycenaean Greeks, the famed Greek poet Homer views Helen of Troy, the unwitting catalyst for that epic conflict, as innocent of any suffering she might have caused others because of her indescribable physical beauty:

> "…There's nothing shameful about the fact that Trojans and well-armed Achaeans have endured great suffering a long time over such a woman—just like a goddess, immortal, awe-inspiring. She's beautiful."[5]

Following the fall of Troy, Menelaus is about to exact his revenge upon the faithless Helen, but is unmanned when he once again witnesses her beauty, and he drops his sword.

In the classic myth of the Judgment of Paris, Aphrodite persuaded the young Trojan prince, Paris, who was judging a heavenly beauty contest, to award the prize of *kalliste* (most beautiful) to her, passing over her Olympian rivals Athena and Hera. She promised him that, if he awarded her the victory, Helen, the "most beautiful woman in the world," would be his bride. Although Helen was, in fact, the bride of the influential Spartan, Menelaus, Paris, while visiting Sparta under the guise of a diplomatic mission, connived to abduct Helen under cover of darkness, taking her back to Troy. Menelaus, seeking revenge, quickly assembled a huge fleet in retaliation. With favorable winds, they sailed across the Aegean Sea in short order, laying siege to Troy. The long and bitter conflict eventually led to the complete destruction of the Trojan civilization.

Philosophers Weigh In …

The pursuit of beauty is not motivated solely by a romantic or erotic impulse. Great philosophers through the ages have sought to explain the allure of the beautiful in a variety of ways. Like many in the ancient world, Pythagoras and his followers sought the eternal truth of beauty in the celestial symmetries of the heavens, the home of the gods. They established principles of the orderly proportions of musical tone and the Apollonian purity of numerical archetypes so that this celestial perfection could be experienced by human beings here on Earth.

The Classical Greek idea of the Golden Mean, which was derived from the study and replication of the proportions of natural objects, such as the nautilus shell, flowers, and the human body, became an organizing principle in architecture, sculpture, and all areas of art.

Heraclitus, another pre-Socratic philosopher, believed that the elements existed in a state of dynamic balance, and that this perpetual tension created harmony and equilibrium, a philosophy echoed in the Yin and Yang theory of Chinese medicine, in which these seeming polarities support, oppose, overact and become each other.

The revered Chinese philosopher Lao Tzu wrote about the musical intervals as the sound of universal harmony between Yin and Yang. Harmony between apparent dualities can be a hallmark of beauty, and equilibrium between contradictory poles of energy is indispensable to the creation of great art, whether it be music, poetry, architecture, literature, or dance.

For example, in the Italian singing style called *bel canto*, or beautiful singing, the concept of *chiaroscuro* is paramount. This merging of light (*chiaro*) and darkness (*scuro*) refers to the harmonious blending of the Yin and Yang dimensions of an individual voice. A perfectly balanced voice, united in these polarities, flows through the entire vocal range in an effortless dance of unfettered expression and supreme lyricism. The result is a vocal expression that can only be termed beautiful.

The Emanation of Spirit

From the Western perspective, modern words for beauty come from two principal streams: the Latin adjective *bellus* in the Romance languages – Italian, Spanish, French, English – and Teutonic words resembling the modern German word *schönheit*, found in Dutch, Danish, Norwegian, and Swedish usage. *Schönheit* descends from Old German *skôni,* which means 'gleaming' or 'bright.'[6]

This equating of beauty with luminescence suggests that the concept could be associated with celestial radiance. Of all the natural phenomena that ancient humans could have observed, only heavenly bodies appear to emit their own light. Chief among these is the Sun, which, as the ultimate source of all life on Earth, was invariably worshipped for its spiritual essence.

In contrast to 'beauty,' the less common English word 'pulchritude' stems from the Latin adjective 'pulcher.' While 'pulcher' was later supplanted by 'bellus,' scholar Dr. Pierre Monteil wrote in his book *Beau et Laid en Latin* ("Beautiful and Ugly in Latin"), reviewed online in the *American Journal of Philology*, that based on its usage through the centuries, 'pulcher' appears to have referred to a type of beauty that transcends physical form.[7] Hence it might be more properly applied to an ethereal expression of the soul, that is anything but superficial.

The Dictates of Fashion: Personal Taste and Commercial Profitability

Throughout the centuries, feminine loveliness has invariably been a slave to the dictates of fashion. Culture produces a vision of beauty according to social conventions of each era, the individual predilections of a certain artist or poet, or religious dogma. In his book, *The History of Beauty*, Italian author and semi-otician Umberto Eco recounts how standards of beauty have changed through the ages; he documents quite vividly how, as the centuries have passed, the definition of beauty, especially for women, takes on different meanings, connotations and qualities, because of social standards and spiritual underpinnings.

For example, one of the stylistic fingerprints of the 16th century Flemish Baroque painter Peter Paul Rubens, was a depiction of woman as slightly plump, *zaftig*, even voluptuous, certainly if compared to contemporary models. Rubens' conception of these lush, rosy-cheeked, dimpled, earthy goddesses was so influential that today we describe certain women as *Rubenesque*.

In ancient Chinese face reading, it was considered not only a sign of good fortune, but also physically desirable, for both men and women to have firm pouches, called 'money bags,' below the curves of the mouth (St-4 Dicang Earth's Granary). This indicated that the person possessed a reserve of Earth Qi, and had enough stored energy to be able to forage for food, if necessary, and to eat regular meals. According to Lillian Bridges, the ancient Chinese considered this to be:

> "… one of the most important areas of the face, and was very lucky to have. It was considered best when it looked like a peach – soft, plump, pink and fuzzy. The ancient Chinese considered money bags to be the primary warehouse of the face, and it showed someone could accumulate energy or money."[7]

The Gibson Girl was a pen-and-ink drawing created by Charles Dana Gibson in the late 1890s. She was every woman's ideal and every man's dream. Charles Gibson was quoted as describing her as "the American girl to all the world."[8] The Gibson Girl ideal of beauty was characterized by a bouffant hairdo, upswept into a chignon, sexy eyes with thick lashes, high, arched eyebrows, pronounced cheekbones and a strong jaw line. Her figure was full, hourglass-shaped and well formed. The Gibson Girl created the perfect woman, combining traditional female beauty with the spunk and wit of American youth, and was the spirit of the early 20th century.[9]

In the Roaring Twenties and early 1930s, this preference for feminine ripeness completely flipped to the flapper. In contrast to the architectural constructions and prominent bustles of the Victorian era, the flappers wore simple, beaded, short, form-fitting dresses. In spite of their slender, almost boyish figures, they did not surrender their femininity.

In the 1940s and '50s, fashion models were aristocratic and aloof-looking, especially when photographed by Richard Avedon. Hollywood actresses were glamorous, funny, feminine and very much women, shapely and juicy. While they may have occasionally portrayed ingenues, they were in no way adolescent or androgynous, as has been the norm in mainstream cinema for some time.

Goddesses of the silver screen, such as Greta Garbo, Rita Hayworth, Ingrid Bergman, Myrna Loy, Norma Shearer, Vivien Leigh, Olivia de Havilland, Joan Fontaine, Rosalind Russell, Grace Kelly and countless others, are indelible examples of artistic craft and refinement, coupled with an ideal of femininity that celebrated its paradoxical mystery and allure – erotic yet vulnerable, womanly and innocent.

In the 1960s and early '70s, the trend moved to a younger, more casual look, yet still feminine and not wholly youth-driven, exemplified by Audrey Hepburn. However, in the last 20 years, the bar has dropped almost a decade in the fashion world. Adolescence is celebrated at almost every turn, in countless magazine spreads and celebrity gossip rags. The faces are plump with the blossoming of the teen years, featuring pouty lips, and bodies that are more angular and muscled, a paradigm of desirability without precedent.

Some commentators have gone on record as saying that current standards of female beauty violate women's collective self-image. Young women are especially vulnerable to this subtle manipulation, and struggle to conform to the unrealistic standards imposed by the fashion industry and relentlessly reinforced in advertising, movies and television.

Striving to emulate the emaciated appearance of models, the consequences are a plethora of health imbalances related to eating disorders, such as anorexia and bulimia, and overconsumption of diet soda, caffeine and other stimulants. The Internet is also beginning to play a significant role in communicating this disinformation; a new study from the University of Haifa has found that teenage girls who are more active on social networking sites are at a higher risk of developing a negative body image.[10]

In my opinion, this commoditization of beauty masks a thinly veiled misogyny, one in which women are victimized by fashionistas whose principal motivation is to increase the market share for their clothing designs, shoes, perfumes, and other products.[11]

Beautiful = Young and Thin

Prompted by the dual manipulations of fashion and advertising, women of all ages seek the next hot trend or cosmetic procedure that will make them more beautiful – desired and loved. While younger women are stressed in the relentless pursuit of the latest fads so that they may look sexy in every situation, older women submit themselves to cosmetic procedures in order become more youthful.

But this narrow focus is contrary to current demographics worldwide, with aging baby boomers in the vast majority. The baby boomers will create a massive elder population that will have greater longevity than any comparable group throughout recorded history.

And yet, we continue to be controlled by the unreasoning dictates of a youth-obsessed culture that worships young and thin as the *sine qua non* of beauty. These subliminal messages are bad for our health, well-being and self-esteem. Older women are considered invisible unless they have a youthful appearance and are trim and tight from lifting weights at the gym. Men are affected to a lesser extent, but they are still not immune to this skewed perception, and their desirability is greatly enhanced if they do not appear old, tired, or overweight.

> *"How pleasant is the day when we give up striving to be young – or slender."[12]*
> — *William James*

The modern pursuit of the fountain of youth negates the gift of age, wisdom born of experience. The focus on achieving the appearance of unblemished adolescent perfection at the expense of celebrating sage maturity has begun to impact other cultures. Now we witness similar marginalization of people, and particularly women, in their middle and senior years occurring around the world.

I think it is a tragedy that an individual whose face exhibits traces of emotional self-expression and a life well-lived, such as smile lines around the eyes as testimony to a lifetime of laughter and joy goes unnoticed, and the presence of brilliant *Shen* radiating from those eyes is not recognized as beautiful.

My hope is that with education and increased awareness we may transcend these limited conceptions of beauty, and recognize, as the ancients did, that beauty belongs to individuals from every decade. Authentic beauty is ageless and embodies tolerance, compassion, balance and humor. It is an outpouring of the soul beneath the skin.

Two Archetypes of Timeless Beauty

Timeless beauty is the dominion of the collective unconscious, and far removed from any contemporary notion of beauty as the latest fashion trend. Mythological feminine archetypes that embody an ideal of beauty withstand the test of time. These resonant symbols of women's primordial potency remind us that beauty includes in its purview qualities of beneficence, compassion, and wisdom.

> *"Age cannot wither her, nor custom stale Her infinite variety ..."*
> *— William Shakespeare; from* Antony and Cleopatra, *act 2, scene 2*

In turning to these myths for insight, it is important to distinguish between Eastern and Western concepts of beauty. We will examine two embodiments of the divine feminine, the Greek goddess of love, Aphrodite, or Venus, and the bodhisattva Kuan Yin, who is a principal figure in East Asian Buddhist practices that features most prominently in Oriental symbolism, particularly in China and Japan. How do these ancient stories color our psyches, consciously and unconsciously?

Venus: Goddess of Love and Passion

Throughout human history, the planet Venus has been recognized as the brightest star in the heavens, except, of course, for our Sun. Because of its variegated appearance, Venus was seen as an avatar of the triple goddess. She is Maiden who rose every morning renewed in youth and virginity, who waxes into full womanhood as the Mother, and then wanes in power and strength to become the Crone and fade into the darkness of eternal night. The goddess Venus has had many names in many cultures – Inanna, Ishtar, Astarte, Aphrodite – representing love, beauty, fertility, and also war. In her dual nature, Venus encompasses the polarities of birth and death.

Beauty is in the Eye ... Or Perhaps It Isn't

The goddess Venus represents a complex archetype in human consciousness, and it is perhaps because of this complexity that human beings have an ambiguous relationship with her most obvious attribute – physical beauty.

The account of Venus' birth is one of the most striking of Greek myths. Its central image of a goddess emerging from sea foam has captured the imagination of Western man for centuries (Figure 1.1). The physical perfection of female divinity in this myth is a haunting ideal of feminine pulchritude, tantalizing, infinitely desired for its erotic allure. This birth moment presents to

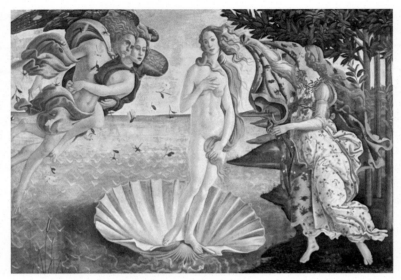

Figure 1.1 The Birth of Venus, Botticelli. Venus' gaze is slightly cross-eyed, which lends her more charm and mystery. She is even more beautiful for her unique imperfection referred to in Italy as the "strabismus di Venere." *Botticelli, Nascita di Venere, Galleria degli Uffizi Botticelli, The Birth of Venus, Uffizi Gallery 1486, tempera on canvas. Reproduced by permission of the Ministero dei Beni e delle Attività Culturali e del Turismo, not be reproduced or duplicated in any media without permission.*

us the *beauty of the eye*, a ravishing vision forever floating just beyond our reach, uncorrupted by the passing of years, a quality to which we can only aspire, infinitely elusive and ephemeral.

We should contrast this artistic rendering of the birth of Venus with her mythic biography, in which she repeatedly demonstrated that she was the least standoffish of the Olympian goddesses. She is characterized by an unambiguous and refreshing eroticism, and gifted with both generous and carnal affection and a complete lack of ambivalence about sex.

Beauty as the Revelation of Inner Life

Unlike most of her divine female relations, Venus/Aphrodite was invariably depicted in the nude, representing a second component of her beauty, that of *revelation*. Her nudity represents the opposite of artifice – it is the simple, direct loveliness of the natural world, all embracing and constantly changing. It is likewise indicative of extreme vulnerability, and ultimately, a manifestation of the inner being, the soul. Venus' radiance, the rays of the Morning Star, is the outpouring of her spiritual essence, the *Ausstrahlung*,[13] which Oriental medicine terms the Shen.

Venus' outer beauty reveals to us something of the inner radiance of the soul. Such luminescence is far removed from a sterile and remote beauty of the eye.

It emanates from the Heart, which is ruled by the Sun, the bright star at the center of our solar system, and the actual source of Venus' light.

Kuan Yin: Beauty Resounds in the Heart

Compared to Venus, Kuan Yin might seem at first to present a very different notion of feminine beauty. Kuan Yin is traditionally viewed as the embodiment of compassion and loving kindness, a bodhisattva who forswore Nirvana, taking a vow to save all sentient beings. She was a goddess who chose to live on Earth until every inhabitant had achieved enlightenment. Unlike her Olympian counterparts, she was free of pride or vengefulness, but like Venus, she mediated between Earth and the heavens (Figure 1.2).

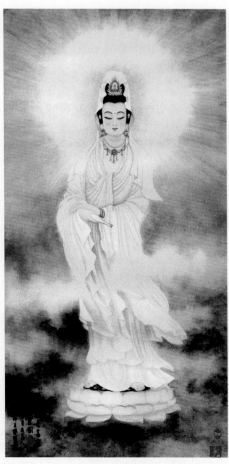

Figure 1.2 Kuan Yin, Goddess of Compassion. Kuan Yin is a benevolent bodhisattva, who is receptive, hearing the troubles of humanity. With her kindness and consciousness, she helps eliminate attachment and suffering. *Reprinted with kind permission of Tanya Sydney, Illumine Arts.*

Kuan Yin's loving compassion was accessible to everyone without dogma or ritual, just as Venus embraced god and mortal alike, qualities that are alluded to in her name, which refers to her ability to be receptive as well.

Embracing Yin and Yang

Kuan Yin was portrayed as her male component Avalokitesvara into the 10th century. The feminine form gradually assumed greater prominence with the introduction of tantric Buddhism into China in the 8th century, during the T'ang Dynasty, and she was invariably depicted as a beautiful bodhisattva in a shimmering white robe. By the 9th century, Kuan Yin's familiar female likeness could be found in every monastery in China.

The seeming contradiction arising from Kuan Yin's hermaphroditic nature, as both god and goddess, is explained in the Lotus Sutra as the capacity to take many forms, and to enter the physical world to bring enlightenment to everyone.

Iconography depicts her in a variety of ways, and each aspect reveals a unique facet of her beautiful and merciful presence. In fact, her beauty, grace and compassion present to us an ideal of womanhood for the East, as does Venus for the West.

Kuan Yin is depicted standing on a tall rock holding a child, which emphasizes her motherly love. She is depicted riding a dragon, with a willow twig in one hand and a bowl filled with the dew of immortality in the other. Sometimes she appears as the thousand-armed goddess, demonstrating her mercy and consolation for all mankind. Most often, though, she is shown as a slender woman in flowing white robes, representing purity, holding a lotus in her left hand. And, while the Oriental esthetic traditionally refrained from illustrations of feminine nudity, Kuan Yin's luminous white robe is almost translucent in some representations, revealing the outlines of her form in a manner similar to Aphrodite's unabashed golden-hued splendor.[14]

Kuan Yin and Venus each symbolize beauty in their unique way, but also have much in common. A synergy of the two forms a bridge between the ancient and modern world, and perhaps more importantly, between the prevailing attitudes of modern Western society and the philosophy that lies beneath Oriental medicine.

Conclusion

How do these two goddesses meet within us on our personal life's journey? I believe that they would reveal themselves to us as a light in the eyes, shining Shen, a spirit of compassionate wisdom, a life lived completely in lusty enjoyment, with a willingness to learn, to be creative, receptive, and to listen with openness and impartiality to others. Most of all, we, as avatars of these goddesses, would not be afraid to walk in the path of maturity, to laugh, to express joy and sorrow, to have smile lines around the eyes, to be expressive, juicy, loving, to age gracefully and beautifully!

In the West, and on a global scale, the pursuit of beauty has become the quest for eternal youth. Increasingly, we perceive life principally with our eyes, always at a safe and comfortable distance from the object of our scrutiny. We have become a civilization of observers, transfixed by the unrealistic images that flood our screens, television, cell phones, iPads, and personal computers.

Saturated with these idealized, carefully manipulated and artificial objects and people, we have little tolerance for reality, with its myriad flaws; consequently, physical perfection is to be maintained at all costs. The slightest wrinkle upon the face, as indicative of character or sign of maturity, is to be erased immediately.

We are a bored, restless culture that fears our own emotions, the chaos of transformation and the possibility of surrendering ourselves to the fierce beauty of the aging process. If we examine the world around us though, we can see that there is beauty in all stages of growth. Are the fiery leaves of autumn any less splendid because they are in the last throes of their death? A star blazes with the intensity of 1000 suns before it winks out of existence.

Oriental medicine reminds us that life is a journey. Without Shen fueling the heart's compassion, animating the spirit, and enlivening the countenance, we are not in harmony with ourselves. To paraphrase the poet Madeleine L'Engle in a poem from her cycle, *The Weather of the Heart*, it is with "our own souls" that we are "out of tune."[15] With our faces frozen by Botox and the natural beauty of our smiles distorted by collagen, we graphically portray our fear of aging and surrender to death, the great void. Ironically, we have all-too-willingly subjected ourselves to the embalmer's art long before the inevitable hour of our mortality. Our unlined faces are mute testaments to an unlived, fearful existence.

Let us, as practitioners, seek out and inhabit a middle ground between these polar attitudes. Let us capitalize on the advances of Western medical science and technology to enhance the quality of individual existence without sacrificing our souls. In embracing the tenets of Oriental medicine, we recognize that our progress on the path is inherently meaningful, and that we are renewed in the continual unfolding of our spiritual destiny. Let us share our vision of aging as an organic pilgrimage, unique to each person, rich with experience and wisdom, and infused with gratitude for the gift of life.

REFERENCES

1. *Webster's 7th New Collegiate Dictionary*. Springfield: G. & C. Merriam Company; 1972. p. 76.

2. Kuczynski A. Beauty Junkies: Inside Our $15 Billion Obsession with Plastic Surgery. New York, NY: Doubleday Books; 2006. p. 103–4.

3. http://www.quotationspage.com/search.php?3Author=George+Orwell@file=other.

4. Eco U. History of Beauty. New York, NY: Rizzoli International Publications; 2004. p. 37.

5. Eco, op. cit., p. 37.

6. Nietzsche FW. The Birth of Tragedy and Other Writings, translated by Ronald Speirs. London, UK: Cambridge University Press; 1999. p. 154.

7. Braunlich AF. Excerpt from American Journal of Philology, vol. 88, no. 1, found at http://links.jstor.org/sici?sici=0002-9475(196701)88%3A1%3C114%3ABELEL%3E 2.0.CO%3B2-0; Internet, accessed 12/12/06 (original unavailable).

8. Bridges L. Face Reading in Chinese Medicine. 2nd ed. London, UK: Churchill Livingstone; 2012. p. 193.

9. Quote found at: http://www.loyno.edu/~kchopin/new/women/gibsongirl.html.

10. Jeffreys S. Beauty and Misogyny: Harmful Cultural Practices in the West. New York, NY: Routledge; 2005.

11. http://www.jpost.com/Health-and-Science/Link-found-between-Facebook-use-and -eating-disorders.

12. James W. The Principles of Psychology. Chapter X, The Empirical Self (1890), found at http://psychclassics.asu.edu/James/Principles/prin10.htm.

13. See http://www.dictionarist.com/Ausstrahlung; this is a German noun that means "radiation, energy radiated in the form of waves or particles, act of beaming or glowing, radiance."

14. In the very first line of his Hymn to Aphrodite, the Greek poet Homer says, "Sing to me, O Muses, of golden Aphrodite!" She is almost invariably described as golden throughout Greek literature. This radiance is almost certainly that of the Sun, without which the planet Venus would have no luminescence.

15. L'Engle, M. To A Long Loved Love: #3, "I know why a star gives light", The Weather of the Heart. Wheaton, IL: Harold Shaw; 1978, p. 12.

CHAPTER 2

Bodyscapes

"Tell me, I'll forget, show me, I will remember; but, involve me, and I'll understand."
— *Chinese proverb*

The Three Levels of Constitutional Treatment

What distinguishes Constitutional Facial Acupuncture from other treatment modalities is the strong constitutional component. I do not refer to my system as cosmetic, or describe it as a 'face lift,' because those words do not take into account the constitutional roots and fundamental principles of Chinese medicine.

The term 'face lift,' for instance, confuses patients, giving them unrealistic expectations about the possible outcome of a single treatment. They will expect, even demand, to experience instantaneous results, like they would with cosmetic surgery.

Constitutional Facial Acupuncture is an organic process that is cumulative in nature, and consequently it works more effectively in a series of sessions. The body needs time to heal and to reabsorb the signs of aging.

The clarity and energy involved in the naming of this protocol is highly significant. Describing a facial acupuncture treatment as a 'face lift' may strike practitioners as a savvy marketing strategy, because the general public will, most likely, be attracted by those words, and immediately book an appointment. However, they will not understand that this constitutional approach to the facial landscape is in no way comparable to a procedure performed by a plastic surgeon.

Some years ago, I was advertised as a facial acupuncturist, without my knowledge, in a magazine in a busy city. My contact information was also provided, without my consent, at the end of a brief article on facial acupuncture. This pamphlet had a huge circulation in the area, because it was readily available in subway stations, on buses, on the river ferries, etc.

In due course, my office phone began to ring off the hook; I would estimate that 150 prospective patients all wanted to make appointments. However, most of them were astonished to learn that I would be treating the body, as well as the face, and that these treatments would involve an investment of time and money.

My assistant and I repeatedly explained to all 150 callers that Constitutional Facial Acupuncture is a unique modality, based upon Chinese medicine principles, and not similar to an esthetician/cosmetologist's treatment or to plastic surgery. To be effective, and to see change, it would be necessary for me to insert needles into their body, as well as their face. This was a rather simple explanation, but I found that more detailed information was simply not understood.

This experience provided me with a learning curve in a number of ways: (1) I wasn't aware that there was so much interest in facial acupuncture at that time; (2) nor did I realize how little the average person knew about Chinese medicine and the constitutional aspects of these treatments; and (3) I was reminded of the importance of clear communication, education and maintaining one's personal integrity in dealing with the general public.

It is crucial to be as accurate as possible in advertising your services, and make certain to emphasize facial acupuncture's constitutionally grounded approach.

In this chapter, we will explore the three constitutional levels of treatment that are featured in the Constitutional Facial Acupuncture protocol. The idea of 'grounding' a facial acupuncture treatment by incorporating these three levels is not a new one. Notable acupuncturists, such as Jeffrey Yuen, Tran Viet Dzung, and his Vietnamese teacher, the late venerable Nguyen van Nghi, are purported to use these multiple levels to support the Jing, ancestral Qi, Ying, post-natal Qi and the Wei, in order to release the exterior.

The number 3 is one that has a great deal of significance from a symbolic perspective. 1 and 2 can be viewed as the archetypal polarities of existence, whether you describe them as Yin/Yang, masculine/feminine, darkness/ light, consciousness/unconsciousness, energy/matter, spirit/body, etc. Three-ness represents a union of these two primal opposites, and thus, at its core, it describes a creative fusion of contraries that results in the birth of something new.

'3' is also regarded as a number of completion for much the same reason; it presents us with a bridge between different realms, as in Heaven, Earth and Humanity. We human beings are very much children of earth, but contained with us is a spark of divine fire. Our feet are firmly planted on the ground, and despite this, through the powers of our intellect and the motivations of our desire to connect with something beyond our everyday existence, we cannot help but reach for the stars. Throughout ancient mythology, we find triumvirates in which the various aspects of the divine are given expression, the Holy Trinity, the Triple Goddess, each of which encodes an essential attribute of the whole.

When you utilize this approach to the constitutional component of facial acupuncture treatments, incorporating the Jing, Ying and Wei, you will be addressing the entirety of your patient's being.

In Constitutional Facial Acupuncture treatments, the acu-points for the three levels – Jing, Ying, and Wei – are selected according to the patient's diagnostic results, and the meridians intrinsic to each. Specific Traditional Chinese Medicine (TCM) patterns and Five Element meridian imbalances are taken into consideration in this diagnostic analysis.

We will begin by examining the Jing level of these treatments, which targets the Eight Extraordinary Meridians, hereditary factors, and their relationship to the endocrine system. In a treatment, the Eight Extraordinary Meridians are the initial factor taken into consideration, because they operate at the level of ancestral Qi and relate to individual genetic heritage. Opening a treatment with the Eight Extraordinary Meridians will help you to more thoroughly anchor your patient's Yang Qi prior to the facial needling.

The Jing Level

In Chapter 3, I go into considerable depth about the Eight Extraordinary Vessels and their general properties, functions, usage, contraindications and cautions, guidelines, and how each individual vessel connects to the face and the emotions constitutionally.

Accordingly, I will not repeat that information here, but, instead, will explain why I utilize these vessels as the principal grounding component in Constitutional Facial Acupuncture treatments.

The Eight Extraordinary Meridians address pre-natal level Qi, promote increased longevity, 'healthy aging,' and also spark cellular memory connected to our genetic blueprint. They are related to Jing and Yuan Qi, both of which are stored in the Kidneys.

Jing, the clearest distillation of essence, is fundamentally linked to the core of our individual identity. A person can increase the level of Jing through healthy consumption of food and nutrition, as it relates to growth and development on a day-to-day basis. However, this is a gradual organic process.

Nevertheless, according to Chinese medicine, you cannot build Yuan Qi – congenital Qi. Although Yuan Qi is similarly housed in the Kidneys, it

15

provides the energy or catalyst that contributes to the manifestation of Jing Qi. A good analogy might be that Jing Qi is the core of an individual's nuclear reactor, specifically, the fuel rods, which provide the energy necessary to sustain a controlled chain reaction, while Yuan Qi is the reactor itself.

Jing Qi flows in cycles of 7 years for women, and 8-year cycles for men. These particular cycles are intrinsically linked to the reproductive life of both the sexes, and their cycles of aging. Consequently, the Eight Extraordinary Meridians have a significant impact upon the endocrine system, and the waxing and waning of hormonal levels throughout an individual lifetime.

Jing is comprised of both pre-natal and post-natal Qi, and therefore it can be slowly enhanced by a balanced lifestyle – diet, exercise, meditation, and acupuncture and herbs, among other treatments.

In treating patients constitutionally, observing their genetic predispositions toward, and attitudes about, aging, it is beneficial to work with them at a deeper level to support Kidney Qi and essence.

The opening/coupling points of these vessels, when needled contralaterally, are sufficient to support and ground the Jing level of the treatment. This approach considers both their intrinsic natures and emotional/energetic and psychospiritual implications.

The English acupuncturist, Royston Low, in his book *The Secondary Vessels of Acupuncture* states "the Eight Extraordinary Meridians, which work at the genetic level, influence and control the production of hormones in the body."[1] Much of the significant research on hormonal balance is the result of the "marriage of Western and Eastern approaches," although little is documented in traditional Chinese medicine.

Significant contributions have been made by adherents of the French acupuncture school – in particular, Jacques Lavier and his colleagues. Other studies have been conducted in Germany and Japan.

Chong Mai/Yin Wei Mai: The Hormonal Effect

This meridian pair is used to address hereditary imbalances. In Chinese medicine, ancestral Qi is considered to be stored in the Kidneys and Chong Mai has its point of origin in this organ. However, according to Low, due to its symptomatology, Chong Mai may, in fact, arise in the adrenal medulla. Low says that "the hormone concerned is adrenalin, which has sympatheticomimetic action, and its use is, therefore, indicated in cases of organ insufficiency, especially in the Heart."[2] Yin Wei Mai has two actions: hormonally, it affects both the thyroid gland and the nervous system, via Ren-22 Tiantu Celestial Chimney. Other recommended points are Liv-14 Qimen Cycle Gate and Sp-13 Fushe Bowel Abode, Sp-15 Daheng Great Horizontal and Sp-16 Fuai Abdominal Lament.

In the Ling Shu, the Chong Mai is described as the 'Sea of Blood.' The points are Bl-11 Dazhu Great Shuttle, St-37 Shangjuxu Upper Great Hollow and St 39 Xiajuxu Lower Great Hollow. Symptoms of these points embrace a subjective feeling of fullness in the body (excess blood) and a 'smallness' in the body (deficient blood).

Chong Mai clearly relates to blood; it has a strong effect on the digestive system, as seen by the association with St-37 Shangjuxu Upper Great Hollow and St-39 Xiajuxu Lower Great Hollow. In the Ling Shu, there is an interesting discussion about Chong Mai's blood and Qi relationship, and the fact that the pathway encircles the lips and mouth:

> "When Blood and Qi are abundant, it causes a flow to the skin and a warming of the flesh. When the blood only is abundant, it pulsates and seeps to the skin and produces fine hairs. So, women at birth have an excess of Qi and an insufficiency of Blood because they have been stripped of Blood in the Penetrating and Conception Vessels, so that the mouth and lips are not nourished, and hair does not grow. Eunuchs have lost their generative muscles (penis and testicles) and have been injured in the Penetrating Channel; the Blood has been stripped from it and not returned, the lips and mouth are not nourished, and consequently facial hair does not grow."[3]

I have included this quote because it relates to hormonal function and illustrates the relationship of Chong Mai and other Eight Extraordinary Meridians to the endocrine system.

Hormonal Effects of Du Mai/Yang Qiao Mai

The Yang Qiao vessel acts on the production of adrenocorticotropic hormone (ACTH), a hormone that impacts the adrenal cortex. The Chinese concept of the Kidney organ relating to the Yin and Yang of the entire body recognizes that this organ system also includes the adrenals. According to Low, the Yang Qiao also acts upon the somatotrophic hormones.

Du Mai, which controls the spinal cord and brain via Du-4 Mingmen Life Gate strengthens the kidney adrenal function, benefits Kidney Yang and nourishes source Qi. A prescription for stimulating cortisone production via acupuncture treatments is to tonify Bl-1 Jingming Bright Eyes.

This acts directly on pre-pituitary to stimulate the production of both gonadotrophic and somatotrophic hormones. SI-3 Houxi Back Ravine, the master point of Du Mai, is a pituitary point, according to Kiiko Matsumoto.

Hormonal Effects of Ren Mai/Yin Qiao Mai

Edema or fluid metabolism in women can be treated by the Yin Qiao Mai via Kid-2 Rangu Blazing Valley, Kid-6 Zhaohai Shining Sea, and Kid-8 Jiaoxin Intersection. The secretion of renin from the adrenal cortex can be affected by these points as well, which also impacts the gonadotrophic center of the pituitary gland.

In menopause, an excess of gonadotrophic hormones is associated with waning sex hormones; the Bl-1 Jingming Bright Eyes point on the Yin Qiao meridian connects the anterior pituitary with the gonads and adrenal cortex.

Royston Low stipulates that the Ren Mai corresponds to aspects of the pelvic parasympathetic ramifications. The use of Ren-9 Shuifen Water Divide, Lu-7 Lieque Broken Sequence and Kid-6 Zhaohai Shining Sea can be especially effective in treating edema.

Hormonal Effects of Dai Mai/Yang Wei Mai

This pairing regulates migraines caused by menstrual imbalances. The Yang Wei Mai affects the nervous system via the Gallbladder and Liver meridians, and the points on the cranium, while the Dai Mai affects the hormonal system. Liv-13 Zhangmen Camphorwood Gate, the front Mu of the spleen, and influential point of Zang, is important because "unemployed sex hormones are neutralized in the Liver."[4] Severe migraines often occur as a result of excess gonadotrophic hormones.

In addition to the above specific applications in the realm of hormonal response, the Eight Extraordinary Meridians are considered to encode fundamental hereditary aspects of the individual, what Oriental medicine terms the Jing; therefore, employing them in the context of a facial acupuncture treatment can have profound impact upon both the visible and implicit symptoms of the aging process, promoting healthy aging, greater quality of life and harmony.

The Ying Level

The Ying level, which targets post-natal Qi and utilizes the Twelve Regular Meridians in the Constitutional Facial Acupuncture protocol, is the second constituent of Constitutional Facial Acupuncture's three-pronged constitutional approach.

The focus here is on nutrition, diet, exercise, sleep patterns, rest and relaxation, creative and emotional expression, and spiritual awareness.

Post-natal Qi is also expressed through the Kidney Qi and essence, which can be slowly cultivated and nurtured, until it flowers into a well-being that radiates throughout the entire system.

While TCM diagnostics focus on Qi, blood and fluids to address this level (the Ying), I also integrate it with the Five Elements and their interaction with the pathology of the Twelve Regulars.

In a typical treatment, I first examine the intake form, and ask the patient all the appropriate questions. I also pay particular attention to whether they have written down their diet – breakfast, lunch, dinner and snacks. It is very telling when the patient leaves this area of the form blank, or only provides me with a few entries. I know that they are not making nutrition a priority, or they are too busy, on a diet, or not eating for some other reason. It is then apparent to me that the Constitutional Facial Acupuncture treatments will not be as effective.

I had an elderly patient several years ago who had just lost her husband of many years. They had been together constantly – working, sleeping and sharing their meals every evening.

An examination of her intake form revealed virtually no details of her diet; upon inquiring further, she told me that she had lost interest in food since her husband's passing. She had shared all of her meals with her husband, and dining together had been one of their enjoyable daily rituals. Understandably, not eating was her way of grieving for him.

Given this lack of sustenance, I knew that I could not help her if she didn't replenish her Qi and blood by eating regular meals. Despite these diminished expectations, I agreed to treat her for a while, and encouraged her to make contact with her circle of friends and permit herself to enjoy meals in a social setting, which she did, briefly.

However, this beneficial change was short-lived, and she went back to her solitary routine without nourishment. Subsequently, because she was essentially depriving herself of vital nutrients, she became so depleted energetically that her body would simply not respond to the treatments.

In continuing to deny herself all but the most minimal sustenance, she was exhausting her natural Jing essence, and not reinforcing her post-natal Qi. I recommended that she consult some other therapists to help her navigate the grieving process, but she showed no inclination to do so. Shortly thereafter, she abandoned her facial acupuncture treatments.

This is a sad story, but it illustrates the necessity for patients to have proper nutrition in order to experience optimum results from facial acupuncture treatments. Without replenishing their Qi and blood, you cannot effect changes in either their constitution or their face.

The Twelve Regular Channels have many functions, but one of the most important is the circulation of Qi and blood. Acupuncture is an art and a craft, one which practitioners can cultivate and perfect in order to treat their patients in the most effective way possible. It balances and restores health by eliciting a dynamic response that re-establishes this vital movement of Qi and blood.

However, repetitive patterns and deeply engrained habits that undermine our innate vitality will eventually drain Jing and negatively impact the organ systems. The external pathways of the Twelve Regulars house the acupuncture points, but the internal pathways connect to the organs. It is important not to overlook this aspect in the treatment process.

In Chapter 4, I will review the Twelve Regular Meridians, emphasizing in particular the internal pathways and their indications. A chart which illustrates the constitutional implications of TCM and Five Element imbalances, and how they impact the process of aging, will be provided, as well as a list of suggested acupuncture points and their indications.

The Wei Level

The Wei Level releases the exterior and is within the purview of the tendino-muscular meridians (TMM). These particular vessels are referred to as tendino-muscular because they travel in the depressions and planes between the muscles and the tendons.

The TMMs are superficial and related to, and named for, the Twelve Regular Meridians. Their pathways can be discerned from the Twelve Regulars by superficial palpitation of the large, band-like muscle areas over the Regular Meridians. When palpated, they may elicit pain or achiness.

They are repositories of Wei Qi and form the body's first line of defense against pathogenic influences. Wei Qi cycles differently in the TMM; it flows in the Yang meridians during the day and the Yin meridians at night.

These are superficial channels and their symptoms are usually limited to muscle, ligament and joint problems. The signs and symptoms of the TMM can manifest as either excess or deficiency. Excess may exhibit itself as pain, spasms, or contracture, whereas deficiency may present as dull achy pain, muscle atrophy, paleness, or possible cold in the affected area.

In the treatment of the Wei Qi level in Constitutional Facial Acupuncture, tight tender, trigger, motor or 'Ashi' points are identified through an assessment of the patient's symptoms, and through palpation. It is possible to release a tight shoulder, which I refer to as 'hanger' syndrome – with tension localized around the GB-21 Jianjing Shoulder Well area – either locally or distally. However, this depends upon what I have ascertained through palpation and my interpretation of the patient's symptoms. I call another presentation 'Wandering Skirt' syndrome, which presents as bloating and tightness around GB-26 Daimai Girdle Vessel.

This and other Wei level treatments will be outlined in Chapter 6. In the meantime, it is important for you to be able to distinguish between trigger, motor and 'Ashi' points. All of these points and areas are effective in releasing the surface and address imbalances in the muscles, ligaments and tendons.

Definition of Motor Points, Trigger and 'Ashi' Points

Motor Points: a motor point is a specific location where nerves enter into muscles. When these sites are needled, the muscle 'fires' and resets its spindles, which is accompanied by a grabbing/gripping action. Information concerning this stimulation of the muscle spindle is then transmitted to the patient's central nervous system (CNS), which then instructs the muscle either to relax, if contracted, or tighten, if flaccid or weak. The patient may feel a subjective sensation that is similar to 'De qi' – an achy feeling, a sensation of heat, or a grabbing of the needle. However, this response has been evoked by the stimulation of the neuromuscular junction, and should not be confused with the arrival of Qi.

Trigger Points: a trigger point is located in tissue that is compressed and tender, and can give rise to referred pain. They are customarily activated when a muscle remains in a shortened position for a long period of time, or has been subjected to repetitive strain or stress.

Dr. Janet Travell recommended the use of a 'snapping palpation'[5] or rolling the trigger point under the fingertips to ascertain whether it elicits a jump, when it refers back to the attachment at the end of the muscle. A special needling technique called 'pecking' stimulates the trigger point in the shortened muscle. The muscle then ripples, or fasciculates, which can release the accumulated tension.

Motor Points vs. Trigger Points
A motor point is usually treated when either a muscle has become atrophied, or it is very tight. As it is a neuromuscular junction, it is needled via an acupuncture point or points; however, it should be recognized that it is an anatomical area characterized by the innervation of muscle. Each area can be in a slightly different place, and the associated 'entry' points will not be the same on both sides of the body or face. It is imperative that the practitioner searches for the motor point, and likewise, recognizes that an individual patient's reaction to the stimulation of motor points may differ from one side of the body to the other. It should also be noted that some patients have slower nervous system reactions to motor point needling.

Some practitioners suggest that motor points and trigger points are identical, but, in my experience, I have not found this to be the case. A trigger point can be located at the site of a motor point, and thus appear to be the same; however, not all trigger points are situated in neuromuscular junctions. Usually, trigger points are located more superficially than motor points when palpated.

The term 'Ashi' refers to a painful point that is tight and tender; these points may not be either trigger points or motor points, and they are palpated locally or distally in the area of pain, aching or tightness.

The Twelve Cutaneous Regions

Prior to our discussion of the Wei level of treatment in Chapter 6, I feel that it is appropriate to include a brief summary of the Twelve Cutaneous

Meridians, because they traverse the most superficial area of the body and represent the skin.

These areas share the same names with the Twelve Regular Meridians, and aid in the circulation of Qi and blood in the skin and the superficial surfaces of the body; however, they have no points of their own. Their more important functions include the circulation of Wei Protective Qi, opening and closing the pores, and supporting immune response. Thus, it can be seen that they relate to Lung Qi.

They prevent the invasion of the body by external pathogens, and act as a defensive barrier between the deeper-lying Twelve Regular Meridians and the outside world. Although the ancient texts do not provide information regarding their role as part of the body's protective arsenal, any skin disorder, such as eczema, psoriasis, acne, hyperpigmentation, growths or urticaria can be included in their particular pathology.

The superficial nature of these skin areas means that they are responsive to therapeutic techniques, like shallow traverse needling, as in threading a needle in the face, plum blossom, cupping, Gua Sha, intradermal needling, moxibustion, massage, medicinal salves, topical herbal masks and poultices, creams and essential oils.

The Cutaneous Regions follow the areas associated with the Six Divisions or Energies, which delineate specific pathological factors derived from climatic changes, such as cold, wind, heat, damp, dryness, and fire. In other words, they are the first line of defense, and circulate Wei Qi throughout the skin and tissue level.

REFERENCES

1. Low R. The Secondary Vessels of Acupuncture: A Detailed Account of their Energies, Meridians and Control Points. New York, NY: HarperCollins; 1984.

2. Ibid.

3. Wu J-N. Ling Shu or the Spiritual Pivot. Honolulu: University of Hawaii Press; 1993. p. 213-214.

4. Low, op. cit.

5. Travell JG, Simons DG. Myofascial Pain and Dysfunction: The Trigger Point Manual, Vol. 1. Baltimore, MD: Williams and Wilkins; 1983.

CHAPTER 3

The Eight Extraordinary Meridians

"The path comes into existence only when we observe it."
— *Werner Heisenberg*

In the past few years, The Eight Extraordinary Meridians have received more attention from the Chinese medicine community and we have witnessed a rekindling of interest, not only in the physical properties, but also the psychoemotional aspects of these vessels.

The idea of fostering physical transformation has a long tradition in Taoist alchemical practices, which preceded the birth of Traditional Chinese Medicine (TCM). In general, alchemical theories worldwide postulate that spiritual essence has become trapped in physical form. The goal of alchemy is to liberate the spirit from matter, and to refine the dross of everyday existence into the gold of the Philosopher's Stone, or the Golden Elixir in Taoist philosophy. In this process, it was believed that the alchemist would achieve immortality.

While in the West this alchemical process involved cooking unrefined matter, such as lead in a furnace called a retort, in Taoist alchemy, the body became the transformational vessel. In the Han Dynasty, 3rd century BCE, *weidan*, or external alchemy, involved consuming toxic minerals, such as sulfur and cinnabar, to transform Shen spirit. Ge Hong, a famous Chinese alchemist, believed that minerals contained the seeds of transformation and immortality.

Later, in the Sung dynasty, 11th century BCE, *neidan*, or inner alchemy, developed from these earlier practices. Toxic minerals were not ingested to the same degree – instead, the redemption of spirit was sought via internal disciplines, such as acupuncture, breath, meditation, and cultivation of the Three Jiaos or the Three Elixir fields.

The rise of Mao Tse Tung and the Chinese Communist Party in 1949 spawned the modern herbalized form of Chinese medicine, which came to be called Traditional Chinese Medicine (TCM). Taoist philosophy and healing practices, including the use of the Eight Extraordinary Meridians, were no longer considered important.

TCM developed after approximately three centuries of Westernization in China, which was initially instituted by missionaries in the Ching Dynasty (AD 1636–1912). Since Western medicine employed more drugs in treating illness, it was only natural that, over time, the use of Chinese herbs was more readily embraced.

As herbal medicine gained in popularity, the more esoteric aspects of Chinese medicine, such as the Five Phases, the 13 Ghost Points of Sun-Si-Miao, the Windows of the Sky points, and other Taoist acupuncture theories – were accorded less respect.

During the Cultural Revolution, Mao Tse Tung attempted to unify the Chinese health system. It is well documented that he exiled valued acupuncturists, scholars and free thinkers, whose beliefs and practices did not conform to his new system. He also burned scholarly books and precious ancient documents. Many of these individuals escaped to Japan, Vietnam, Taiwan, and to the West, transporting their knowledge and documents with them in hopes of preserving the ancient roots and venerable teachings of Chinese Medicine.

In reality, there had never been a traditional practice of Chinese Medicine. Westerners, in their effort to define the new Maoist medicine, assumed it was traditional. Chinese medicine textbooks translated into Western languages erroneously identified Mao's medicine as 'Traditional' Chinese Medicine (TCM).

In the 1970s, the newly instituted Academy of Traditional Chinese Medicine translated *The Barefoot Doctor's Manual, An Outline of Chinese Medicine* and *The Essentials of Chinese Medicine* into other languages, and with these books, the TCM style of acupuncture came to dominate the instruction and practice of Chinese medicine in Western countries.

TCM is only a part of the entire practice of Chinese medicine and treatment but has had a strong presence in our schools and institutions for the past few decades, despite the existence of fine schools that focus on Five Element theory and Taoist traditions.

However, an awareness of the nature and significance of the Eight Extraordinary Meridians and Taoist transformative practices has been preserved with recent concerns about aging and longevity, Western society's fascination with Buddhism, an increase in Western tourists and spiritual seekers visiting Asian countries, and the influence of Chinese medicine masters who escaped from China with their rich knowledge of the original Five Element medicine and its roots.

I personally use TCM in my facial acupuncture practice and in my teaching, because I find it practical and effective in working with my patients and students. However, I also make it a priority to integrate Taoist philosophy, Japanese acupuncture, the Five Elements and especially the Eight Extraordinary Meridians into my treatments, because they address questions of longevity, genetic imbalances, hormones, and problematic conditions that cannot be treated successfully with the Twelve Regular Meridians. These vessels anchor the Jing essence that circulates at a deep level in the body and ground the patient's Yang Qi, which has a tendency to rise to the face in a treatment.

By needling the appropriate master/couple points first, you not only access the Reservoir of Qi, but also can prevent headaches or an exacerbation of pre-existing conditions like hypertension or hot flashes.

The Extraordinary Meridians are a very important constitutional level treatment in my facial acupuncture protocols. I needle the Extraordinary Meridians first, contralaterally, to promote increased longevity, foster healthy aging, and support the patient's genetics.

Some schools of thought advocate needling bilaterally, using two sets of master/couple points; others employ ion pumping cords, which are used in Japanese acupuncture, and some manipulate the needles to tonify, sedate, or to get 'De qi.'

I honor and respect these protocols, but my own personal experience in facial acupuncture leads me to recommend that practitioners needle these vessels sparingly. In ancient Chinese medicine theory, the right Kidney was considered to be the Life Gate, or Mingmen Fire, and the left was the physical kidney. Later, in the Ming Dynasty, Chinese doctors no longer adhered to this theory, and considered Mingmen to be in the 'space between the Kidneys.' Our essence is housed in this 'space between the Kidneys,' and Extraordinary Meridians tap directly into our pre-natal Qi. Therefore, I recommend that the Extraordinary Meridians be used with knowledge of their potential benefits and contraindications, which will be explored later in this chapter.

In Chinese embryology, the Eight Extraordinary Meridians are the first vessels to be formed in the womb at the conception of a child. As the *Wu Chi*, the Oneness of the Universe, separates itself into the duality of Yin and Yang, light and dark, the subsequent union of these two primal polarities engenders the manifestation of everything in the realm of matter, from the largest galaxies – even the Universe itself – to the smallest microbes and beyond that into the realm of subatomic particles. These dual energies, the Cosmic Mother and Father, are present at the birth of each and every human being, and connect us on an alchemical level with the Wu Chi, the stillness and origin of all things.

It is important to remember that these vessels contain our genetic blueprint, and function as a repository for Jing essence, the life spark that reflects our healthy DNA, our destiny and potential in life.

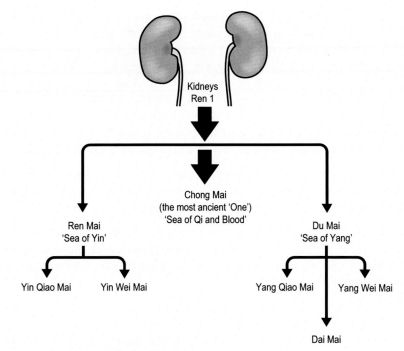

Figure 3.1 Embryological order of the Eight Extraordinary Meridians.

In Figure 3.1, Kidney essences create the Eight Extraordinary meridians, starting with Chong Mai, which is the progenitor, or the oldest, of these vessels. Chong Mai facilitates the birth of Ren Mai and Du Mai, and the other Eight Extraordinary Meridians follow.

Master/Couple Points

Since these vessels influence Jing and are powerful opening points for my Constitutional Facial Acupuncture treatments, I needle the master/couple points with fine 40 gauge 30 mm Japanese needles, with shallow insertion and without manipulation.

I needle with intention and respect; I am grounded and aware of my breath, and I encourage my patients to breathe into their Dantien, as well. I do not force the 'De qi' sensation, but, most of the time, the Qi arrives.

My students are always curious as to whether I needle the Eight Extraordinary Vessels according to gender. Every teacher has a different opinion on this topic, depending on his or her training and studies. Personally, I am not dogmatic, because I know that the ancient texts provide contradictory information on this topic, and their interpretation is further complicated by the particular translation being used.

Also, many authors were involved in writing these documents, over a period of centuries, which further confuses the issue. For me, choosing the master point depends upon the results of my diagnosis, signs and symptoms, the patient's immediate needs, and my intuition, knowledge and experience as a practitioner.

I do needle the master point first, in order to open the Qi of the channel, and then I follow with the couple point. I do not needle the master point according to gender, which, traditionally, is said to be on the right side for women, and the left side for men.

In his book, *The Channels of Acupuncture*,[1] Giovanni Maciocia points out that Sun Si Miao, in his *Thousand Ducat Prescription* (*Qian Jin Yao Fang*), does mention needling by gender, but he did not specifically indicate that this practice should be followed with the Eight Extraordinary Meridians.

The Great Compendium of Acupuncture also recommends needling the master point first and then the couple point, but needling by gender is not discussed. Maciocia further states that the classics do not prescribe the use of master and coupling points according to male and female principles.[2]

I find this information to be liberating, because it frees us from stereotypical considerations of gender in our treatment of these vessels. It is also enlightening to know that, given their profound genetic significance, they are not rigidly defined as being either male or female. As they represent pre-natal Qi, they are formed in the womb even before the sex of the child is determined.

My patients present to me a unique picture of constitutional balance or imbalance each time I see them for an appointment. Of course, there are TCM patterns that manifest constitutionally and which may persist throughout a series of treatments.

Constitutional Facial Acupuncture, while including a consideration of these patterns, addresses each patient as an individual; therefore, I do not treat my patients in the same way every time they come for an appointment. Some acupuncture points may be repeated, but this protocol does not follow a set prescription in which each patient receives the same treatment approach, contrary to their needs. Consequently, it is important for the practitioner to be present, perceptive, and to make intuitive and conscious treatment choices, both constitutionally and facially, each time they see a particular patient.

The Infinity Symbol ∞

In needling the master/couple points contralaterally, i.e., on the opposite side, an infinity symbol, a sacred geometry pattern, is created on your patient's body. For example, by first needling Du Mai SI-3 Houxi Back Ravine as the master point on the right side and the couple point Yang Qiao Mai Bl-62

Shenmei Extending Vessel on the left, and by viewing the patient's navel as the center of a figure eight configuration, the other half of the symbol is energetically completed by the patient's own Qi on the other side of the body.

This completed energetic circuit is specifically related to ancestral Qi and the genetic blueprint of the patient. The number eight has a particular significance in Oriental numerology, and is considered to relate to longevity. In general, by itself, we can view a figure eight as a geometric configuration that has no beginning and no end; hence, it is infinite. Once again, it relates to the alchemical pursuit of immortality.

However, if we lay a figure eight on its side, ∞, it becomes a specialized mathematical symbol known as the lemniscate, which is commonly used to designate infinity. The lemniscate is frequently utilized in esoteric iconography to indicate a certain numinosity, the idea being that the person or thing adorned with it possesses spiritual power and transcendence. Usage of a similar figure has been found in Tibetan rock carvings, and the antecedents of the symbol itself date back to ancient Greece. Some sources suggest that it is analogous to the final letter of the Greek alphabet, omega. It is often compared, as well, to the ancient image of the uroboros, a snake devouring its tail, which has considerable significance in alchemical tradition, and is a potent symbol of death and rebirth. Thus, the invocation of the lemniscate pattern through this contralateral needling of the Eight Extraordinary Meridians is powerfully resonant and transformative.

The fact that a patient will follow through energetically with the completion of the figure 8 on the side of the body that was not needled is a testimony to the intelligence of the human organism, and the natural flow of Qi which self-heals and self-harmonizes. This is why I do not recommend needling both sides of the body, except in rare circumstances, such as injuries on both sides of the body, an imbalance of Yin and Yang Qiao, and the right and left sides of the body, or if there is an indication for bilateral needing in the diagnostics.

Cellular Memory

Because these vessels house inherited ancestral Qi and are related to Jing essence and Kidney Yin and Yang, they also affect cellular memory in the body. I have observed in my practice that when there is a genetic predisposition toward certain illnesses inherent in the family line through the perpetuation of intergenerational patterns, the Eight Extraordinary Meridians may either prevent this illness or keep the symptoms from manifesting.

For example, one of my patients had a tendency to be asthmatic, which she had inherited from her mother. When under stress, she manifested symptoms like wheezing, coughing and dyspnea. This caused fear and panic, and, because she had just lost her mother, grief exacerbated her symptoms.

By opening with the master point Lu-7 Lieque Broken Sequence, and the couple point, Kid-6 Zhaohai Shining Sea, of the Ren channel, at the beginning of the treatment, she was able to keep the asthmatic symptoms from further manifesting, which allowed her to more easily handled the grieving process.

Ren Mai is the Conception Vessel, which governs and opens the Yin of the entire body, and energetically represents the Mother archetype. In the Five Element correspondences, Lu-7 Lieque Broken Sequence relates to the Metal element and may be used to treat grieving issues. To further ameliorate her suffering, I applied cypress essential oil on this point with a Q-tip after I needled it.

Cypress Essential Oil (Cupressus sempervivens)

Cypress is a stately tree of ancient origins and was a familiar sight in cemeteries throughout the Mediterranean region, particularly in Greece and Rome. The oil extracted from the cypress tree was also once an important ingredient in preparations used to treat children with whooping cough. Ancient Chinese physicians would often prescribe an ocean voyage to the isle of Crete for their patients with respiratory ailments, where they would inhale the salubrious aroma of the cypress.

Cypress essential oil is a wonderful restorative for the Lung, and also a sedative, anti-spasmodic, and diuretic. In addition, it has an astringent quality, which reduces excessive phlegm and fluid in the body.

Cypress is a tonic for the Lung, Spleen and Kidney, and is especially effective in the treatment of pulmonary issues like eczema, bronchitis, and tuberculosis. Since time immemorial, the cypress tree has been associated with death and dying; it was invariably found in Greek and Roman graveyards. Cypress wood is virtually indestructible once it is harvested; it does not decay. The ancient Egyptians fashioned their sarcophagi from cypress wood. Cypress invokes the qualities of long life and it is beneficial for those in states of grief, and, similarly, for individuals with weak Lung Qi.

For my asthmatic patient referred to above, I of course used other constitutional body points, Chinese herbs, topical and internal, Kidney spirit points, and some facial points, based upon her needs at the time. However, the constant factor in her treatment was my use of the Ren Mai, the nurturing mother, which evoked deep healing at a cellular level.

The Eight Extraordinary Meridians may also be used to treat past abuse issues stored in the cellular memory. When patients are ready to relinquish these unconscious blockages, the Eight Extraordinary Meridians are very effective in helping them remember the trauma. I view these submerged memories as an emotional pathogen stored in the Reservoir of Qi, which lies deep under the Twelve Regular Meridians. This function protects the patient from extreme distress, if they are not yet ready to remember past violations.

The Chong Mai is the oldest and the progenitor of the Eight Extraordinary Meridians, and can be most effective when used in the treatment of re-emergent abuse or addiction issues. Because Chong Mai rules blood, which is the strongest link between our immediate family members, and past and future generations, it is especially potent in dealing with our genetic blueprint, DNA and cellular memory.

The Meaning of the Eight Extraordinary Meridians

The Eight Extraordinary Meridians (*Qi Jing Bai Mai*) were named for the first time in the *Yellow Emperor's Classic of Internal Medicine* (*Nan Jing*). It is difficult to translate Chinese characters and terms into English because the symbols have many meanings, and interpretation depends largely on context. In Chinese medicine, the words used to describe the Eight Extraordinary Meridians represent both their functions and their individual identity. For example, the word *qi* is used to describe the functional flow of energy in other meridian pathways, but the Qi of the Eight Extraordinary Vessels is unique and exceptional, belonging only to them.

Therefore, I have given you multiple words to describe and explain the special nature of these vessels.

Qi Jing Ba Mai

Qi: Qi represents something unusual, different, exceptional, strange, rare, wonderful, miraculous – something extra, a phenomenon beyond the mundane aspects of reality. This Qi pertains specifically to these meridians. There is a mystery involved in ancestral Qi, in the creation of life, our genetic heritage, and in the birth of a child.

Jing: Jing refers to a channel, an enclosed tubular passageway, a conduit, through which the natural ancestral waterway of Kidney essence flows.

Ba: Ba represents the number eight and specifically relates to longevity, the eight directions of the compass, the Bagua, and to the universal symbol for infinity.

Mai: Mai is a vessel that is not only a pathway, but also a canal, likened to an artery, which allows Jing to circulate through the body.

According to chapter 27 of the *Nan Jing*, the Eight Extraordinary Meridians exist beyond the scope of the Twelve Regular Meridians, and that is the reason why they are called referred to as extraordinary. They have been well

TABLE 3.1 THE EIGHT EXTRAORDINARY MERIDIAN MASTER/COUPLE POINTS

Chong Mai

Master: Chong Mai, Penetrating Vessel; Sp-4 Gongsun Yellow Emperor

Couple: Yin Wei Mai, Yin Linking Vessel; PC-6 Neiguan Inner Gate

Du Mai

Master: Du Mai, Governing Vessel; SI-3 Houxi Back Ravine

Couple: Yang Qiao Mai, Yang Heel Vessel; Bl-62 Shenmei Extending Vessel

Ren Mai

Master: Ren Mai, Conception Vessel; Lu-7 Lieque Broken Sequence

Couple: Yin Qiao Mai, Yin Heel Vessel; Kid-6 Zhaohai Shining Sea

Dai Mai

Master: Dai Mai, Belt Vessel; GB-41 Zulinqi Foot Overlooking Tears

Couple: Yang Wei Mai, Yang Linking Vessel; TH-5 Waiguan, Outer Gate

documented in ancient Chinese texts, such as the *Ling Shu*, the *Nan Jing*, and the *Qi Jing Ba Mai Kao*, written by Li Shi Zhen, among others.

In Table 3.1, master and couple points of the Chong Mai, Du Mai, Ren Mai and Dai Mai are highlighted. Traditionally, the master point is needled first to open up the vessel's Qi, and then followed by the couple point.

General Properties

The Eight Extraordinary Meridians have specific attributes and properties that distinguish them from the Twelve Regular Meridians.

1. They interact with the Twelve Regular Meridians, but do not have an internal/external organ relationship with them, nor do they affect the Zang/fu directly, though they do influence the internal organs. For example: the Lung/Large Intestine meridians are related to the Lung interiorly and to the Large Intestine exteriorly. The Eight Extraordinary Meridians do not have this Yin/Yang relationship.

2. The Eight Extraordinary Meridians have no points of their own, but they borrow points from the Twelve Regular Meridians. The Du Mai and the Ren Mai are exceptions and do have their own acupuncture points.

3. The Eight Extraordinary Meridians are conduits of pre-natal Yuan Qi and derive from Kidney essence.

4. Each Eight Extraordinary Meridian has a master and a couple point. They open and activate two different Twelve Regular Meridians, and treat the indications of these meridians, as well as the Eight Extraordinary Vessel indications. For example, Du Mai SI-3 Houxi Back Ravine treats the symptoms and indications of the Small Intestine meridian, while Bl-62 Shenmei Extending Vessel treats the Bladder meridian's indications. Therefore, Du Mai not only addresses its own meridian imbalances, but it can also address more complicated issues manifesting in the Small Intestine and Bladder meridians.

5. The Qi of these extraordinary vessels does not flow in one direction, but ebbs and flows like the tides. The Ren Mai and Du Mai are exceptions to this tidal movement because their Qi flows up to communicate at the end of their respective pathways when they merge at the frenulum of the upper lip at Du-28 Yinjiao Gum Intersection.

6. The names of the Eight Extraordinary Meridians are indications of their special function, as opposed to the Twelve Regular Meridians whose names relate to organ systems and their Qi functions.

Table 3.2 outlines the names for the Eight Extraordinary Meridians and summarizes their related functions. For example, Chong Mai is called the 'Sea of Blood,' which explains its functional connection with menstrual imbalances, heart issues and blood stasis.

Meridian Functions

The Eight Extraordinary Meridians have specialized functions that distinguish them from the Twelve Regular Meridians:

1.   Reservoir and Storage of Qi

In chapter 27 of the *Nan Jing*, the Eight Extraordinary Meridians' unique reservoir/storage of Qi function is compared to the natural waterways or vessels of the body. In case of an emergency, when pathogenic Qi, like heavy rain, overflows and fills the Twelve Regular Meridians, the Eight Extraordinary Vessels come to the rescue by receiving, containing, and storing this perverse energy. In this way, it no longer circulates in the regular meridians and cannot harm the body.

2.   Protective/Wei Qi

This important function maintains the body's inherent homeostasis by regulating, balancing, and maintaining body temperature, Qi and blood

TABLE 3.2   NAMES AND FUNCTIONS OF THE EIGHT EXTRAORDINARY MERIDIANS

Vessel	Name(s)	Function
Chong Mai	The Penetrating Vessel, Vital Passage, the Sea of Blood	Regulates the flow of Qi and blood in the regular meridians; relates to blood, the Heart, gynecological and digestive issues, as well as imbalances of the front of the body
Du Mai	The Governing Vessel, the Directing Vessel, the Sea of Yang meridian	Governs the Qi of all Yang meridians; related to the brain, spinal column and the back of the body
Ren Mai	The Conception Vessel, which fosters responsibility; the Sea of Yin meridian	Receives and carries the Qi of all Yin meridians; related to reproductive, urogenital and breathing functions, and the front of the body
Dai Mai	The Belt or Girdle Vessel	It binds up all the Regular Meridians; the only channel that horizontally binds all the meridians together. It relates to damp heat issues such as leucorrhea, and rules opposite side, lower and upper extremity imbalances
Yin Wei Mai	The Yin Linking Vessel, which means connection or network	Maintains the balance of Yin throughout the body; dominates the interior of the body
Yang Wei Mai	The Yang Linking Vessel; connects and networks	Maintains the balance of Yang throughout the body; dominates the exterior of the body
Yin Qiao Mai	The Yin heel vessel; relates to movement of the lower extremities, and the left and right sides of the body	Agility and motion of the lower limbs, on the inside of the heel; also balances sleep cycles by closing the eyes
Yang Qiao Mai	The Yang heel vessel; relates to movement of the lower extremities, and the left and right sides of the body	Agility and motion of the lower limbs, on the outside of the heel; controls sleep cycles by opening the eyes

circulation, metabolism and other transformational processes that ensure health and well-being.

Wei Qi externally activates the space between the Kidneys and between the muscles to warm the organs and protect them from external pathogens; the body is then fortified with Protective/Wei Qi and nutritive Ying Qi.

Wei and Ying Qi work in tandem with the Reservoir of Qi function to isolate pathogenic Qi, drain it into the reservoir, and then store it to keep the body safe from harm.

3. Pre-Natal Yuan Qi and Jing Essence

The Eight Extraordinary Meridians are derived directly or indirectly from Kidney Jing, and circulate essence throughout the body. There is a Chinese saying that it takes 40 parts of blood to replenish one part of Jing. Hence, it takes quite a bit of time to generate this distilled essence, and a little drop of Jing is a precious commodity indeed. Both Yuan Qi and Jing Qi represent ancestral Qi. However, in my understanding, there is a slight difference between these two pre-natal Qi essences.

a. Yuan Qi is considered more static, resides in the lower Dantien, and regulates the embryo's development before birth.

b. Jing Qi is more vibrant, is stored in the Kidneys, and regulates the baby's development after birth. Jing Qi also circulates in the vessels, but is beneficially influenced by proper diet and food intake.

In other words, Jing Qi relates to Ying post-natal Qi, and can eventually be replenished by food, drink, a healthy diet, rest, exercise, and balanced emotions. According to Chinese medicine philosophy, Yuan Qi cannot be augmented or fundamentally altered. The good news is that the Eight Extraordinary Meridians are comprised of Jing Qi, which can slowly be replenished by life style changes. We are not totally controlled by our genetics, or pre-natal Qi, but have a choice in how we live our lives.

4. Regulates Life Cycles and Aging

The life cycles of 7 years for women and 8 years for men are described in chapter 1 of the *Su Wen, Simple Questions*. These cycles pertain to the endocrine glands and maturation of the reproductive cycle in both sexes. They specifically relate to the Chong, Du and Ren Mai vessels, because these channels all originate in the lower abdomen, or in the uterus or prostate.

5. The Curious Organs

The Eight Extraordinary Vessels have a connection to the internal organs via the Curious Hollow organs, which store and nourish essence and blood. Because the Eight Extraordinary Meridians are fed directly by Kidney Jing and circulate Jing throughout the body, they also supply the Curious Organs.

The circle in Figure 3.2 illustrates the powerful connection between the Curious Organs and the Eight Extraordinary Meridians as repositories of Kidney essence.

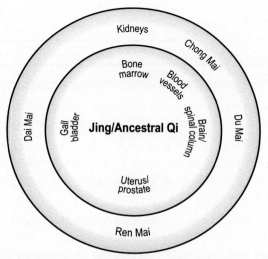

Figure 3.2 The Curious Organs' connection to Eight Extraordinary Meridians and Kidney Jing.

6. Hereditary Imbalances

The Eight Extraordinary Vessels can lessen, or even heal, inherited imbalances or patterns through their linkages with pre-natal Qi, Kidney Jing, and the endocrine system via the principle of Qi, blood and fluids.

In the treatment of children, the Eight Extraordinary Vessels can be used to promote growth, and address deep-seated constitutional issues. Du Mai is especially recommended for physical and mental retardation.

7. Trauma and Shock

The Eight Extraordinary Vessels maintain homeostatic balance in the body by storing, regulating and receiving excess pathogenic Qi, balancing body temperature and metabolism, and supporting Qi, blood and fluids. Because of these functions, they prevent dispersion of Qi in the body during trauma and severe shock, or an invasion of toxins, poisons and other environmental pollutants.

SUMMARY OF GENERAL FUNCTIONS

- Reservoir and storage of Qi
- Wei Qi protection
- Yuan Qi vs. Jing essence
- Life cycles of 7 and 8
- Connection with Curious Organs
- Hereditary imbalances
- Trauma and shock

General Usage

It is important to have guidelines and cautions regarding the use of the Eight Extraordinary Meridians in a treatment protocol. There are a number of different schools of thought on the use of the Eight Extraordinary Meridians and I do not profess that my particular philosophy and approach is the only one that is appropriate.

However, in the context of my treatment protocols in Constitutional Facial Acupuncture, and drawing upon many years of experience in this particular modality, I am happy to share my own insights, and give you some helpful guidelines about usage:

1. Use the Eight Extraordinary Meridians when the Regular Meridians are not working, i.e., you've treated the patient many times and nothing is changing. When a patient isn't responding to treatment with the Regular Meridians, use an Eight Extraordinary Meridian associated with similar symptoms and has points related to those of the Regular Meridian in question. You can also drain an excess Regular Meridian into the Eight Extraordinary Meridian's Reservoir of Qi. This will permit the Eight Extraordinary Meridians to either store, move, regulate or hold pathogenic Qi in check.

2. Use the Extraordinary Meridians when a patient manifests many symptoms throughout the body and these symptoms are connected to many different meridians. The Extraordinary Meridians are also indicated when excess Yang and excess Yin manifest simultaneously, or the patient's pulses seem balanced and normal, but they are still unhealthy.

3. Use the Extraordinary Meridians when the patient has chronic imbalances and deficiencies and the Twelve Regular meridians are not having any effect on these symptoms. For example, the Extraordinary Meridians are indicated if a patient has chronic Qi deficiency with a metabolic imbalance, or has long-term psychoemotional issues. Stress has a direct impact on the Jing level, and using these vessels can create a shift in the patient's chronic problems. However, lifestyle changes and post-natal Qi support are important in ameliorating such long-term stress-related conditions.

4. Use the Extraordinary Meridians to address endocrine imbalances. Because they relate to Kidney Qi and essence, hormonal imbalances can benefit from treatments that incorporate the Extraordinary Vessels. Each respective master/couple point relates to particular hormones and the nervous system. Therefore, menopause, andropause, menarche, and metabolic conditions like hypo- and hyperthyroidism, can all be treated with the Extraordinary Meridians (see Chapter 2, The Jing Level).

5. Use the Extraordinary Meridians for issues of aging and longevity. Because of their connection to Kidney Jing and Yuan Qi, the Extraordinary Meridians can effect substantial change at a deep genetic level, supporting

inherited pre-natal and post-natal Qi. Therefore, congenital imbalances and aging tendencies can be addressed by the Extraordinary Meridians. As we age, the Kidney, root of Yin and Yang of the entire body, tends to become deficient. Using the Eight Extraordinary Vessels therapeutically in treatment can support Kidney essence and healthy aging.

6. Use the Extraordinary Meridians for emotional issues. For example, Yin Wei Mai treats depression, anxiety and dream-disturbed sleep; Ren Mai relates to the reproductive cycle and the attendant emotions of frustration and anger; and Chong Mai addresses rebellious Qi, which causes restlessness and abdominal urgency, which manifests as anxiety.

SUMMARY: GENERAL USAGE OF THE EIGHT EXTRAORDINARY MERIDIANS

- Regular meridians are not working
- Many symptoms
- Chronic imbalances
- Endocrine imbalances
- Longevity and aging issues
- Emotional issues

Contraindications and Cautions

- Do not use on a severely immune compromised or ill patient.

- Do not use when patients have colds, flu or fever, or are in the early stages of an illness.

- Do not use on patients younger than 5 years of age.

- Do not use on severely exhausted or weakened patients.

- Do not use in cases of excessive bleeding.

- Use sparingly on patients with severely deficient Kidney Qi.

- Be cautious using during trauma or shock

- I recommend caution in using electrostimulation on these vessels because we live in a culture in which electrical energy is pervasive, and in my opinion, using electrostimulation on the master/couple points could subject your patient to an overdose of current that would deeply penetrate their pre-natal Kidney Qi.

Guidelines

- Do treat patients who have good Qi and are healthy.

- Do treat patients of any age, except for children under 5 years of age.

- Be aware that sometimes treating these vessels can precipitate a healing crisis, which can manifest as colds, flu or excess mucus.

Since there are many fine books that cover the Eight Extraordinary Meridians in detail (see Bibliography), it is not necessary for me to do so here. Instead, I will highlight and summarize their master/couple point locations and indications, the pathways for each vessel, and their crossing points.

A summary table for each meridian includes the pathway, functions, syndromes and most importantly, the effect that each of these signs and symptoms has on the face, complexion and emotional expression.

Please refer to Table 3.1, the Eight Extraordinary Meridian Master/Couple Point Table, and note that any given master point can serve as a couple point for the paired meridian. For example, while Sp-4 Gongsun Yellow Emperor would normally be the master point, which is needled first, sometimes, based on diagnostics, PC-6 Neiguan Inner Gate may be considered the master point, and Chong Mai Sp-4 Gongsun Yellow Emperor the couple point.

Each of these points can open the Qi of the Eight Extraordinary Meridians. Please discern your patient's individual needs prior to choosing which master/couple points to use in your treatment.

In the following summary, tables for each Extraordinary Meridian connect constitutional imbalances with facial syndromes and their emotional manifestations. Constitutional Facial Acupuncture is a unique modality that does not take a purely cosmetic approach to beauty. Please note that if there are no indications for the face or emotions based on constitutional symptoms, that area of the table will be left blank.

Chong Mai
The Penetrating Vessel or the Vital Passage
The Sea of Blood
The Sea of the Twelve Regular Meridians

Master point	Sp-4 Gongsun Yellow Emperor
Couple point	PC-6 Neiguan Inner Gate
Location	Sp-4 Gongsun Yellow Emperor is located on the medial aspect of the foot, in the depression anterior and inferior to the base of the first metatarsal bone, at the junction of the red and white skin
Needling	perpendicular 0.5–0.8 cun

Indications	Luo point of the Spleen meridian, opens and regulates Chong Mai channel
	Harmonizes the Spleen and Stomach
	Moves damp and stagnant Qi, and blood stasis, and treats both excess and deficient digestive issues, such as borborygmus, distention, diarrhea and pain around the navel (the navel is the Earth element diagnostic area for Japanese *hara* palpation)
	Gynecological and menstrual issues, such as irregular menses and retention of the placenta
	Edema in the face and leg
	Shen issues, such as manic depression, insomnia, heart pain
Psychospiritual	Chong Mai's master point Sp-4 Gongsun Yellow Emperor relates to the Earth element; an imbalance can manifest as nurturance issues, which can negatively impact self-acceptance and self-esteem
	The Chong Mai master point Sp-4 Gongsun Yellow Emperior is used in combination with its couple point, PC-6 Neiguan Inner Gate on the Yin Wei Mai channel. This pair of points affects the heart, chest, uterus and stomach. In regulating the flow of Qi and blood in the Twelve Regular Meridians, this vital passage is significant in treating gynecological disorders, digestive issues, prolapses and heart problems. As the Sea of Blood, Chong Mai influences all aspects of blood, including heart and uterine blood, and the circulation of blood in the vessels
Comments	Because it relates to blood, DNA, genetics and pre-natal Qi, the Chong Mai can energetically affect intergenerational illness or patterns that are passed down through the family via the ancestral blood line
	Chong Mai mirrors the Three Treasures of Taoist philosophy. It is a fusion of Yin and Yang, and represents the space between Heaven (Yang) and Earth (Yin), thus it contains the seed of humanity. As the progenitor and the oldest of the Eight Extraordinary Vessels, it represents our genetic blueprint

Chong Mai Pathway (Figure 3.3)

1. The Chong Mai originates in the uterus/prostate and emerges at the perineum at Ren-1 Huiyin Meeting of Yin.

2. One branch ascends inside the sacrum and the lumbar spine.

3. Another branch ascends from Ren-1 Huiyin Meeting of Yin and emerges at St-30 Qichong Surging Qi; this branch connects with the Kidney channel and travels upward from Kid-11 Henggu Pubic Bone through Kid-21 Youmen Dark Gate, where it disperses in the chest and breast.

4. From the chest, a third branch ascends to the throat, curves around the lips, permeates the face, and terminates below the eyes.

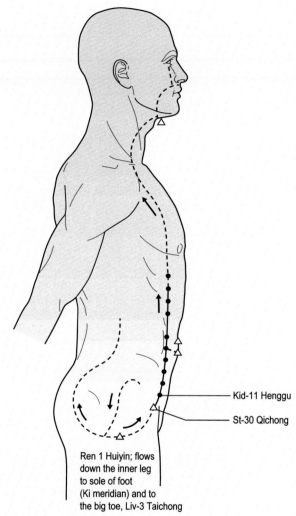

Kid-11 Henggu

St-30 Qichong

Ren 1 Huiyin; flows
down the inner leg
to sole of foot
(Ki meridian) and to
the big toe, Liv-3 Taichong

Figure 3.3 Chong Mai pathway.

5. A fourth branch emerges at St-30 Qichong Surging Qi, which descends along the medial aspect of the leg to the medial malleolus, and separates at the heel.

   a. One branch descends to the sole of the foot and connects with the Kidney meridian.

   b. The second branch descends to the big toe, and connects with the Liver meridian at Liv-3 Taichong Great Surge.

Please note that since Liv-3 Taichong means Great Surge, and because it carries the name of Chong, I have included this point in the descending branch of the meridian. However, not all sources agree that this point is part of the Chong Mai.

Liv-3 Taichong Great Surge can also be used to diagnose excess or deficiency in the Chong Mai channel, simply by palpating the pulse of the point. The *Ling Shu*, chapter 62, states that Chong Mai begins in the uterus or womb, and facilitates the moving Qi between the Kidneys, which is the root of ancestral Qi, the spark of life that ignites essence, and the stimulus for the birth of a child.

However, there is also some question as to whether Chong Mai follows the route of the Kidney meridian, or whether it has its own pathway. In the *Su Wen*, Chong Mai is said to travel up the body just lateral to the Kidney line. This makes sense to me because then Chong Mai would be situated between the Kidney and Stomach pathways, both of which it affects and rules.

CHONG MAI PATHWAY SUMMARY

- Starts in the uterus/prostate and emerges at Ren-1 Huiyin
- Ascends inside the spinal column
- Emerges from St-30 Qichong, travels up the throat to the face and lips, and ends at the eyes
- From St-30 Qichong, it descends down the leg to the medial malleolus, and separates at the heel
- One branch descends to the sole of the foot
- The other branch descends to the big toe

Crossing Points

Ren-1 Huiyin Meeting of Yin

Kid-11 Henggu Pubic Bone

Kid-12 Dahe Great Manifestation

Kid-13 Qixue Qi Hole

Kid-14 Siman Fourfold Fullness

Kid-15 Zhongzhu Central Flow

Kid-16 Huangshu Vital Shu

Kid-17 Shangqu Shang Bend

Kid-18 Shiguan Stone Pass

Kid-19 Yindu Yin Metropolis

Kid-20 Tonggu Open Valley

Kid-21 Bulang Dark Gate

St-30 Qichong Surging Qi

Liv-3 Taichong Great Surge

TABLE 3.3 CHONG MAI SIGNS AND SYMPTOMS

Pathway	Pattern	Syndromes	Face/Emotion
1. Originates in the uterus/prostate	Sea of Blood; all blood issues, excess and deficiency	Reproductive and gynecological imbalances	
		Amenorrhea (blood deficiency)	Pale complexion; mental unrest
		Menopause (blood deficiency)	Red face/hot flashes; anxiety
		Painful menses, fibroids (stagnation)	Lines between the eyebrows; possible suspended sword
2. Ascends the spine	Sea of Blood	Menstrual cramps; lower back	Contorted face (pain); irritable
3. St-30 to Kid-11-21; disperses in chest	Rebellious Qi	Gastrointestinal; tight and tense abdomen, 'abdominal urgency'	Pale face (cold); frozen expression (pain)
		Acid reflux, constipation, flatulence, tenesmus (stagnation)	Red face (heat rising); impatient, irritable, angry
		Painful breasts, premenstrual syndrome (PMS) (stagnation)	Suspended sword lines between eyebrows; irritable
		Lump in throat, sighing, thyroid issues, goiter	Saggy, lined neck; anxious or no energy
		Lung issues, copious phlegm	Edema, puffy eyes; damp, foggy mentally, possible mania with heat
4. From the chest up to the throat, circles around the lips and up the face to the eyes	Rebellious Qi	Heart pain, palpitations, headaches, 'Xu Li' syndrome	Hot and red chest and face; restless, anxious

Continued

TABLE 3.3   CHONG MAI SIGNS AND SYMPTOMS—cont'd

Pathway	Pattern	Syndromes	Face/Emotion
Circles around lips and mouth	Blood and Qi deficiency	Poor nourishment in digestive system (Sp/St); hormones, menopause (cycles of 7 and 8)	Thin lips, pale color, possible mustache (women); worried, fatigued
Up to eyes	Blood and Qi deficiency	Sunken, discolored area under eyes	Lines, bags and wrinkles under the eyes; sad, adrenally exhausted, grief, aging
5. From St-30 down the medial aspect of the leg to the sole of the foot and the big toe	Rebellious Qi, Wei syndrome	Cold feet and hands (Reynaud's syndrome), edema, numbness	Heat rising, red face or cold, pale face; frustrated, agitated, tired, exhausted

In Table 3.3, the meridian pathway, specific patterns, their associated syndromes, how they relate to facial wrinkles, sagging tendencies and emotional expression are outlined. Chong Mai presents as rebellious Qi and heat rising from the nipples to the face. The patient has a red face, and is irritable and impatient.

CLINICAL NOTE

'Xu Li' sydrome relates to Chong Mai's rebellious Qi function and manifests as excess Stomach heat with a red face, neck and chest upward from the nipples. Over time, the Stomach heat may injure the Heart.

Yin Wei Mai

The Yin Linking Vessel

The Yin Connecting Vessel

The Yin Networking Vessel

Master point	PC-6 Neiguan Inner Gate
Couple point	Sp-4 Gongsun Yellow Emperor
Location	PC-6 Neiguan Inner Gate; 2 cun above the transverse crease of the wrist, between the tendons of the palmaris longus and the flexor carpi radialis
Needling	Perpendicular 0.5–0.8 cun; be careful of the meridian nerve, which lies directly under PC-6 *Neiguan* Inner Gate. Do not manipulate the needle once you have inserted it, because it causes an electric feeling due to the nerve placement

Indications	Luo point of the Pericardium Channel; opens and regulates Yin Wei Mai
	Calms Shen, balances, and regulates Heart Qi, and treats blood deficiency. Therefore, it is a good point for emotional issues like depression, sadness and mania
	Harmonizes the Stomach and treats nausea and vomiting, such as in morning sickness and motion sickness
	Treats heart pain, and symptoms like palpitations, arrhythmia and fright
	Helps with insomnia, epilepsy, wind stroke, aphasia, hypertension and memory loss
	Treats both cold and Qi deficiency in the Stomach/Spleen
	Distention or fullness with borborygmus
	Abdominal pain and masses
	Rectal prolapse, fever, jaundice and malaria
	Painful and irregular menses
	Post-partum syndrome
Psychospiritual	Because the heart rules the Blood and Shen, emotional imbalances, such as anxiety, depression, worry, sadness and obsession can arise. It also opens the chest and treats painful obstructions
Comments	The master point of Yin Wei Mai is PC-6 Neiguan Inner Gate, which is used in combination with its couple point Sp-4 Gongsun Yellow Emperor. Yin Wei Mai connects and gathers together all of the Yin channels. It mainly affects the Heart, chest, Stomach and inner leg area
	Yin Wei Mai nourishes blood and Yin, and especially nourishes Heart blood to alleviate pain in the heart, not only on a physical, but also a psychospiritual level

Yin Wei Mai Pathway (Figure 3.4)

1. Yin Wei Mai originates at the medial aspect of the lower leg and at Kid-9 Zhubin Guest House.

2. It ascends along the medial aspect of the leg, knee and thigh, to the lateral abdominal area and meets at Sp-13 Fushe Bowel Abode, Sp-15 Daheng Great Horizontal and Sp-16 Fuai Abdominal Lament.

3. It then traverses the hypochondrial region to meet at Liv-14 Qimen Cycle Gate.

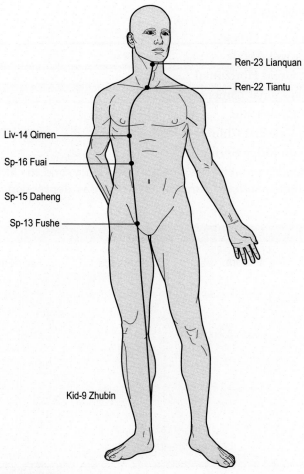

Ren-23 Lianquan

Ren-22 Tiantu

Liv-14 Qimen

Sp-16 Fuai

Sp-15 Daheng

Sp-13 Fushe

Kid-9 Zhubin

Figure 3.4 Yin Wei Mai pathway.

4. It continues ascending to the diaphragm, chest, and throat, where it meets the Ren Mai Channel at Ren-22 Tiantu Celestial Chimney and Ren-23 Lianguan Ridge Spring. There, it terminates at the root of the tongue. Please note, the Nan Jing suggested that the Yin Wei Mai originated at Sp-6 Sanyinjiao, the meeting point of the three Yin channels.

YIN WEI MAI PATHWAY SUMMARY

- Starts at Kid-9 Zhubin
- Ascends the inner leg to Sp-13 Fushe, Sp-15 Daheng and Sp-16 Fuai
- Continues to ascend to Liv-14
- Continues to ascend to the diaphragm, chest and throat to Ren-22 Tiantu and Ren-23 Lianguan
- Terminates at the root of the tongue

Crossing Points

Kid-9 Zhubin Guest House

Sp-13 Fushe Bowel Abode

Sp-15 Daheng Great Horizontal

Sp 16 Fuai Abdominal Lament

Liv-14 Qimen Cycle Gate

Ren-22 Tiantu Celestial Chimney

Ren-23 Lianguan Ridge Spring

In Table 3.4, Yin Wei Mai relates to blood deficiency, and the attendant emotional issues that manifest in menopause, such as depression, anxiety and irritability.

TABLE 3.4 YIN WEI MAI SIGNS AND SYMPTOMS			
Pathway	**Pattern**	**Syndromes**	**Face/Emotion**
1. Starts at Kid-9	Blood deficiency	Achy, numb joints (Bi syndrome)	Face contorted with pain
	Yin deficiency	Sore, dry, female genitalia; menopause	Dry skin, small lines/ wrinkles; restless, anxious
2. Inner leg to Sp-13, 15, 16	Hypochondriac fullness	Sp/St issues; borborygmus, hemorrhoids, prolapses	
	Rebellious Qi	Hiccups, hot flashes, motion sickness	Menopause (hormones); dry skin lines and wrinkles; mental unrest
		Morning sickness	Pregnancy (hormones)
3. Diaphragm and chest	Blood and Yin deficiency (Shen disturbance)	Heart pain, angina, palpitations, chest oppression emotional issues, insomnia, headache	Mouth turns down, nasolabial fold droops; sadness, depression, anxiety
		Post-partum syndrome	Worry, weeping
4. Connects with throat at Ren-22 and Ren-23, and ends at root of tongue	Yin deficiency	Loss of voice, thyroid/parathyroid imbalance (hormones)	Sagging neck with lines; sadness, inability to express emotions, especially anger
	Blood deficiency		Low self-esteem and will power, discouragement

Ren Mai

The Conception Vessel

The Directing Vessel

The Sea of Yin

Master point	Lu-7 Lieque Broken Sequence
Couple point	Kid-6 Zhaohai Shining Sea
Location	Lu-7 Lieque Broken Sequence is 1.5 cun above the transverse crease of the wrist in a depression between the tendon and the bone, on the styloid process of the radius
Needling	Perpendicular insertion 0.5–0.8 cun

Indications	Luo Point of the Lung Channel
	Command Point of Head and Face
	Releases the exterior and circulates Protective Qi
	Controls the skin's action of opening and closing the pores
	Stimulates descending and dispersion of Lung Qi
	Tonifies Lung Qi
	Treats colds, sore throats, flu and asthma
	Opens nasal congestion
	Treats grief and sadness
	Alleviates pain and stiffness in the head and neck; headaches
	Expels wind, facial paralysis and phlegm
Psychospiritual	Ren Mai regulates the reproductive system, and can be used to address irregular menses, dysmenorrhea, infertility, impotence and leucorrhea, blood stagnation, manifesting as fibroids cysts and masses, and Yin deficiency issues like menopause, hot flashes, excessive sweating and anxiety
	Facial imbalances, such as puffiness and skin discoloration can be treated effectively with Ren Mai. It is also helpful in addressing Lung imbalances, such as asthma, childhood asthma and cough

Comments | The master point of the Ren Mai is Lu-7 Lieque Broken Sequence, and the couple point is Kid-6 Zhaohai Shining Sea on the Yin Qiao channel. Ren Mai controls all the Yin meridians of the body, and is known as the Sea of Yin. The name Conception Vessel highlights the Yin aspect of ancestral Qi that relates to fertility, hormones and the Yin fluids of the body. The other name, Directing Vessel, emphasizes its function as the director of this Yin Qi in the entire body

Ren Mai connects with the Mu/Alarm points of the Urinary Bladder, Small Intestine, Heart, Pericardium, Stomach and the Three Jiaos, which links the Zang/Fu organs, controls the cycles of 7 and 8, and the endocrine system

Yin Qi, blood essence and fluids circulate throughout the body, and this movement lubricates all the organs and channels

Ren Mai Pathway (Figure 3.5)

1. Ren Mai originates in the uterus/prostate, and then emerges from the perineum at Ren-1 Huiyin Meeting of Yin.

2. It ascends the midline of the abdomen, chest, throat and jaw, connecting with The Three Jiaos in respective order.

3. The outer pathway terminates at Ren-24 Chengjiang Supporting Liquid below the lips, then circles around the lips and mouth internally and meets the Chong Mai channel.

4. From there, it internally connects with Du Mai at Du-28 Yinjiao Gum Intersection, ascends the face to St-1 Chengqi Tear Container and enters the eyes.

5. A branch arises in the pelvis, enters the spine and travels upward along the spine.

6. The Luo Connecting Channel of Ren Mai separates at Ren-15 Jiuwei Turtledove Tail, and sends fan-like branches all over the abdominal area.

Please note that the Ren Mai, Du Mai and Chong Mai all arise from the uterus/prostate, which facilitates the moving Qi between the Kidneys; then they break off at Ren-1 Huiyin Meeting of Yin to follow their respective pathways.

REN MAI PATHWAY SUMMARY

- Originates in the uterus/prostate and emerges at Ren-1 Huiyin
- Ascends to the abdomen, chest, throat and jaw
- Terminates at Ren-1 Huiyin
- Internally curves around the lips and mouth
- Connects with Du-28 Yinjiao internally
- Ascends the face to St-1 Chengqi internally, and enters the eyes
- A branch from the pelvis enters the spine
- Luo channel at Ren-15 Jiuwei sends additional branches over the abdominal area

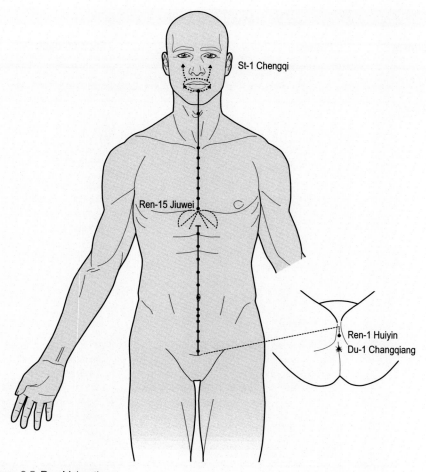

St-1 Chengqi

Ren-15 Jiuwei

Ren-1 Huiyin
Du-1 Changqiang

Figure 3.5 Ren Mai pathway.

Please note that the Ren Mai, Du Mai and Chong Mai all arise from the uterus/prostate, which facilitates the moving Qi between the Kidneys; then they break off at Ren-1 Huiyin Meeting of Yin to follow their respective pathways.

Master point: Lu-7 Lieque Broken Sequence

Couple point: Kid-6 Zhaohai Shining Sea

Luo Connecting point: Ren-15 Jiuwei Turtledove Tail

Beginning point: Ren-1 Huiyin Meeting of Yin

While Ren Mai and Chong Mai both address gynecological issues, Ren Mai treats Qi and Yin deficiency, and Chong Mai treats more excess conditions, such as blood stasis and Qi stagnation (see Table 3.5).

TABLE 3.5   REN MAI SIGNS AND SYMPTOMS

Pathway	Pattern	Syndromes	Face/Emotion
1. Originates in uterus and prostate		Reproductive and gynecological imbalances	
	Qi and Yin deficiency	Irregular, painful menses, endometriosis, vaginitis	
	Yin deficiency	Menopause: hot flashes, night sweats, insomnia (hormones)	Flushed, red face; agitated, mental restlessness
	Qi stagnation with damp	Fibroids, masses, cysts, polycystic ovary syndrome	
	Qi stagnation	Hernia (men)	
	Regulates life cycles of 7/8; endocrine systems, supports transitions	Puberty, menstruation, conception, pregnancy, childbirth, menopause, infertility, impotence	All reproductive cycles; emotional hormonal responses, anxiety, restlessness, outbursts of anger, impatience, weeping, sadness, depression
			From pregnancy: rosy complexion (full of hormones) to menopause: flushed face, dry skin, lines above the mouth, wrinkles (waning hormones)

The Three Jiaos; Internal Organ Imbalances

Pathway	Pattern	Syndromes	Face/Emotion
2. Ascends to the lower abdomen (Lower Jiao)	Damp and stagnation	Kidney: pain and edema	
	Qi stagnation	Bladder: urine retention	
	Qi deficiency	Incontinence	
	Qi deficiency and stagnation	Intestines: diarrhea, flatulence, abdominal distention/pain, constipation	

Continued

TABLE 3.5   REN MAI SIGNS AND SYMPTOMS—cont'd

Pathway	Pattern	Syndromes	Face/Emotion
3. Middle Jiao	Nutritive Qi Qi deficiency and stagnation	Epigastric area; Stomach/Spleen: indigestion, nausea, vomiting	
4. Ascends to the chest (Upper Jiao)	Lung Qi not descending; Wei Qi deficiency	Lung: asthma, cough, shortness of breath	Dry, pale complexion; cautious, fearful
	Yin deficiency	Heart: angina, heart pain, palpitations, insomnia	Broken capillaries on the tip of the nose; anxiety, depression
5. Ascends to the throat, and circles around the lips	Yin deficiency (Qi sensation rising to the throat)	Dry, swollen throat, aphasia, stiff tongue (facial paralysis)	Lines on neck/droopy; wry mouth, facial paralysis (stress-connected)
	Yin Qi (hormones)	Menopause	Dry skin, lines above upper lip; anxiety, agitated, frustrated, anger, adrenal stress
6. Internally connects with Du-28; ascends the face to St-1, and enters the eyes	Qi stagnation	Hyperpigmentation, puffiness (damp), eczema (dry, flaky)	Anger (Liver imbalance), frustration, grief/stress
	Yin deficiency (Lung)	Malar flush, chronic eye imbalances, myopia and hyperopia (near/far-sighted)	Red cheeks, anxiety, lines around the eyes, squinting
7. Enters the spine and connects to Ren-15, Luo Connecting Vessel	Connects to Du Mai (Ren-15); blood issues	Memory issues, emotional disorders	Anxiety, worry, fear, mania, depression (all of these emotions can be viewed on the face)

Yin Qiao Mai

The Yin Heel Vessel

The Yin Stepping Vessel

The Sea of Yin

Master point	Kid-6 Zhaohai Shining Sea
Couple point	Lu-7 Lieque Broken Sequence
Location	Kid-6 Zhaohai Shining Sea is 1 cun below the medial malleolus in the depression between the two tendons
Needling	perpendicular insertion 0.3–0.5 cun

Indications	Nourishes Yin and essence, i.e., Kidney Yin deficiency
	Benefits throat and vocal cords; sore throat and asthma
	Clears heat and cools blood
	Menstrual issues; heavy periods and uterine prolapses
	Calms the spirit
	Treats insomnia and somnolence, epilepsy at night, sadness
	Frequent dribbling urination
	Chronic eye diseases
Psychospiritual	Both Qiaos control brain function and emotions; imbalances in Yin Qiao manifest as apathy, lassitude, a sense of defeat and poor will-power
Comments	The master point of Yin Qiao Mai is Kid-6 Zhaohai Shining Sea, and the couple point is Lu-7 Lieque Broken Sequence. Yin Qiao Mai is considered a branch of the Kidney meridian. When the medial muscles of the legs are tight, and the foot is inverted, the lateral leg muscle will be weak or atrophied
	Yin Qiao also regulates the involuntary closing of the eyes, as in somnolence. Since the channel travels up to Bl-1 Jingming Bright Eyes, eye disorders manifest, such as inflammation of the eye, optic nerve atrophy, and glaucoma, to name a few
	Lower abdominal pain and disorders in the intestine, urinary and gynecological issues, such as hernia, uterine bleeding, dribbling urination, borborygmus, diarrhea, constipation and abdominal masses, cause imbalance in the body. Also prevalent are throat issues, such as laryngitis, nodules on vocal cords, and Plum Pit Qi
	When the Yin Qiao Mai channel is imbalanced, there will be somnolence, epilepsy and muscle spasms on the medial part of lower legs, while the outer portion of the leg could be atrophied. The foot will turn in (pigeon-toed), there will be pain in the lower abdomen and external genitalia, hernia, leucorrhea, sore throat and laryngitis

Yin Qiao Mai Pathway (Figure 3.6)

1. Yin Qiao Mai starts at the inside of the medial aspect of the heel, and travels to the navicular bone at Kid-2 Rangu Blazing Valley, and then to Kid-6 Zhaohai Shining Sea.

2. It then ascends the inner aspect of the leg to Kid-8 Jiaoxin Intersection Reach, the Xi-cleft point of the Kidney meridian.

3. It continues up the medial aspect of the thigh to the genitalia.

4. Then it traverses the abdomen and chest via the Kidney meridian to the supraclavicular fossa.

5. It continues up the throat to connect with St-9 Renying Man's Prognosis.

6. It then moves up the face along the zygomatic arch to join Yang Qiao Mai at Bl-1 Jingming Bright Eyes, and enters the brain.

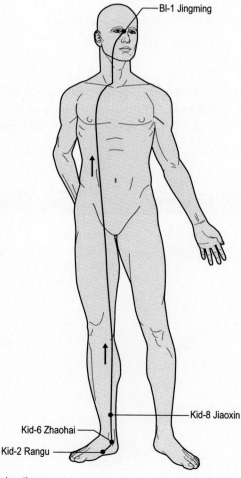

Figure 3.6 Yin Qiao Mai pathway.

YIN QIAO MAI PATHWAY SUMMARY

- Starts in the heel at Kid-2 Rangu and travels to Kid-6 Zhaohai
- Ascends to Kid-8 Jiaoxin, and ascends to the genitals
- It travels up to the abdomen, chest and supraclavicular fossa
- It continues up the throat to St-9 Renying
- It moves up the face to Bl-1 Jingming, then enters the brain

---

Crossing Points

Kid-2 Rangu Blazing Valley

Kid-6 Zhaohai Shining Sea

Kid-8 Jiaoxin Intersection Reach; Xi Cleft Point

St-12 Quepen Empty Basin - Supraclavicular fossa

St-9 Renying Man's Prognosis

Bl-1 Jingming Bright Eyes

In Table 3.6, the Yin Qiao Mai pathway ascends the face to Bl-1 Jingming, and controls the closing of the eyes. The patient may have narcolepsy and sleeps after dinner, while driving a car, or spontaneously throughout the day.

TABLE 3.6   YIN QIAO MAI SIGNS AND SYMPTOMS

Pathway	Pattern	Syndromes	Face/Emotion
1. Starts in the heel, ascends to Kid-2, Kid-6 and Kid-8	Wei atrophy syndrome	Inversion of foot, medial leg tight, lateral side of leg flaccid/atrophied, multiple sclerosis (MS)	
2. Ascends to external genitalia	Excess Yin; blood stasis or damp issues	Vaginitis/itching, swollen scrotum, genital pain	
	Qi stagnation, blood stasis	Urinary tract problems, retention of urine, blood in urine	

Continued

TABLE 3.6   YIN QIAO MAI SIGNS AND SYMPTOMS—cont'd

Pathway	Pattern	Syndromes	Face/Emotion
3. Ascends to abdomen, chest, and to the supraclavicular fossa	Stagnation of Qi and blood	Gynecological and reproductive issues; abdominal masses, fibroids	Depression
	Bi syndrome	Supraclavicular fossa, shoulder pain	
	Blood stasis	Uterine bleeding, irregular menses, retention of placenta, difficult labor	
4. Continues up to the throat, St-9	Stagnation and stasis	Plum Pit Qi, laryngitis, vocal cord nodules, sore throat	Blotchy throat, neck lines, sagging; suppressed anger, unexpressed grief, cannot speak
5. Ascends to the face and medial cheek to the eye, Bl-1	Yin deficiency; eye disorders	Somnolence, red, painful eyes (inner canthus), glaucoma, optic nerve atrophy	Can't keep eyes open
6. Enters the brain	Balances emotions/mind	Hypoactivity, low will power, Shen-less, depression, epilepsy (at night)	All emotions can be seen in the face; low self-esteem, apathy

Du Mai
The Governing Vessel
The Sea of Yang Meridian

Master point	SI-3 Houxi Black Ravine
Couple point	Bl-62 Shenmai Extending Vessel
Location	SI-3 Houxi Black Ravine is on the ulnar side of the hand in the depression proximal to the head of the fifth metacarpal bone, located by making a fist
Needling	perpendicular insertion 0.5–0.7 cun

Indications	Shu Stream Wood point of the Small Intestine Meridian
	Regulates Du Mai channel and eliminates internal wind, including convulsions, epilepsy and trismus
	Clears heat and damp, treats jaundice, malaria, chills, fever and night sweats
	Benefits the eyes, throat and sensory organs, deafness, tinnitus, red and painful eyes, aphasia after wind stroke
	Supports the muscles and tendons, and alleviates stiff neck, back and headache pain
Psychospiritual	Du Mai connects to the brain, and treats emotional, mental and nervous system issues, such as schizophrenia, depression, anxiety, poor memory, epilepsy, neuromuscular diseases and nervous tension
Comments	The master point of Du Mai is SI-3 Houxi Black Ravine and the couple point is BI-62 Shenmai Extending Vessel. Du Mai governs all the Yang channels and is called the Sea of Yang. When Yang Qi is overactive, it can cause a stiff spine, headache, and pain in the eyes. Du Mai also warms all the organs and meridians with Yang Qi, and particularly supports Kidney Yang. Because it houses the back Shu points, it treats all imbalances in the internal organs, such as Heart palpitations and arrhythmias
	Du Mai also nourishes bone marrow and Kidney Jing, and aids congenital and degenerative disorders, immune deficient conditions, slow growth, chronic fatigue and a poor constitution. The sense organs and urogenital system are also within the purview of this comprehensive vessel

Du Mai Pathway (Figure 3.7)

1. Du Mai originates in the uterus/prostate, and then flows to the perineum at Ren 1 Huiyin Meeting of Yin, as do the Chong Mai and Ren Mai.

2. From there, Du Mai moves to the coccyx, where it joins the Kidney and Bladder channels.

3. It then follows the spine to the back of the neck, to Du-16 Fengfu Wind Mansion, where a branch enters the brain.

4. It continues up to the vertex, down over the forehead to the nose and ends at Du-28 Yinjiao Gum Intersection, where it meets with the Ren Mai.

5. Another branch follows the Ren Mai's pathway and starts at the perineum, ascends the midline to the navel up through the Heart, throat, chin, circles around the lips and ends below the eyes.

6. The Luo Connecting Vessel ascends from Du-1 Changqiang Long Strong in parallel lines up the back to the nape of the neck, where it spreads all over the occiput.

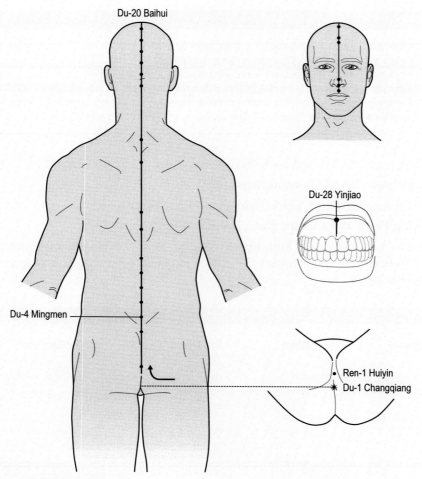

Du-20 Baihui

Du-28 Yinjiao

Du-4 Mingmen

Ren-1 Huiyin
Du-1 Changqiang

Figure 3.7 Du Mai pathway.

Please note that the Du Mai and Ren Mai intersect at Du-28 Yinjiao Gum Intersection, the frenulum of the lip, and that they have subsidiary branches that run in parallel. For example, the Ren Mai has a branch that travels up the spine, and the Du Mai has a pathway that ascends the front of the body.

Ren and Du form two halves of a continuous energetic circuit, and yet, within this unitary structure, they have their own individual indications and personalities. In Taoist alchemical traditions, the microcosmic orbit breathing meditation called the Water Wheel focuses on uniting these pathways with a seamless, unending stream of breath in order to connect with pre-natal Qi, longevity and awareness.

DU MAI PATHWAY SUMMARY

- Originates in the uterus/prostrate, and then flows to the perineum
- Moves to coccyx and joins the Kidney/Bladder meridians
- From the perineum, ascends the spine to Du-16 Fengfu, and enters the brain
- Ascends to the vertex, over forehead and ends at Du-28 Yinjiao
- Starts in perineum, ascends to Heart and throat, then around the lips and under the eyes
- Another branch ascends from Du-1 Changqiang up the back to the occiput

---

Master point: SI-3 Houxi Back Ravine

Couple point: Bl-62 Shenmai Extending Vessel

Luo Connecting Point: Du-1 Changqiang Long Strong

Starting Point: Du-1 Changqiang Long Strong

In Table 3.7, because Du Mai supports Kidney Jing, it addresses birth defects, growth hormone and pituitary deficiency in children, as well as osteoporosis and arthritis.

TABLE 3.7   DU MAI SIGNS AND SYMPTOMS

Pathway	Pattern	Syndromes	Face/Emotion
1. Originates in uterus and prostate	Kidney Yang deficiency	Gynecological disorders; impotence, infertility, low sexual drive	Pale face; no vitality, fatigue, depression, cold
	Kidney Yang and Qi deficiency	Regulates menstrual cycles	Hormonal acne; low self-esteem
	Kidney Yin deficiency	Menopause; hot flashes, etc.	Dry skin, acne (flux/ flow of hormones)
2. Moves to the coccyx and joins Kidney/Bladder channels	Kidney Yang deficiency	Incontinence, frequent urination	
	Lifts Yang Qi	Prolapses; uterus, bladder, hemorrhoids, excessive menstrual bleeding	Prolapse of facial muscles, especially sagging neck (platysma muscle)
3. From the perineum, travels up the spine to Du-16 and connects with the brain	Calms mind, tonifies Heart Yang	Mental disorders; depression, mental restlessness, poor memory, insomnia, palpitations/fright, schizophrenia, manic/ depressive, hysterical laughing, incessant talking, disoriented	All emotions and mental disorders are seen in the face

Continued

TABLE 3.7   DU MAI SIGNS AND SYMPTOMS—cont'd

Pathway	Pattern	Syndromes	Face/Emotion
4. Ascends to the the vertex (Du-20) over the forehead and ends at Du-28	Nourishes brain and brain marrow	Dizziness, tinnitus, blurred vision, weak legs	
	Nervous system disorders	Neuromuscular disease, neuropathies, nervous tension	Pain shows in the face; tight and tense, agitated
	Expels internal wind (heat)	Bell's palsy, epilepsy, windstroke, aphasia, convulsions (infantile), coma, dizziness, vertigo	Wry mouth, droopy eyelids, facial paralysis; fear, anxiety, stress
	Kidney Yang and Jing deficiency	Congenital disorders; birth defects, slow growth (children), joint degeneration	
	Internal Organs		
5. Follows the Ren Mai channel; from the perineum, it ascends the midline to the Heart, throat, chin, circles around the lips and ends below the eyes	Kidney Yang deficiency	Bladder; damp, edema	Puffy eyes in Bl-1 area
		Spleen/Stomach; diarrhea, cold limbs	Facial lines; fatigue, poor nourishment
	Kidney not grasping Lung Qi	Lung; shortness of breath, asthma, cold hands	Pale face, dry face; fear
	Kidney Qi and Yang deficiency	Heart; mental issues	Mouth turned down/ not smiling; unhappy, depressed
	Sense Organs		
	Kidney Yin deficiency	Thyroid issues; swollen painful throat	Lines in throat area
	Opens the nose	Sinusitis/rhinitis	Puffy in sinus/eye area
	Kidney Yin and Jing deficiency	Circles around lips	Lines above lips (fear); thin lips (worry)
	Kidney Qi and Jing deficiency	Below eyes	Dark circles and puffiness around eyes
6. Ascends to Du-1, travels up the Bladder channel to the occiput	Expels external wind	Fever/headache, occipital neck pain and stiffness	Back of neck refers to front throat area – sagging, lines, wrinkles; irritated, impatient
	Kidney Yang deficiency	Acute lower backache	Pain seen in face; cold feeling, fear

Yang Qiao Mai

The Yang Heel Vessel

The Sea of Yang Meridian

Master point	Bl-62 Shenmai Extending Vessel
Couple point	SI-3 Houxi Back Ravine
Location	Bl-62 Shenmai Extending Vessel is located in the depression directly below the lateral malleolus
Needling	perpendicular insertion 0.3–0.5 cun

Indications	Bl-62 Shenmai Extending Vessel is a ghost point
	Alleviates internal and external wind, with symptoms such as dizziness, headache, daytime epilepsy, windstroke, aphasia and facial paralysis
	Benefits and moistens red, painful eyes; nosebleeds, and tinnitus
	Clears heat and calms Shen; mania, depression and insomnia
	Relaxes and alleviates low back and hip pain
Psychospiritual	Both Qiaos control brain functions and emotions; imbalances in Yang Qiao manifest as a feeling of being overwhelmed, out of synch with personal cycles, and a tendency to blame others for their problems.
Comments	The master point of Yang Qiao Mai is Bl-62 Shenmai Extending Vessel and its couple point is SI-3 Houxi Back Ravine. When Yang Qiao Mai is out of balance, there can be insomnia, daytime epilepsy, or muscle spasms in the lateral part of the lower leg, and the medial aspect of the leg may be atrophied. The foot may evert, or turn out, and often there is pain in the hip and lower back
	The Yang Qiao Mai is related to the Bladder; it can be used to treat rheumatoid arthritis and joint conditions, especially red, swollen, painful joints
	If the entire pathway is affected, there is general stiffness in the body and in the lower limbs, trunk, shoulder and neck, and the patient's left and right sides are out of balance

Yang Qiao Mai Pathway (Figure 3.8)

1. Yang Qiao Mai originates in the lateral heel and intersects with Bl-62 Shenmai Extending Vessel, Bl-61 Pucan Subservient Master and Bl-59 Fuyang Instep Yang.

2. From there, it ascends the lateral aspect of the thigh and hip to GB-29 Lower Juliao Squatting Bone Hole, and passes through the lateral aspect of the abdomen to the hypochondriac area.

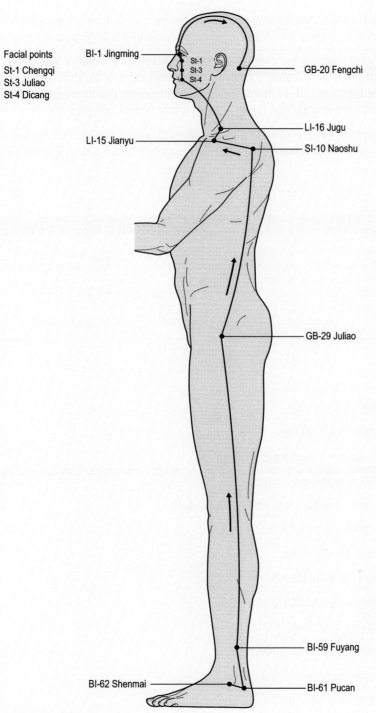

Facial points
St-1 Chengqi
St-3 Juliao
St-4 Dicang

BI-1 Jingming

St-1
St-3
St-4

GB-20 Fengchi

LI-16 Jugu

LI-15 Jianyu

SI-10 Naoshu

GB-29 Juliao

BI-59 Fuyang

BI-62 Shenmai

BI-61 Pucan

Figure 3.8 Yang Qiao Mai pathway.

3. It then ascends to the scapula and shoulder and intersects with SI-10 Naoshu Upper Arm Shu, LI-16 Jugu Great Bone, and LI-15 Jianyu Shoulder Bone.

4. It travels up the lateral side of the neck to the corner of the mouth at St-4 Dicang Earth's Granary; it then continues to climb the face (St-3 Juliao Great Bone Hole and St-1 Chengqi Tear Container) to the inner canthus of the eye (Bl-1 Jingming Bright Eyes) where it joins Yin Qiao Mai.

5. It ascends the forehead and goes laterally along the side of the head, where the pathway intersects with GB-20 Fengchi Wind Pool, and enters the brain.

YANG QIAO MAI PATHWAY SUMMARY

- Originates in lateral heel and meets Bl-62 Shenmai/Bl-61 Pucan and Bl-59 Fuyang
- Ascends the lateral leg to GB-29 Lower Juliao, and up to abdomen and hypochondriac
- Continues up to LI-16 Jugu, and LI-15 Jianyu
- Ascends the face to St-4 Dicang, St-3 Juliao and St-1 Chengqi, and to the eye at Bl-1 Jingming
- Finally, it travels over the forehead to meet GB-20 Jianyu and enters the brain

---

Crossing Points

SI-3 Houxi Back Ravine

Bl-62 Shenmai Extending Vessel

Bl-59 Fuyang Instep Yang

GB-29 Lower Juliao Squatting Bone Hole

SI-10 Naoshu Upper Arm Shu

LI-16 Jugu Great Bone

LI-15 Jianyu Shoulder Bone

St-4 Dicang Earth's Granary

St-3 Juliao Great Bone Hole

St-1 Chengqi Tear Container

Bl-1 Jingming Bright Eyes

GB-20 Jianyu Shoulder Bone

The Yang Qiao Mai is responsible for ocular computer stress syndrome; staring at the computer screen for hours can cause red bloodshot eyes, tight neck and shoulders, headache, irritability and insomnia (see Table 3.8).

TABLE 3.8   YANG QIAO MAI SIGNS AND SYMPTOMS

Pathway	Pattern	Syndromes	Face/Emotion
1. Originates in the lateral heel and intersects with Bl-62, Bl-61 and Bl-59	Wei atrophy syndrome	Eversion of foot, lateral leg tight, medial side of leg flaccid/atrophied	
2. Ascends to the lateral thigh, hip (GB-29) and hypochondrium	Bi syndrome	Lateral hip pain, unilateral backache, sciatica, lateral hypochondriac pain	
	Damp in Bladder	Urinary problems, urinary pain and difficulty, dribbling urine	
3. Ascends to the shoulder and meets at SI-10, LI-16 and LI-15	Bi syndrome	Lateral shoulder pain and stiffness, joint/ bone pain	
4. Travels to the lateral neck, then ascends to the face at St-4, St-3, St-1, and to the eye at Bl-1	External wind	Aversion to wind, headache, fever, stiff neck, runny nose	
	Internal wind	Windstroke, hemiplegia, aphasia, convulsions, epilepsy (daytime), facial paralysis from Bell's palsy, stroke, neuropathies	Wry, droopy mouth, saggy eyelids and cheek; stress, anxiety
5. It continues up to the forehead and side of the head, to GB-20, and enters the brain at Du-16	Internal wind	Insomnia, red, painful eyes (inner canthus), glaucoma, optic nerve atrophy	Can't shut eyes, bloodshot eyes, dark circles and bags under the eyes from no sleep; irritable, exhausted
	Balances emotions/ Shen	Manic/depression, schizophrenia, agitation, overexcitement, hyper-activity, restlessness	All emotions and mental issues can be seen in the face; violent, depressed, angry

Dai Mai

The Belt Vessel

The Girdle Vessel

Master point	GB-41 Zulinqi Foot Overlooking Tears
Couple point	TH-5 Waiguan Outer Gate
Location	GB-41 Zulinqi Foot Overlooking Tears is located in the depression distal to the junction of the fourth and fifth metatarsal bones, on the lateral side of the tendon of m. extensor digiti minimi of the foot
Needling	Perpendicular insertion 0.3–0.5 cun

Indications	Shu Stream Wood point/Horary Point of the Gall Bladder
	Releases damp in the genitalia; vaginal itch, cystitis, leucorrhea and irregular menses
	Promotes free flow of Liver and Gall Bladder; migraine headaches due to Liver Yang Rising, and Qi stagnation
	Eye disorders such as dry, painful eyes and night blindness
	Dispels internal wind; vertigo, dizziness, deafness and tinnitus
	Pain in the hip and knee
Psychospiritual	Dai Mai refers to the Gall Bladder's function of decision making, and patients with an imbalance in the Dai Mai are invariably 'sitting on the fence,' holding on to resentments, and not prepared to make a difficult decision
Comments	The master point of Dai Mai is GB-41 Zulinqi Foot Overlooking Tears, and its couple point is TH-5 Waiguan Outer Gate. Dai Mai is called the Belt or Girdle Meridian, because it is the only vessel that flows horizontally and wraps around the waist. In the classical texts, Dai Mai symptoms are described as sitting in cold water, bloated abdomen and saggy waist. This meridian is particularly good for treating damp issues, such as vaginal discharge and cystitis, leucorrhea, and gynecological problems such as irregular menses, metorrhagia, fibroids and uterine prolapse
	It can also be used to address Gall Bladder channel conditions like migraine headaches, red and painful eyes, deafness and tinnitus, upper and lower one-sided pain and injuries
	Other symptoms may include low back pain, paralysis of limbs, abdominal distension, and flatulence

Dai Mai Pathway (Figure 3.9)

1. Dai Mai originates at Liv-13 Zhangmen Camphorwood Gate.

2. Then it connects with GB-26 Daimai Girdling Vessel, GB-27 Wushu Fifth Pivot and GB-28 Weidao Linking Path, where it circles around the waist like a belt.

3. From there, it connects with the Kidney Divergent Channel on the back at the level of Du-4 Mingmen Life Gate.

DAI MAI PATHWAY SUMMARY

- Begins at Liv-13 Zhangmen
- Circles around the waist at GB-26 Daimai, GB-27 Wushu and GB-28 Weidao
- Connects with Du-4 Mingmen on the back

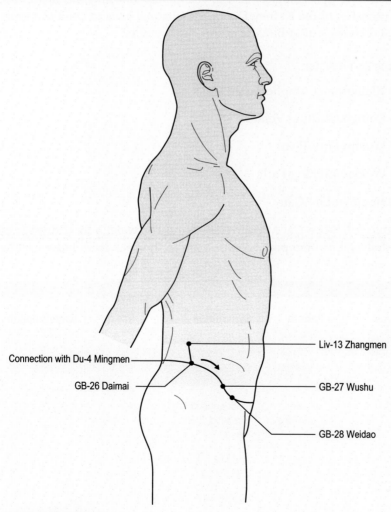

Figure 3.9 Dai Mai pathway.

Please note: Yitian Ni[3] cites the ancient text *Qi Jing Ba Mai Kao* (*Research on the Eight Extraordinary Channels*), in which the author Li Shi Zhen stipulates that Liv-13 Zhangmen Camphorwood Gate is the starting point of Dai Mai.

Kiiko Matsumoto and Stephen Birch[4] also note that according to the *NanJing*, the Dai Mai begins at the rib cage, and in the same chapter, Wang Shu He's *Commentary on the Nan Jing* clarifies that the rib cage means Liv-13 Zhangmen Camphorwood Gate.

I personally feel that this is correct, and have included this as the original starting point of the vessel.

Dai Mai also receives pre-natal Qi from the Kidney (Liver/Gall Bladder Channel) Divergent Meridian, which treats issues of damp heat in the lower Jiao, including gynecological issues, yeast infections and endometriosis. One of the branches of the Kidney Divergent Channel goes to Du-4 Mingmen Life Gate, and comes out at Bl-23 Shenshu Kidney Shu.

Crossing Points

Liv-13 Zhangmen Camphorwood Gate

GB-26 Daimai Girdling Vessel

GB-27 Wushu Fifth Pivot

GB-28 Weidao Linking Path

Du-4 Mingmen Life Gate

See Table 3.9. Since Dai Mai circles around the waist and addresses cold in the Kidneys, it can temporarily ease pain in the back from kidney stones.

TABLE 3.9 DAI MAI SIGNS AND SYMPTOMS

Pathway	Pattern	Syndromes	Face/Emotion
1. Originates at Liv-13, Spleen Mu	Liv/GB Qi stagnation	Hypochondriac pain, distention, painful breasts, chest tightness, difficulty breathing	
	Liv/GB overacting on Sp/St	Diarrhea, borborygmus, poor digestion, food retention, belching, flatulence	
2. Connects to GB-26, GB-27, GB-28	Liv/GB Qi stagnation (phlegm)	Abdominal fullness/distention/obesity; Abdominal masses, tumors, fibroids	

Continued

TABLE 3.9   DAI MAI SIGNS AND SYMPTOMS—cont'd

Pathway	Pattern	Syndromes	Face/Emotion
3. Connects with Du-4, then Bl-23	Damp heat in GB	Urogenital: vaginitis, leucorrhea, genital herpes, eczema, irregular menses, uterine prolapsed, urine retention/incontinence	
	GB channel disorders	Migraines, painful red eyes, lymph gland swelling, deafness, tinnitus, night blindness, upper/lower opposite side injuries, pulling sensation on the side of the body	
	Mental/ emotional disorders	Damp heat in GB	Two lines between eyebrows; frustration, resentment, anger, impatience

Yang Wei Mai

The Linking Vessel

The Connecting Vessel

The Fastener Vessel

Master point	TH-5 Waiguan Outer Gate
Couple point	GB-41 Zulinqi Foot Overlooking Tears
Location	TH-5 Waiguan Outer Gate is located 2 cun above TH-4 Yangchi Yang Pool, on the forearm, in the depression between the radius and the ulna
Needling	perpendicular insertion 0.5–1 cun

Indications	Relieves the exterior and expels dampness
	Expels heat to treat sore throat and fever
	Treats arm, shoulder and neck pain, and stiffness and spasms in the body by invigorating the channel
	Treats ear infections from Wind Heat or Liver Fire; deafness, tinnitus
	Treats migraines due to Liver Yang Rising

Continued   67

	Protects the Wei Qi; chills, fever, irritability, hypochondriac pain, bitter taste in mouth, constipation
	Calms the Shen
	Red and painful eyes, tearing when exposed to wind
Psychospiritual	Symptoms of both chills and fever, plus hypochondriac and chest distention, can manifest when Yang Wei Mai is imbalanced. Yang Wei Mai treats both excess and deficient Yang Qi, and is effective in addressing Shen disturbances, such as manic depression, obsessive-compulsive behavior, anger and frustration
Comments	The master point of Yang Wei Mai is TH-5 Waiguan Outer Gate, and its couple point is GB-41 Zulinqi Foot Overlooking Tears. The Yang Wei Channel controls all the Yang meridians and regulates the protective Wei Qi; when both Yin and Yang Wei are weak, there is a loss of body strength, as well as willpower. One of the main symptoms is chills and fever, because it balances the Wei Protective Qi in the body
	The Yang Wei Mai dominates the exterior, and regulates the Qi in the Taiyang and Shaoyang Channels. It is related to both the Bladder and the Gall Bladder

Yang Wei Mai Pathway (Figure 3.10)

1. Yang Wei Mai begins at the lateral aspect of the foot at Bl-63 Jinmen Metal Gate.

2. It then ascends the Gall Bladder meridian to GB-35 Yangjiao Yang Intersection, to the hip joint, and further along the hypochondriac and intercostal area to the posterior aspect of the shoulder, where it passes through SI-10 Naoshu Upper Arm Shu, TH-15 Tianliao Celestial Bone Hole and GB-20 Fengchi Wind Pool.

3. From there, it ascends the side of the neck to the forehead to arrive at GB-13 Benshen Root Spirit and GB-14 Yangbai Great White.

4. Then, it circles back on the head and around the ear, connecting GB-15 Toulinqi Head Overlooking Tears and GB-20 Fengchi Wind Pool.

5. The pathway ends at the nape of the neck, where it meets Du-15 Yamen Mute's Gate and Du-16 Fengfu Wind Mansion.

YANG WEI MAI PATHWAY SUMMARY

- Begins at Bl-63 Jinmen
- Laterally ascends the hip to GB-35 Yangjiao
- Passes up the lateral hypochondrium and ribs to the shoulder and meets at SI-10 Naoshu, TH-15 Tianliao and GB-20 Fengchi
- Ascends the side of the neck to the forehead and intersects with GB-13 Benshen and GB-14 Yangbai
- Circles back and around the ear, connecting with GB-15 Toulingqi and GB-20 Fengchi
- Terminates at Du-15 Yamen and Du-16 Fengu

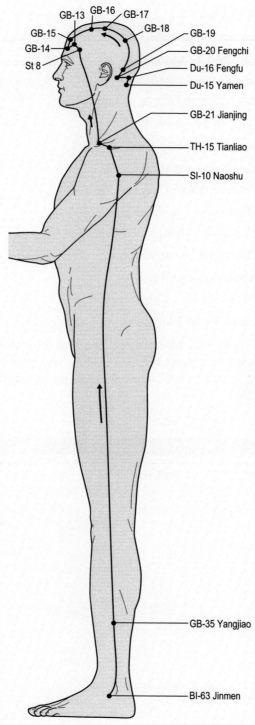

Points on the head
GB-13 Benshen
GB-14 Yangbai
GB-15 Toulingqi
GB-16 Muchuang
GB-17 Zhengying
GB-18 Chengling
GB-19 Naokong

GB-13
GB-16
GB-17
GB-15
GB-18
GB-14
St 8
GB-19
GB-20 Fengchi
Du-16 Fengfu
Du-15 Yamen
GB-21 Jianjing
TH-15 Tianliao
SI-10 Naoshu
GB-35 Yangjiao
Bl-63 Jinmen

Figure 3.10 Yang Wei Mai pathway.

Crossing Points

BL-63 Jinmen Metal Gate

GB-35 Yangjiao Yang Intersection

SI-10 Naoshu Upper Arm Shu

TH-15 Tianliao Celestial Bone Hole

GB-20 Fengchi Wind Pool

GB-13 Benshen Root Spirit

GB-14 Yangbai Great White

GB-15 Toulinqi Head Overlooking Tears

GB-16 Muchuang Eye Window

GB-17 Zhengying Upright Construction

GB-18 Chengling Spirit Support

GB-19 Naokong Brain Hollow

Du-15 Yamen Mute's Gate

Du-16 Fengu Wind Mansion

Because Yang Wei Mai protects the Wei Qi and treats Shaoyang syndrome, which is the last stand before a pathogen penetrates the interior of the body, its pathway can be used to treat AIDS, cancer and more serious illnesses (see Table 3.10).

TABLE 3.10 YANG WEI MAI SIGNS AND SYMPTOMS			
Pathway	**Pattern**	**Syndromes**	**Face/Emotion**
1. Begins at Bl-63	Bi syndrome	Pain in lower back, knee, legs and external malleolus, one-sided backache on lateral side of the body	Face contorted due to pain; irritability
	External wind (Wei Qi)	Shivering/aversion to cold/intermittent chills and fever (Shaoyang syndrome), bitter taste in mouth	
2. Ascends to GB-35 (Xi Cleft point), passing up to the hip joint	Bi syndrome	Swollen, painful knee	
	Wei syndrome	Lower leg atrophy (cold and painful)	

Continued

TABLE 3.10	YANG WEI MAI SIGNS AND SYMPTOMS—cont'd		
Pathway	**Pattern**	**Syndromes**	**Face/Emotion**
	Bi syndrome	Lateral hypochondriac distention, hip pain, sciatica (GB channel), hypochondriac pain	
3. Ascends to the shoulder, SI-10, TH-15, GB-21	Bi syndrome	Scapular, shoulder, arm, neck pain	
4. Travels up the side of the neck to the forehead, GB-13, GB-14	Liver Yang Rising	Unilateral headache, pain in forehead, neck, red eyes	Two lines between eyebrows (damp heat in GB)
	Internal wind	Dizziness, facial paralysis due to Bell's palsy or stroke	Droopy eyelid, deviation of mouth; stress, frustration, anger, trauma
	Calms Shen (mind)	Schizophrenia, multiple personalities, obsessive/compulsive	Jealousy, suspicion, excessive anger
5. Circles around ear at GB-15 – GB-20	Liver Yang Rising	Tinnitus, deafness	
	Damp heat (GB)	Discharge from ears	
6. Ends at the back of the head at Du-15, Du-16 (brain)	Internal wind	Epilepsy, convulsions, sudden blurred vision	Contorted facial expressions; Fear/ fright, anxiety

Conclusion

The Eight Extraordinary Meridians carve out a singular and marvelous network of energetic pathways deep within the human body. As we have seen, while some of them share certain acupuncture points and pathways with the Twelve Regular Meridians, they nevertheless display their own individual character – pathways, indications, functions and usages.

They also resonate very profoundly at an archetypal level, and play a decisive role in the determination of our individual character and the forging of our particular destiny.

For example, Ren Mai controls all the Yin meridians of the body, but it also represents the archetypal feminine (Earth), and relates to issues of nourishment that arise from bonding or not bonding with Mother (Yin).

Du Mai controls all the Yang meridians, and relates to the archetypal masculine (Heaven) and issues involving standing upright, risk taking and becoming independent in life.

Chong Mai, the Sea of Blood, the progenitor of Ren and Du Mai, represents our genetic blueprint, and relates to intergenerational patterns passed down through a family's bloodline.

Dai Mai, or the Belt Meridian, represents archetypal shadow issues, manifesting as Shaoyang imbalances, which can lead to an inability to make a challenging decision, and a tendency to store unwanted 'stuck' life issues under the belt as damp heat and phlegm.

The Yang and Yin Qiao Mai (Heel) Vessels facilitate movement of the lower limbs on the right (Yang) and the left (Yin) sides of the body, and they characterize our different interactions with the world. The Yang Qiao personality blames others for their problems (wind) and can't sleep, while the Yin Qiao personality turns their anger inward, and sleeps all of the time.

The Yin and Yang Wei Mai (Linking Vessels) maintain the balance of Yang and Yin throughout the body, and relate to the Du and Ren Mai, respectively. They govern the reproductive cycles of 7/8, and archetypally represent how we choose to relate to aging.

In our exploration of these meridians, we retrace the steps of our life's journey and the challenges we may encounter when bonding with Mother (*Ren*), taking risks (*Du*), and interacting with the world (the *Qiaos*). Depending on our ancestral heritage and conditioning (*Chong*), we may have problems digesting and assimilating new experience; when we encounter these obstacles, we may stuff them under the belt to avoid making a decision (*Dai*).

How we respond to this experiential life process and the inescapable fact of our own aging (*Weis*) is ultimately revealed to us in the way we choose to live our lives. Let us navigate this passage with integrity, dignity, and sufficient wisdom to realize that every season of life can be filled with hope, joy, and the potential for continued transformation.

REFERENCES

1. Macioia G. The Channels of Acupuncture: Clinical Use of Secondary Channels and Extraordinary Vessels. London, UK: Elsevier Press; 2006. p. 401.

2. Ibid., p. 346.

3. Ni Y. Navigating Channels of Traditional Chinese Medicine. San Diego, CA: Oriental Medical Center; 1996. p. 120.

4. Matsumoto K, Birch S. Extraordinary Vessels. Brookline, MA: Paradigm Publications; 1986. p. 46.

CHAPTER 4

The Twelve
Regular Meridians

"Wisdom is sweeter than honey, brings more joy than wine, illuminates more than the Sun, is more precious than jewels. She causes the ears to hear, and the heart to comprehend."
— *Makeda, Queen of Sheba, 1000 BCE*

This chapter focuses on fundamental Five Element constitutional treatments for facial acupuncture. I have organized this information according to the pathology of the Five Phases and integrated it with the corresponding Twelve Regular Meridian pathway indications. Each Five Element section includes a Recommended Constitutional Treatment Protocol, featuring an Eight Extraordinary Meridian pair, a root supporting treatment with locations, functions and both physical and psychospiritual indications. Based upon my years of personal experience with Traditional Chinese Medicine (TCM), and Japanese and Vietnamese acupuncture, I have selected and presented treatment protocols, targeting specific syndromes that I feel are particularly relevant to your work as facial acupuncturists. You will learn specialized point locations, needling and palpation protocols, and also find suggestions regarding moxibustion and magnet therapy.

I have done my best to acknowledge the fine Japanese teachers who have created these protocols and transmitted their wisdom to subsequent generations of practitioners – Kiiko Matsumoto-sensei, Nagano-sensei, Manaka-sensei, Kawai-sensei and Dr. Hukaya. I am also grateful to my teacher, Carolyn Bengston, who kindly taught me Bac-si Truong Thin's Vietnamese Back Treatment and other Vietnamese treatment protocols.

In working with touch and palpation, Japanese acupuncture treatments rely upon the detection of tight tender areas that may not necessarily coincide with

TCM locations, but vary from treatment to treatment. For example, Nagano-sensei's Stomach Qi points manifest in different locations on the Stomach meridian for each patient.

Japanese acupuncture also employs hara palpation, and the Five Element reflex points, which are palpated for tight tenderness, pain or knotty, rope-like, sensations. This tenderness may change when the acupuncture treatment points are held for 30–60 seconds. If this occurs, then these points are needled on the body. The reflex area is checked again during the treatment to see if it has cleared; if not, another set of points is selected, and, of course, the pulse is re-checked. The patient's body communicates what it needs, in the form of a shout or a whisper, and the Japanese acupuncture practitioner is receptive to the incoming signals. This is a living, vital and intricate system with an extended tradition of blind acupuncturists, whose sense of touch is so refined that their fingers act as little ears, sensitively attuned to the shifts and changes in the patient's Qi.

While there are many different lineages and schools within Japanese acupuncture, I offer you these protocols and other techniques that I have found to be not only useful, but also very effective in the successful treatment of patients with Constitutional Facial Acupuncture.

The Metal Element: Lung, Hand Taiyin, and Large Intestine, Hand Yangming Pathways

The Lung Meridian Pathway: Hand Taiyin

- The Lung Meridian originates in the middle Jiao at Ren-12 Zhongmen Central Venter, and flows downwards to connect with the Large Intestine.

- Winding back, it goes along the upper orifice of the Stomach, through the cardiac orifice and the diaphragm, then penetrates the Lung. From the Lung, it communicates with the throat at Ren-22 Tiantu Celestial Chimney, and emerges at Lu-1 Zhongfu Central Treasury.

- Then it travels continuously downward along the antero-lateral aspect of the forearm, and enters the 'cunkoa' or radial artery at the wrist at Lu-9 Taiyuan Great Abyss.

- Traversing the thenar eminence, the pathway ends at the radial side of the top of the thumbnail at Lu-11 Shaoshang Lesser Shang.

- A branch proximal to the wrist emerges at Lu-7 Lieque Broken Sequence and runs directly to the radial side of the tip of the index finger, where it links with the Large Intestine Meridian at LI-1 Shangyang Lesser Yang.

Symptoms of Lung Hand Taiyin Meridian

- Pain in shoulders, back and supraclavicular fossa; aversion to cold.
- Pain along course of meridian, e.g., tennis elbow, stiff forearm.
- Wrist disorders, carpal tunnel syndrome.

Internal Branch Disorders

- Disorders of throat, trachea, vocal chords and voice.
- Shortness of breath, spontaneous sweating, bronchitis, asthma, chest tightness, palpitations and emphysema.
- Diaphragmatic tightness.
- Frequent urination, incontinence, edema.
- Diarrhea, constipation.

The Large Intestine Meridian: Hand Yangming

- The Large Intestine Meridian starts from the tip of the index finger at LI-1 Shangyang Lesser Yang.
- It then travels upwards along the radial side of the index finger between the 1st and 2nd metacarpal bones to the wrist joint.
- From there, it ascends the forearm to the lateral aspect of the elbow.
- Then it travels up the lateral aspect of the upper arm to the highest point of the shoulder LI-15 Jianju Shoulder Bone.
- It continues along the anterior border of the acromion to the 7th cervical vertebra, Du-14 Dazhu Great Hammer, and descends to the supraclavicular fossa, where it enters the body cavity and connects internally with the Lung.
- It then passes through the diaphragm and enters the Large Intestine at St-25 Tianzhu, Celestial Pivot.
- A branch from the supraclavicular fossa runs upward to the neck, passes through the cheek and enters the gums of the lower teeth.
- From there, the left meridian goes to the right, and the right meridian to the left, and to both sides of the nose LI-20 Yingxiang Welcome Fragrance, where the Large Intestine Meridian links with the Stomach Meridian of Foot Yangming.

Symptoms of Large Intestine Hand Yangming Meridian

- Neck stiffness and swelling.
- Pain in shoulder, bursitis, arm, tennis elbow and index finger.
- Sinusitis, epistaxis, toothache, red, painful eyes and throat, facial paralysis, rashes, itching and hyperpigmentation.

Internal Branch Disorders

- Intestinal disorders, abdominal pain and swelling, borborygmus, flatulence, diarrhea.

- Epigastric pain, vomiting, facial edema, constipation, belching.

- Associated Lung complaints; asthma, bronchitis, cough.

The Metal Element: Communication

Lung, Hand Taiyin, and Large Intestine, Hand Yangming, represent the minerals, ores, metals and beautiful gems of the earth. For example, the diamond symbolizes endurance and longevity, because it cannot be destroyed, except by very high temperatures. Metal and crystals have substance, strength and conduct electricity, which makes them the main component in communications technology. They form a network in the Earth, as does the meridian system within our bodies.

The Lung takes in energy from the air, while the Large Intestine lets go and eliminates unwanted substances from the body. Functionally, the Metal element governs Qi and breathing, as well as the distribution of Qi and fluids throughout the body. When it is balanced, a person is positive, has abundant Qi, communicates freely and is vital. When the Metal element is imbalanced, they are sad, pessimistic and remote.

The Lung is the only Zang organ that connects to the inner and outer worlds of heaven, Tian, and Earth, Tu. Taking in a breath, 'inspiration,' links us to heavenly Qi, creativity and vibrancy, while letting go and releasing the breath, 'expiration,' connects us again to Earth, the physical aspect of the Lung, which represents the Po, or the corporeal soul.

Letting go of resentments and pre-conceived ideas about reality allows us to be fully alive in the moment. This process of breathing in Heaven, and relinquishing the old engenders reverence and simplicity, according to the ancient Chinese.

Our first breath of life belongs to the Lung, which not only provides us with the ability to be in relationship with others, but also the integrity to stand alone.

METAL ELEMENT PATHOLOGY	
Immune system	Frequent colds and influenza, low immunity, deficient Qi, lassitude, asthma, emphysema, cough, shortness of breath (SOB), palpitations, chest pain
Lymphatic system	Chronic swollen lymph nodes

Continued

Head, nose and throat	Nasal obstruction, rhinitis, sinusitis, pharyngitis, laryngitis, tonsillitis, epitaxis, frontal headache
Fluid imbalances	Body and facial edema, urine retention, enuresis, incontinence, yellow urine
Digestive tract	Diarrhea, constipation, abdominal fullness and distention, epigrastic pain
Pathogenic influences	Aversion to cold, fever without perspiration, sinus, headache, sneezing
Allergies	Sneezing, watery, itchy eyes, nose and throat; craves milk products
Weak connective tissue	Tendonitis, 'tennis elbow,' frequent ankle sprains, arthritis
Complexion	Rashes, itchy, painful skin, hyperpigmentation and discolorations, acne, eczema, boils and psoriasis
Emotions	Extreme grief and sadness

Recommended Constitutional Treatment Protocol

Open the Ren Mai contralaterally with the Eight Extraordinary meridians; Lu-7 Lieque Broken Sequence and Kid-6 Zhaohai Shining Sea.

Root Treatment

Lu-10 Yuji Fish Border (Right Side)
Lu-9 Taiyuan Great Abyss (Left Side)
Ying Spring Fire Point

Location	At the midpoint of the thenar eminence of the 1st metacarpal bone, at the border separating the red and white skin
Functions	Clears Lung heat
	Benefits throat
	Sescends rebellious Qi
	Shen disturbances
Indications	Dry, sore throat, loss of voice
	Asthma, cough, shortness of breath (SOB)

	Coughing up and vomiting blood, hiccoughs
	Agitation, fear, anger and mania
	Pain and heat along the meridian
Psychospiritual	This fire point on the Metal element warms and encourages metal to become more malleable, less cold and sharp like a knife
	It fosters the qualities of abundance, generosity, recognition and love
Comments	Ying Spring points clear heat, and Lu-10 Yuji is an excellent distal point to treat Lung heat and throat issues, such as swelling, dryness and loss of voice
	It helps descend Lung Qi and calms coughing and also addresses
	bleeding imbalances due to rebellious Qi
	Its internal pathway originates at Ren-12 Zhongwan Central Venter, and, as a result, stomach issues like vomiting blood can manifest. Lung heat upsets the chest area, causes Shen disturbances, as well as pain and heat in the joints, especially arthritis in the thumb joint. Due to both an aversion to cold and Lung heat, there can be skin disorders. Tonify this point for cold, silvery and flaky skin, and sedates it for hot, red and inflamed skin

Lu-9 Taiyuan Great Abyss
Shu Stream Earth Point
Yuan Source, Tonification Point
Influential Point of the Vessels

Location	On the palmar aspect of the transverse wrist crease, in the depression at the lateral side of the radial artery
Functions	Tonifies Lung Qi and Yin
	Transforms phlegm
	Regulates and descends Lung Qi
	Regulates and harmonizes blood circulation in the vessels
	Alleviates pain in the meridian
Indications	Cough, cold, asthma, wheezing, dyspnea, shortness of breath (SOB)
	Hemoptysis, sore throat, chest pain

Continued

	Agitation, manic behavior
	Belching, red painful eyes
	Pain and weakness in the wrist, shoulder and back
Psychospiritual	Lu-9 Taiyuan is particularly useful when a person is in despair and deep depression
	When everything in their life seems chaotic, this point provides stability, security, nourishment and loving support. It is an Earth Yuan Source point on the Metal element, which directly tonifies the spiritual aspect of the Lung, and gives hope to a person who feels like they are falling into an abyss
Comments	Lu-9 Taiyuan is the most important point on the Lung meridians. As a Shu Stream Earth point, and the Mother of the Earth element, it allows Qi to flow abundantly forth from this deep abyss. It is also a Yuan Source point and directly treats the Lung organ. Lung rules Qi flow in the body, and Qi commands and moves blood, which allows the Lung to gather and tonify Qi in the heart and chest, in the area of Ren-17 Danzhong Chest Center. It is also the Influential Point of the Vessels, which affects the pulses and circulation of blood in the arteries and veins

Japanese Acupuncture Treatments

The Lung is described as the tender organ, and it rules protective Wei Qi and the immune system. Patients with lowered immunity tend to catch colds and flu more readily than others, and they lack the ability to shake these illnesses once they have contracted them. If the pathogen penetrates deeper into their bodies, imbalances such as asthma, bronchitis and strep throat can manifest. Usually a previous tonsillectomy, which includes removal of the adenoids, negatively impacts the immune system, and they may have chronic issues of swollen lymph nodes in the throat, groin and armpits.

Since weak connective tissue also relates to the strength of the immune system, they could have loose ligaments and collagen disorder. Metal element-related immune imbalances manifest as neck pain in the area of the scalene muscle at TH-16 Tianyou Celestial Window, along the levator scapula muscle, and also at the patellar ligament of the knee.

As a result of these imbalances, the complexion tends to be pale, and, due to the correspondingly weak connective tissue, the skin is delicate, dry and more prone to wrinkles and sagging.

With the involvement of the Large Intestine, there can be associated constipation and diarrhea, and focal infections in the sinuses with nasal obstruction and discharge.

Asthma

Treatment points	Japanese Lu-5 Chize Cubit Marsh plus Japanese Kid-3 Taixi Great Ravine, or:
	Japanese Lu-5 Chize Cubit Marsh plus Japanese Sp-4 Gongsun Yellow Emperor
Locations	Dr. Hukaya's Lu-5 Chize is more lateral than the TCM Lu-5 Chize. It is located in the cubital crease midway between the TCM Lu-5 Chize and LI-11 Quchi, Pool at the Bend. Palpate it 1 cun above or below for tight tenderness. Japanese Kid-3 Taixi is found closer to the TCM Kid-4 Dazhong Large Goblet, in the depression 0.5 cun below and slightly posterior to Kid-3 Taixi. The TCM location for Sp-4 Gongsun is on the medial aspect of the foot in the depression distal and inferior to the base of the 1st metatarsal bone. The Japanese Sp-4 Gongsun may be needled more distal and inferior to the 1st metatarsal bone, depending upon palpation for tight tenderness. The Japanese Asthma Shu is 0.5 cun superior and 0.5 cun lateral to Bl-17 Geshu Diaphragm Shu. This Influential Point of Blood is located 1.5 un on either side of the spine under the 7th thoracic vertebrae
Palpation and needling protocol	First discern what pattern you are treating, and then couple Japanese Lu-5 Chize and Japanese Kid-3 Taixi with the Asthma Shu, or Japanese Lu-5 Chize and Japanese Sp-4 Gongsun with the Asthma Shu. Needle the Japanese Lu-5 Chize 15 degrees toward Lu-9 Taiyuan in the cubital crease or 1 cun above or below the point, depending upon palpation. Add Japanese Kid-3 Taixi, and needle toward the Achilles tendon. Palpate the Asthma Shu for pressure pain or knottiness and needle it bilaterally downward toward the patient's feet. If the knot is large, the asthma is chronic, and the area needs to be warmed with moxa. Burn 6–7 direct moxa cones bilaterally on this point, and make sure that your patient feels the heat with each cone. You can apply a Japanese ointment called Shiunko under the moxa to provide a protective barrier between the skin and the burning moxa. The ingredients are Dang Gui *Radix angelicae sinensis,* which tonifies blood, and Zi Cao Gen *Radix arnebiae seu Lithospermi,* for cooling the blood, sesame oil and beeswax. Needle Japanese Sp-4 Gongsun at a 90-degree angle into the patient's foot. Needle all of these points bilaterally, or use moxibustion
Indications	Difficulty inhaling; Japanese Lu-5 Chize and Japanese Kid-3 Taixi
	Difficulty exhaling; Japanese Lu-5 Chize and Japanese Sp-4 Gongsun
	Wheezing, dyspnea, shortness of breath (SOB)
	Fatigue, lassitude
	Cough, tightness in the chest
	Asthma, allergies
Comments	Difficulty inhaling usually indicates constricted bronchi, which impedes the Lung Qi from descending to be grasped by the Kidneys. Problems with exhalation and releasing breath point to dilated bronchi, and indicate Spleen involvement

Loose Ligaments and Weak Connective Tissue

Treatment points	Japanese Stomach Qi, Japanese Kid-6 Zhaohai Shining Sea, TCM BI-62 Shenmai Extending Vessel and Japanese Triple Intestine 10 (T. I. 10)
Locations	Nagano-sensei's Stomach Qi consists of several points located by firm palpation from St-36 Zusanli Leg Three Li, down to St-41 Jiexi Ravine Divide, on the Stomach meridian. Japanese Kid-6 Zhaohai is found lower and further back from the TCM point. When a line is drawn from the posterior and inferior edges of the medial malleolus, the point is at the angle where they meet. There are other non-TCM locations for Zhaohai. My personal favorite for immune deficient patients, who have tenderness and puffiness in the medial ankle area, is a point equidistantly located between a diagonal line drawn from the TCM Kid-6 Zhaohai to the edge of the heel. Palpate for this exquisitely tender spot, and needle it transversely upward toward the location of TCM Kid-6 Zhaohai. The TCM BI-62 Shenmai is in the depression below the lateral malleolus. Nagano-sensei's Large Intestine 10/11 point, called Triple Intestine 10 (T. I. 10) by Kiiko Matsumoto, is between the TCM LI-10 Shousanli Arm Three Li and TCM LI-11 Quchi Pool at the Bend, close to the Triple Heater meridian. If you place your thumb on the patient's radius, and roll it over the bone, in the direction of the body, you will detect tight tender points in this area
Palpation and needling protocol	Palpate Nagano-sensei's Stomach Qi bilaterally by sliding your finger from St-36 Zusanli Leg Three Li down to St-41 Jiexi, and feel for lumps or tight tenderness. Needle these points 45 degrees downward and 45 degrees toward the tibia, then burn 6–7 direct moxa on them. Needle Japanese Kid-6 Zhaohai downward toward the Achilles tendon, and insert TCM BI-62 Shenmai perpendicularly or slightly upward, depending upon your patient's needs. Needles inserted into Triple Intestine 10 (T. 1. 10) are angled 90 degrees toward the Triple Heater meridian. Treat all points bilaterally
Indications	Tendonitis of the elbow; 'tennis elbow'
	Sprained ankles
	A weak patellar ligament of the knee
	Swollen lymph glands
	Low immunity, lassitude and fatigue

Continued

Comments	Connective tissue supports, connects and separates organs and tissues in the body. Fibroblast cells produce connective tissue and are the precursors to collagen elastin production. There are different types of connective tissue which are explained below
	Collagen fibers found in tendons, ligaments, skin and cartilage
	Elastin fiber and type III collagen in the lymphatic organs, Liver and in bone marrow
	This Japanese treatment for loose ligaments is very effective for sprained ankles and tendonitis due to sports injuries. The Qiaos or heel vessels benefit structural or postural problems relating to the lower legs and the right and left sides of the body. They regulate Yin and Yang functions, mobility and the twin hemispheres of the brain.
	To treat a weak patellar ligament which causes pain, swelling and discomfort, add St-44 Neiting Inner Court to this treatment. St-44 indications are covered in the Earth element under the Food Allergy, Food Poisoning and Amebic Dysentery section of this chapter
	Dr. Horiguchi said that weak ligaments are originally caused by focal infections like naso-pharyngitis, due to a compromised immune system

Immune System Imbalances

Treatment points	Nagano-sensei's immune points: Triple Intestine 10
Locations	The location of Nagano-sensei's LI-10/11 point named Triple Intestine 10 was discussed in the previous section on Loose Ligaments and Weak Connective Tissue
Palpation and needling protocol	The Metal element hara is located and palpated on the right side from St-25 Tianshu Celestial Pivot to St-27 Daju Great Gigantic for knots and tight sensations. If the patient has tension in this area, and has Lung symptoms such as a cough, asthma, recurring colds, sinus issues, and a weak or superficial Lung pulse, then it would be good idea to treat them with Nagano-sensei's immune points. Insert the needle bilaterally 90 degrees and angle it toward the Triple Heater meridian. Make sure your patient has their elbows bent, placed over the solar plexus, with the palms facing the body. You can add 6–7 thread moxa cones or use direct moxa with Shiunko ointment. Be aware that you can insert more than one needle if you find multiple knots and tension at this point
Indications	Weak immune system
	Swollen lymph nodes

Continued

Comments	Recurring colds, flu, sore throat
	Weak connective tissue and ligaments
	When a patient suffers from frequent colds, influenza, allergies, a cough, rhinitis, or sinusitis, exhibits a floating or deficient Lung pulse, or complains of tennis elbow or tendonitis, integrate TI-10 into your constitutional treatment protocol
	Low immunity also affects the connective tissue, which is comprised of tendons, ligaments, collagen and elastin fibers. See the Loose Ligaments and Weak Connective Tissue portion of this chapter.
	Needle and/or moxa TI-10 during the treatment, and then apply Japanese magnets to these points after the session to give continued support to the patient's immune system
	You should also educate and instruct your patients how to locate these points for themselves, and how to apply the magnets as a preventative when they feel that they are on the verge of contracting a cold or flu. Have them remove the magnets, if they appear to cause any skin irritation, itchiness or redness. Usually the magnets can remain in place for 3 days

Lu-8 Jingqu Channel Ditch
Jing River Metal Point
Horary Point

Location	The TCM location is 1 cun above the transverse crease of the wrist, in the depression on the lateral side of the radial artery. The Japanese location is ascertained by palpation. Pinch the skin in the area of Lu-8 Jingqu until skin is too thick and cannot be grasped. Needle it obliquely, then transversely, in the direction of the meridian flow or counter to the flow, if there is excess mucus in the chest
Functions	TCM:
	Descends Lung Qi
	Alleviates Lung symptoms
	Clears heat
	Japanese:
	Oxygenates the body
	Horary Master point of the Lung
	Supports organ function
	Treats meridian obstruction

Indications	TCM:
	Asthma, cough, chest fullness, sore throat, shortness of breath (SOB)
	Heat in the palms, fever without perspiration
	Wrist pain and pain in the soles of the feet
	Japanese:
	Brings Qi and oxygen flow to the chest, opens the throat, cleanses and hydrates the skin
	Numbness and tingling in the meridian
	Oxygenates tissues at a cellular level
	After surgery and in treating scars
Psychospiritual	This Jing River point brings fresh Qi and blood to the body, cleanses toxins and revitalizes mind and spirit. It also flushes out hyperpigmentation, boils, mucus, constipation, and addresses chest pain and throat issues
Comments	Lu-8 Jingqu is rarely included in TCM treatments. However, in Japanese acupuncture, it is an important horary point on the Lung meridian. It stimulates circulation of Qi and blood, and transports oxygen throughout the body on a cellular level. Integrate it into treatments for post-operative patients, who not only have blood stasis, but also a general lack of oxygen in their tissues. It is also effective for scar therapy, and in the treatment of meridian obstructions, which contribute to neuropathy, a numb and tingling sensation resulting from certain medications, surgery, a sports injury or an accident. It is similarly excellent for oxygenating and clearing the skin, and alleviating hyperpigmentation, acne or boils

CONSTITUTIONAL TREATMENT SUMMARY
METAL ELEMENT: LUNG AND LARGE INTESTINE

Syndromes	Treatment Points	Indications
Asthma	(J) Lu-5 Chize Cubit Marsh plus (J) Kid-3 Taixi Great Ravine, Asthma Shu	Difficulty inhaling
	(J) Lu-5 Chize Cubit Marsh plus (J) Sp-4 Gongsun Yellow Emperor, Asthma Shu	Difficulty exhaling
Loose ligaments and weak connective tissue	(J) Stomach Qi (J) Kid-6 Zhaohai Shining Sea Bl-62 Shenmai Extending Vessel (J) Triple Intestine 10	Digestive and muscle problems; Yin Qiao Mai imbalance; Yang Qiao Mai imbalance; immune deficiency

CONSTITUTIONAL TREATMENT SUMMARY
METAL ELEMENT: LUNG AND LARGE INTESTINE—cont'd

Syndromes	Treatment Points	Indications
Immune system imbalances	(J) Triple Intestine 10	Weak immune system, swollen lymph glands, recurring colds, influenza
Oxygen point	(J) Lu-8 Jingqu Channel Ditch	Oxygenates body at a cellular level, hydrates skin

(J), Japanese point.

The Earth Element: Stomach, Foot Yangming, and Spleen, Foot Taiyin

The Stomach Meridian Pathway: Foot Yangming

- The Stomach meridian starts at the lateral side of the nose LI-20 Yingxiang Welcome Fragrance.

- It ascends to the bridge of the nose, where it meets the Bladder meridian at Bl-1 Jingming Bright Eyes.

- Traveling downward along the infraorbital ridge to St-1 Chengqi Tear Container, it enters the upper gums.

- Re-emerging, it curves around the lips, and descends to meet Ren Mai in the infraorbital groove at Ren-24 Chengjiang Sauce Receptacle.

- Then, it travels laterally across the lower portion of the cheek to St-5 Daying Great Reception, winds along the angle of the mandible to St-6 Jiache Jawbone, and ascends in front of the ear GB-3 Shangguan Upper Gate. Then it follows the anterior hairline and reaches the forehead at St-8 Touwei Head Corner.

- The facial branch travels in front of St-5 Daying Great Reception, downward to St-12 Quepen Empty Basin, and along the throat to enter the supraclavicular fossa; then it travels posteriorly to the upper back, where it meets Du-14 Dazhui Great Hammer.

- Descending, it passes through the diaphragm, enters the Stomach and connects with the Spleen.

- Another branch arises from the supraclavicular fossa, runs downward to the chest, and passes through the nipples.

- It travels 4 cun lateral to the Ren Mai on the chest, and 2 cun lateral to the abdomen, and descends along the navel to meet at St-30 Qichong Surging Qi.

- An internal branch from the lower orifice of the Stomach descends inside the abdomen, and joins the previous portion of the meridian at St-30 Qichong Surging Qi.

- The meridian continues down to St-31 Biguan Thigh Joint, and further to St-32 Futu Crouching Rabbit, and reaches the knee.

- From there is continues along the lateral aspect of the tibia to the dorsum of the foot, ending at the lateral side of the tip of the second toe (St-45 Lidui Severe Mouth).

- The tibial branch emerges at the St-36 Zusanli Leg Three Li at the lateral side of the middle toe. Another brach from the dorsum of the foot St-42 Chongyang Surging Yang terminates at the medial side of the big toe (Sp-1 Yinbai Hidden White), where it links with the Spleen meridian.

Symptoms of Stomach Foot Yangming Meridian

- Dry nose, front headache, red face and eyes, lip and mouth ulcers, herpes, mouth deviation, painful throat, swollen neck, toothache.

- Muscle spasms, thigh and knee pain.

- Swollen breast, fibrocystic breasts, epistaxis.

Internal Branch Disorders

- Manic depression.

- Gastrointestinal complaints, frequent hunger, gastritis, borborygmus.

- Stomach complaints, ulcers, nausea, vomiting, diarrhea, constipation.

The Spleen Meridian Pathway: Foot Taiyin

- The Spleen Meridian starts from the tip of the great toe, Sp-1 Yinbai Hidden White.

- It travels along the medial aspect of the foot in front of the medial malleolus.

- It follows the posterior aspect border of the tibia up the medial leg, 8 cun above the medial malleolus, and travels in front of the Liver Meridian.

- Ascending the medial aspect of the knee and thigh to the abdomen, it meets Ren-3 Zhongqi Central Pole, Ren-4 Guanyuan Origin Pass, and Ren-10 Xiawan Lower Venter, before entering the Spleen and connecting with the Stomach.

- It emerges from the Stomach area, and ascends lateral to the midline, 4 and 6 cun respectively, meeting GB-24 Riyue Sun and Moon, Liv-14 Qimen Cycle Gate, and Lu-1 Zhongfu Central Treasury.

- The external pathway descends to terminate at the side of the chest Sp-21 Dabao Great Embracement.

- A branch ascends and passes through the diaphragm, along the esophagus, and spreads over the the lower surface of the tongue.

- Another branch from the Stomach passes through the diaphragm and flows into the Heart, and connects with the Heart meridian.

Symptoms of Spleen Foot Taiyin Meridian

- Wei syndrome atrophy of the muscles and extremities.

- Facial puffiness, pain in cheek and jaw.

- Stiffness of tongue, impaired speech.

- Medial leg, knee and thigh pain.

- Swelling of legs, feet and joints.

- Bunions.

Internal Branch Disorders

- Epigrastic pain below the Heart, loose stools, borborygmus, vomiting, nausea, abdominal fullness and distention.

- General fatigue, especially in the limbs.

- Edema, excess phlegm, leucorrhea.

The Earth Element: Nourishment

Stomach, Foot Yangming, and Spleen, Foot Taiyin represent the Yang and Yin aspects of the Earth element. Earth is the center of our existence, and regulates all of the cycles in our lives, from sleeping, breathing and thinking to the menstrual cycle.

Earth is the source of physical nourishment, and refers to our sense of being grounded and rooted within ourselves.

Functionally, the Spleen is in charge of transforming and transporting Qi, as well as controlling and holding blood in the vessels; the Stomach then rots and ripens food, and passes the Qi on to the Spleen for nourishment.

If a person is in harmony with the Earth element, they are grounded, centered, attentive, thoughtful and at home with themselves and the world. If imbalanced, they can be co-dependent, obsessed, uprooted, worried and searching for support or answers outside of themselves. The Yi, Intellect, represents the spirit of the Earth element, and can manifest as creative insights, inspirations or as obsessive thoughts, dogmas or mental inflexibility.

The emotional expression of Earth in an imbalanced state manifests as a constant need for sympathy or an inability to receive any kind of emotional support in troubled times. In my opinion, the balanced state is more akin to empathy. When the internal branch of the Spleen meridian passes through the diaphragm and flows freely and unconditionally to the Heart, caring emotional expressions can be communicated and shared with clarity and compassion, while simultaneously remaining centered in one's own Qi.

EARTH ELEMENT PATHOLOGY

Digestion	Indigestion, food allergies, gas, bloating, belching, duodenal ulcers, loss of appetite, diarrhea, constipation, borborygmus, vomiting, nausea, abdominal fullness and distention, epigastric pain, acid reflux
Eating disorders	Obesity, anorexia, bulimia, binge eating
Blood sugar imbalances	Hypoglycemia, diabetes, sugar cravings, poor memory and concentration
Immunity	Low immunity, lymphatic system imbalances, lassitude and fatigue
Blood pressure	High and low blood pressure imbalances
Organ prolapses	Abnormal smooth muscle function, prolapse of viscera
Menstrual disorders	Irregular menses, menorrhagia, metorrhagia, amenorrhea, dysmenorrhea, leucorrhea
Asthma and bronchitis	Difficulty with exhalation, shortness of breath (SOB)
Edema	Facial swelling, edema in the medial meniscus, lower leg, ankles and feet. Puffiness in the upper half of the abdomen, abdominal masses (phlegm)
Muscular problems	Spasm, cramps, ticklish abdomen and pain in the shoulders, mid-back and lower back, fibromyalgia
Wei syndrome	Atropy of lower extremities
Emotions	Obsessive worry and overthinking, anxiety, manic depression

Recommended Constitutional Treatment Protocol

Open the Chong Mai contralaterally with the Eight Extraordinary meridians; Sp-4; Gongsun Yellow Emperor and PC-6 Neiguan Inner Gate.

Root Treatment

Sp-2 Dadu Great Metropolis (Right Side)
Sp-3 Taibai Supreme White (Left Side)
Sp-2 Dadu Great Metropolis
Ying Spring Fire Point
Tonification Point

Location	On the medial side of the big toe, in the depression distal and inferior to the 1st metatarso-phalangeal joint
Functions	Supports and strengthens Spleen
	Clears Spleen heat
	Moves damp and promotes digestion
	Harmonizes Middle Jiao
Indications	Epigrastric upset, nausea, vomiting, diarrhea, constipation
	Low grade fevers, Heart pain
	Edema, urinary dysfunction
	Cold hands and feet
	Emotions; agitation, obsessive thinking
Psychospiritual	This Fire point on the Earth element provides warmth to the dirt or soil of the Earth. It is a tonification point, which increases a patient's vitality and vibrancy, and dispels physical fatigue and mental lethargy. If the patient has cold hands and feet, moxa this point. Moxa is contraindicated for pregnancy
Comments	The Ying Spring Fire point, Sp-2 Dadu, is one of the best points on the Spleen meridian to clear heat, move damp, and also to strengthen and tonify the function of the Spleen. Emotionally, it addresses agitation, obsessive, constant thinking and worry, which damages digestion. Its name 'Dadu' means Great Metropolis, and refers to a city or center of power and activity. The fact that this point is located on the big toe, and is the Mother, the supporting point of the Earth element, gives it greater significance

Sp-3 Taibai Supreme White
Shu Stream, Yuan Source
Earth Point
Horary Point

Location	On the medial side of the foot, in the depression proximal and inferior to the head of the 1st metatarsal bone
Functions	Harmonizes Spleen and Stomach
	Tonifies the Spleen, resolves damp and damp heat
	Strengthens the spine
	Tonifies Lung and stimulates Wei Protective Qi
	Regulates Qi
	Promotes transportation and transformation of Spleen
Indications	Poor appetite, lower energy, fatigue, abdominal fullness, diarrhea, borborygmus
	Hemorrhoids
	Dysentery
	Bi atrophy syndrome
	Epigastric and Heart pain
	Sensation of heaviness in the body and pain in the bones
	Pain in the knee, thigh, joints, lower back
	Moxa is applicable
Psychospiritual	Sp-3 Taibai Supreme White, when balanced, gives a patient the sense of being centered and abundant. If imbalanced, they feel impoverished, rarely satisfied, and never completely full and whole, no matter how much food or love is given to them. This is a horary point, Earth within Earth, and powerfully reinforces one's sense of identity, self-esteem and grounding in the world
Comments	Sp-3 Taibai is a Shu Stream, Yuan Source point, as well as an Earth point of the Spleen/Stomach meridians. It has a powerful action for directly strengthening and regulating Spleen and Stomach Qi. As a Shu Stream point, it fortifies Spleen Qi and Yang, and, as the Yuan Source point, directly treats the organs and accesses the original Qi in the body. Original Qi is housed in the Dantien, and in the space between the Kidneys, it forms the basis for reproduction of our species, and it is the root of the Twelve Regular meridians. The Spiritual Pivot instructs us to treat the Source points, if any of the 5 Zang Organs are imbalanced or diseased

The Four Corners Abdominal Treatment

This particular treatment is not based upon Japanese acupuncture, but is, rather, a TCM treatment that is very effective for digestive complaints.

Treatment points	St-25 Tianshu Celestial Pivot, Large Intestine Mu point
	Ren-12 Zhongwan Central Venter, Stomach Mu point, Influential Point for the Fu Organs, Meeting Point of the Small Intestine, Triple Heater and Stomach meridians
	Ren-6 Qihai Sea of Qi
Locations	St-25 Tianshu is 2 cun lateral to the center of the navel. Ren-12 Zhongwan is 4 cun above the navel on the abdominal midline. Ren-6 Qihai is 1.5 cun below the navel on the abdominal midline

St-25 Tianshu

Functions	Regulates Large Intestine meridian and organ
	Bi-phasic point; treats both diarrhea and constipation
	Tonifies Yuan Qi; moves and regulates Qi and blood
	Clears heat and damp
	Relieves food stagnation
	Calms Shen
Indications	Constipation and diarrhea
	Abdominal fullness
	Menstrual and reproductive imbalances; irregular menses, dysmenorrhea, infertility, leucorrhea
	Umbilical pain
	Edema; facial swelling
	Mental anxiety
Psychospiritual	This point provides nourishment and grounding for a patient, who is going through life transitions and feels unstable

Ren-12 Zhongwan

Functions	Tonifies Stomach and Spleen Qi
	Resolves damp
	Descends rebellious Qi
	Alleviates pain
	Shen disturbances

Continued

Indications	Epigastric pain, fullness and indigestion, vomiting
	Stomach reflux
	Abdominal distention and pain
	Dysentery
	Heart pain
	Emotions: agitation, overthinking, manic depression
Psychospiritual	This point is useful for patients who have trouble with the process of digestion of both food and emotions. They become stagnant, congested and acidic, manifesting depression and obsessive thinking. It stabilizes and centers people who cannot digest, assimilate, eliminate, or face life's challenges

Ren-6 Qihai

Functions	Tonifies Qi and Yang
	Regulates Qi and blood
	Tonifies original Qi
	Resolves damp
Indications	Poor digestion, constipation
	Exhaustion, collapse of Yang Qi
	Impotence, infertility, seminal emission, uterine prolapses
	Uterine bleeding, irregular menses, leucorrhea
	Dysentery, abdominal pain, diarrhea
	Shortness of breath (SOB), asthma
	Cold sensation below the navel, abdominal masses
	Hernia
	Moxa can be used to warm the lower Jiao, but be careful with pregnant women
Psychospiritual	If this Sea of Qi point is empty, the patient is exhausted, lacks vitality, motivation, and may have Chronic Fatigue syndrome
	Treating this point sparks interest in life, enthusiasm and warms the mind, as well as cold hands and feet

Continued

All Locations

Needling
protocol

The Four Corners is a powerful abdominal treatment for digestive complaints, and it addresses both pre- and post-natal Qi plus deficiency and excess conditions. Use this point combination for patients who have Qi deficiency or heat, diarrhea or constipation, gas, bloating, pathogenic cold in the lower Jiao, and around the navel, as well as Shen disturbances. First, needle St-25 Tianshu bilaterally and perpendicularly. Or, if there is Qi deficiency, angle the needles toward the navel to consolidate the essence back to the center or omphalos.1 If there is excess, angle the needles outward or tonify or sedate these points, by turning the needle clockwise or counterclockwise, depending upon the patient's particular pattern. Use only one of these techniques, not all of them. Ren-12 Zhongwan is needled next, perpendicularly. If there is acid reflux, epigastric or Heart pain, needle this point obliquely downward. This helps descend rebellious Qi and calms anxiety, agitation and obsessive thinking. Ren-6 Qihai is needled last, perpendicularly, for exhaustion, poor digestion, uterine prolapse, infertility or impotence. If the patterns also relate to cold in the lower Jiao, employ thread moxa, pole moxa, or moxa with slices of ginger or aconite to warm this area

Comments

This protocol is called the Four Corners or Four Directions because it traverses four areas of the abdomen, inscribing a diamond shape on the hara with the navel as the focus. St-25 Tianshu is located in the center of the body, and represents the origin of human Qi; according to The Essential Questions, the area above the navel relates to celestial Qi, and below the navel is Earthly Qi. Therefore, with this treatment, the Three Treasures, Jing, Qi and Shen, are effectively mapped out on the hara. St-25 Tianshu and Ren-12 Zhongwan are the Front Mu points of the Large Intestine and Stomach, respectively. The Mu points are places where Original Qi gathers, and the viscera lying beneath the abdomen are easily accessed directly via needles, moxa or hara palpation. Ren-12 Zhongwan is also the Influential Point of the Fu organs, which makes it an important point for treating post-natal Qi, by transforming and transporting food essence and drink throughout the body. Ren-6 Qihai is considered a reservoir, where Qi originates and returns. In Taoist alchemy, breathing techniques and meditation are used to transform the Qi in this area. Qihai treats Qi deficiency, stagnation of Qi and also pathogenic Qi in the lower Jiao

Japanese Acupuncture Treatments

Stomach and Spleen signs and symptoms, such as pain, are usually more pronounced on the left side of the body, and these conditions become better or worse with or without food. Due to the consumption of fast food, excessive sugar intake, the increasing presence of genetically modified products in their diet, and stress, Earth element patients manifest digestive complaints like gas, indigestion and food allergies, in addition to blood sugar imbalances which are associated with hypoglycemia and diabetes.

An imbalance in blood sugar can affect the brain, and the patient becomes unable to concentrate or think clearly. Before a meal, they may develop a headache, feel shaky, irritable and weak; after eating, they usually fall asleep.

Many patients have an authentic desire to lose weight, but have poor, irregular eating habits, food cravings, and lack the willpower to change their diet or lifestyle. There is a tendency to manifest duodenal ulcers.

Often, the immune system is compromised, especially if they have had either an appendectomy or tonsillectomy. When ill, they manifest a sore throat, bronchitis, or asthma and will have difficulty exhaling or releasing a breath.

The Spleen controls the Blood, and when it is irregular, high or low blood pressure may ensue. The muscle tissue, either striated or smooth, which is reflective of blood sugar issues and oxygen flow throughout the body, may be subject to cramping. The abdomen may be overly sensitive and ticklish, and tension and pain accumulates at the top of the shoulder and in the middle and lower back.

Spleen also holds the blood in the vessels, and disharmony can cause blood deficiency, with resulting irregular menses, and excessive bleeding. Spleen's governance of the flesh, in conjunction with the immune system imbalances, contributes to the development of fibromyalgia.

The Spleen meridian lifts Qi to the head and the face, and is responsible for strengthening the smooth muscles of the internal organs; consequently, a weak Spleen contributes to prolapses. There can be fluid imbalances and puffiness at the inner canthus of the eye, medial portion of the knee, and edema in the lower leg and ankles. Bunions that appear in the area of Sp-3 Taibai Supreme White are a sign of Spleen deficiency.

Food Allergies, Food Poisoning, Amoebic Dysentery

Treatment points	Japanese Behind St-44 Neiting Inner Court
Locations	The TCM St-44 Neiting Inner Court is located on the dorsum of the foot in the depression between the 2nd and 3rd toes, proximal to the web margin. The Japanese point St-44 Neiting is behind the TCM location, where the toe crease meets the sole of the foot
Needling protocol	Burn direct moxa on the Japanese location, behind St-44 Neiting, 7–8 times, or pole moxa, which is easier to use when traveling in a foreign country
Indications	Food allergies
	Food poisoning
	Amoebic dysentery

Continued

Comments	This is a powerful point, which promotes bowel movements, releasing toxicity from the body. It alleviates uncomfortable and often severe symptoms almost immediately. When traveling in a foreign country, or even at home, it is a useful and excellent treatment, and should be included in your acupuncture first aid kit for your family, your patients and yourself. The TCM location for St-44 Neiting Inner Court is also an invaluable point for clearing heat in the Yangming meridian, or for Stomach heat or fire, or wind rising to the head and face. It is a Ying Spring point, which treats fever and heat in the Stomach meridian; it is also the Water point on the Earth element. The Control cycle balances the daily circulation of Qi in the Generation cycle, and also controls excess, or the hyperactivity, of the phase controlling it. In this case, Water is kept in check by the Earth element. Therefore, if there are pathological factors, such as stress, climatic changes, emotional imbalances or inherited constitutional weakness, the Earth phase can become overactive, and could harm the function of the Water phase, which it normally controls. Needle this point bilaterally and neutrally, if the patient has any Stomach heat indications, such as hypertension, heartburn, skin rashes or eczema. If, during the Constitutional Facial Acupuncture treatment, a patient who did not initially have Stomach heat begins to exhibit a red face, the pulses become fast, they have hot flashes or the beginnings of a frontal headache, immediately needle St-44 Neiting. Psychospiritually, Inner Court is a peaceful, reflective place, which calms agitated, restless patients, who are uncommunicative or cannot tolerate listening to voices

Fibromyalgia

Treatment points	Japanese Sp-3.2, Liv-3 Taichong Great Surge, Shu Stream, Yuan Source, Earth point, Japanese Stomach Qi, Japanese Oddi Sphincter point
Locations	Nagano-sensei's Sp-3, which was named Sp-3.2 by Kiiko Matsumoto, is 0.5 cun distal to the TCM Sp-3 Taibai Supreme White. Liv-3 Taichong is on the dorsum of the foot in the depression distal to the junction of the 1st and 2nd metatarsal toes. Nagano-sensei's Stomach Qi is firmly palpated from St-36 Zusanli Leg Three Li, down the Stomach meridian on the lower leg, for tight, tender points. Stomach Qi was previously covered in more detail in the section on the Metal element focusing on Loose Ligaments and Weak Connective Tissue. Japanese Oddi Sphincter is on the right side of the hara. If you draw a line on a 45-degree angle from the center of the navel up to the right rib cage, the point is halfway between the navel and the rib cage. Nagano-sensei attributed the right St-22 Guanmen Pass Gate as the Oddi's sphincter reflex point
Palpation and needling protocol	All points are needled bilaterally; Japanese Sp-3.2 is needled 45 degrees toward Sp-4 Gongsun. Liv-3 Taichong is needled perpendicularly in the TCM location. Japanese Stomach Qi is not one point, but can be several tight and tender points discerned by palpation down the Stomach meridian on the lower leg. Needle these points right 45 degrees downward and toward the tibia. Oddi Sphincter is first palpated at the reflex point and tested for pain. To effect a change, needle this point at 90-degrees for 3–5 minutes. A large needle is appropriate for heavier patients. Ask your patients for feedback on the sensation elicited by the needling of this point. It should be slightly uncomfortable. Make sure that you do not needle too deeply

95

Continued

Comments

Fibromyalgia is a chronic illness, more commonly experienced by women from 20–50 years of age. Its symptoms include global body pain in the muscles, tendons, fascia and soft tissue, and it is linked with extreme fatigue, insomnia, headaches, depression, anxiety, stress, and possible trauma. It can become worse with activity, cold damp weather, anxiety and stress. Other reported symptoms include irritable bowel syndrome (IBS), loss of concentration, numb and tingly hands and feet, and tension or migraine headaches. According to Chinese medicine, fibromyalgia relates to the function of the Spleen and the Earth element, with symptoms such as: food allergies, problems with digestion and assimilation, a compromised immune system, resulting from an appendectomy, hypothyroidism, muscle cramps, spasms and pain due to blood sugar imbalances, compromised/diminished oxygenation of the muscle tissues, Bi syndromes, worry, obsessive thinking and stress, all of which contribute to this illness. In my experience, women, in particular, who, due to evolutionary predisposition and societal conditioning, are more adept at multi-tasking, and often cannot say 'no' to others' requests, have difficulty expressing displeasure or anger. The crushing exhaustion and pain, the official diagnosis of fibromyalgia, and the attendant symptoms, force them to rest, and take care of themselves. Occasionally, these patients do not have an investment in getting well, because they are unwilling to addressing the underlying causes of their condition. This commitment requires them to make changes to their lifestyle, diet and emotional responses to stress, and embrace and implement boundaries around their time and energies. Nagano-sensei's Sp-3.2 treats muscle pain and cramping, and promotes blood circulation, by leading blood to the Heart. It is contraindicated for Heart congestion or an enlarged heart. Nagano-sensei's Stomach Qi is an area that is palpated for tight, tender points from St-36 Zusanli, down the lower leg on the tibialis anterior muscle. The acupuncture points in this area may not necessarily be ones you select for needling; however, this is a fertile area of the body, and the functions and indications for a few of them deserve review. I call St-36 Zusanli Leg Three Li the 'everything' point, because it addresses immunity, digestive issues, balances the hydrochloric acid in the Stomach, and grounds the patient, if they are feeling light-headed or overly talkative. It is a Sea of Nourishment point, a horary point, and a lower He-Sea point. St-37 Shangjuxu Upper Great Hollow is the Large Intestine lower He-Sea point, which addresses food retention and aids with the proper functioning of the appendix. St-38 Jiaokou Ribbon Opening is an empirical point for shoulder pain, and regulates the marrow in the Stomach meridian. St-39 Xiajuxu Lower Great Hollow is the Small Intestine lower He-Sea point, and a Sea of Blood point, which helps alleviate pain in the body. St-40 Fenglong Bountiful Bulge is the empirical point for phlegm, and calms the mind. St-41 Jiexi Ravine Divide is a Jing River Fire point which clears Stomach heat and treats joint, ankle and foot problems. Oddi Sphincter is a muscular valve that regulates the flow of bile and pancreatic juices into the descending portion of the duodenum. Oddi Sphincter is responsible for imbalances in the flow of digestive juices in the intestines, and may cause food allergies, muscular problems, indigestion, gas pain, bloating, and and possible duodenal ulcers. Needling this point can beneficially stimulate the pancreas, allowing it to more effectively secrete digestive juices. Liv-3 Taichong Great Surge is a Shu Stream point, which treats joint pain, a Yuan Source point that directly impacts the organs, and an Earth point on the Liver meridian. When the Wood element is overactive, and the Earth element is weak, Liver overacts on Spleen, giving rise to digestive complaints and possible IBS. The Liver is also responsible for the free flow of Qi and blood in the body; it can calm emotions and address tendino-muscular issues

Blood Sugar Imbalances and Sugar Cravings

Treatment points and locations	Huatos of T11; thoracic vertebra next to the Spleen Shu, Bl-20 Pishu
	Huatos of T12; thoracic vertebra next to the Stomach Shu, Bl-21 Weishu
	Du-5, under the spinous process of the 12th thoracic vertebra (T12), next to Bl-21 Weishu
Palpation and needling protocol	Palpate the left Kid-16 Huangshu for a lump the size of a caterpillar. This is considered a sugar lump, and its presence indicates possible imbalances in blood sugar. Needle the Huatos of T11 and T12 bilaterally, angling the needle slightly toward the spinous process, if there are blood sugar imbalances. For intense and obsessive sugar cravings, moxa Du-5
Comments	I have had success treating blood sugar imbalances and the associated sugar cravings, using this simple protocol, integrating it into a full constitutional treatment. The Huatos should be needled every time you see a patient, for a period of several months. Moxa Du-5 only when the sugar cravings are excessive and persistent. I also use kinesiology, muscle testing which is very effective in detecting sugar cravings. For example, one of my patients, who has an Earth element constitution, was overweight and Spleen-deficient, also possesses, not surprisingly, a predilection for excessive amounts of Swiss dark chocolate. I had them bring their favorite chocolate bar to their next appointment and tested them to ascertain the effect that the chocolate had upon their system. While holding it, they were noticeably weak at their left Kid-16 Huangshu, around the navel, and under the left ribs in the area of the Stomach/Spleen. At the end of the session, I tested them again, and there was no discernible weakness without the chocolate bar. They later reported that their cravings for sugar, especially chocolate, had vanished, and they remained sugar-free for 6 months. At the point, I then was able to address the underlying blood sugar imbalances, not merely the manifest symptom of sugar cravings. Unfortunately, after that initial treatment, they left that dark chocolate bar with me, and rather than throw away a perfectly lovely chocolate bar, I ate it myself. Luckily, the resulting sugar cravings were skillfully addressed in a subsequent treatment by one of my colleagues

Organ Prolapses

Treatment points	St-13 Qihu Qi Door, Japanese Inner Yin, St-32 Futu Crouching Rabbit, St-34 Liangqiu, Beam Hill and GB-31 Fengshi Wind Market
Locations	St-13 Qihu is 4 cun lateral to Ren Mai at the lower border of the middle of the clavicle. The Japanese point Inner Yin is one third of the distance upwards from Kid-10 Yingu Yin Valley to the groin on the Kidney meridian. From Kid-10 Yingu, the point is at the end of the first third, or 5 cun above Kid-10 Yingu. St-32 Futu Crouching Rabbit is on the thigh in the rectus femoris muscle, 6 cun above the laterosuperior border of the patella, on the line connecting the anterior superior iliac spine and the lateral border of the patella. St-34 Liangqiu, the Xi Cleft point, is 2 cun above the laterosuperior border of the patella. GB-31 Fengshi is 7 cun above the transverse popliteal crease, on the lateral aspect of the thigh. When the patient is standing with the hands close to their thighs, the point is located where the tip of the middle finger rests
Needling protocol	Treat all points bilaterally; needle St-13 Qihu obliquely and transversely toward the shoulder. Do not needle perpendicularly or deeply, so as to avoid a pneumothorax or puncturing the subclavian artery. Japanese Inner Yin is needled upward toward the ceiling on the Kidney meridian. St-32 Futu, St-34 Liangqiu and GB-31 Fengshi can be needled perpendicularly
Comments	This combination of points is very effective for treating organ prolapses resulting from multiple childbirths, abdominal infections or operations, standing for long periods of time, running downhill or playing basketball. When the Spleen is deficient, it cannot perform its function of holding up the muscles, and prolapses of the uterus, bladder and anus can ensue. I have also used this approach constitutionally, along with Chong Mai, to treat prolapse of the platysma muscle, which is responsible for a sagging, droopy neck with turkey wattles

CONSTITUTIONAL TREATMENT SUMMARY
EARTH ELEMENT: STOMACH AND SPLEEN

Syndromes	Treatment Points	Indications
Four Corners Abdominal Treatment	St-25 Tianshu Celestial Pivot, Ren-12 Zhongwan Central Venter, Ren-6 Qihai Sea of Qi	Digestive problems, gas, diarrhoea, constipation
Food allergies, food poisoning, amoebic dysentery	(J) Behind St-44 Neiting Inner Court	Severe food allergies, food poisoning, dysentery and toxicity in the digestive system

Syndromes	Treatment Points	Indications
Fibromyalgia	(J) Sp-3.2 Liv-3 Taichong Great Surge, (J) Stomach Qi, (J) Oddi Sphincter	Muscle pain and cramps
		Balances emotions
		Digestive complaints
		Gas, bloat, lack of digestive juices in the intestines
Blood sugar imbalances and cravings	Huatos T11 Huatos T12 Du-5	Blood sugar imbalances
		Headache, lack of concentration
		Dizzy when hasn't eaten a meal, sugar cravings
Organ prolapses	St-13 Qihu Qi Door, (J) Inner Yin, St-32 Fuliu Crouching Rabbit, St-34 Liangqu Beam Hill, GB-31 Fengshi Wind Market	Prolapses of uterus, bladder, anus, sagging platysma neck muscle

(J), Japanese point.

The Fire Element: Heart, Hand Shaoyin and Small Intestine, Hand Taiyang

The Heart Meridian Pathway: Hand Shaoyin

- The Heart Meridian originates in the Heart.
- Emerging, it spreads over the 'Heart system,' the pericardium, arteries, nerves and tissues around the heart, and descends through the diaphragm to connect with the Small Intestine.
- The ascending branch separates from the 'Heart system,' and travels upward along the sides of the esophagus to the face and cheek, to connect with the 'eye system,' the tissues, nerves and vessels surrounding and behind the eyes.
- Another branch travels from the Heart through the Lung, then emerges at the axillary fossa.
- From the axilla, the external pathway descends along the medial posterior part of the upper arm, elbow and forearm to the palm of the hand.
- It enters the palm and follows the medial aspect of the little finger to its tip at Ht-9 Shaochong Lesser Surge, where it links with the Small Intestine meridian.

Symptoms of Heart Hand Shaoyin Meridian

- Pain and swelling in chest and upper back, axilla, swollen glands.
- Inner arm pain; stiffness on medial aspect of forearm.
- Weak wrists.
- Hot or cold sensation in medial arm, hypochondria, scapula.
- Hot flashes, night sweats, dry throat, red face.
- Red, swollen eyes, yellow sclera.

Internal Branch Disorders

- Cardiac disorders, chest pain, palpitations.
- Irregular heartbeat, shortness of breath.
- Mental disorders, insomnia, hysteria, dream disturbed sleep.
- Digestive issues, hiatal hernia.

The Small Intestine Pathway: Hand Taiyang

- The Small Intestine Meridian starts at the ulnar side of the tip of the little finger at SI-1 Shaoze Lesser Marsh.
- Following the ulnar side of the dorsum of the hand, it reaches the wrist, where it emerges at the latero-posterior aspect of the elbow.
- From there, it travels along the posterior aspect of the upper arm to the shoulder, circles around the scapula, and meets Du-14 Dazhui Great Hammer on the superior aspect of the shoulder.
- Turning downward to the supraclavicular fossa, it connects with the Heart.
- It descends along the esophagus, passes through the diaphragm to the Stomach, and enters the Small Intestine.
- A branch from the supraclavicular fossa ascends to the neck, and further to the cheek via the outer canthus of the eye, and enters the ear at SI-19 Tinggong Auditory Palace.
- The branch from the cheek travels up to the infraorbital region SI-18 Quanliao Cheek Bone Hole, then to the lateral side of the nose and the inner canthus at Bl-1 Jingming Bright Eyes, where it links with the Bladder Meridian.

Symptoms of Small Intestine Hand Taiyang Meridian

- Swelling, stiffness and pain of cervical region, scapula, shoulders.
- Pain in lateral aspect of arm.

- Pain and stiffness of lateral side of hands and little finger.

- Tongue sores.

- Fever, night sweats.

- Red, painful eyes, yellow sclera.

- Painful, swollen mandible, temporomandibular joint (TMJ).

- Deafness, tinnitus, swollen lymph glands, sore throat.

Internal Branch Disorders

- Yellow urination, urine retention, edema.

- Diarrhea, constipation, abdominal pain and distention.

- Inguinal hernia, distending pain in lower abdomen referring to the back.

The Fire Element: Passion

The Fire element includes the Heart meridian, Hand Shaoyin, and its Yang partner, the Small Intestine meridian, Hand Taiyang, plus the Pericardium meridian, Hand Jueyin, and its Yang pair, the Triple Heater meridians, Hand Shaoyang.

Fire is hot, exciting, dynamic and passionate. It rises up, lifts the spirit, and can be likened to the life-giving rays of the Sun, which unconditionally provide warmth to humans.

A strong Fire element person will be vibrant, enthusiastic, abundant, caring and vital. A person who is deficient in Fire has low energy, is cold, unreceptive, and lacks compassion for the self and others.

In the *Nei Jing*, the Heart is described as the Monarch, who excels in thought, insight and understanding. Functionally, the Heart controls and circulates blood, and houses the Shen spirit. The Small Intestine receives and transforms food and separates the pure from the impure, including unnecessary thoughts and emotions.

Both the Pericardium and the Triple Heater do not house organs; however, their functions are very important in Chinese medicine. The Pericardium is called the Heart Protector, because it wraps around the Heart and guards the heart muscle from shock or trauma.

The Pericardium meridian is also called Circulation Sex. In the *Nei Jing*, it is described as the Official who guides the subjects in the joys and pleasures by encouraging blood flow, the production of sexual fluids, balanced Shen and relationship. The Triple Heater has an important and mystical function in Chinese medicine. The ancient Taoists used alchemical practices to transform the Three Jiaos via meditation, breathing techniques, ingestion of minerals and substances to transform the Three Treasures – Jing, Qi and Shen.

As the Official in charge of irrigation and construction of the ditches, sluices and waterways, functionally it controls the temperature in all the organs, the Three Burners or Jiaos, and connects us to our Yuan original Qi.

FIRE ELEMENT PATHOLOGY	
Shen disturbances	Insomnia, restlessness, dream-disturbed sleep, manic depression, hysteria, anxiety, poor concentration, mood swings, low spirits, poor memory
Cardiovascular system	Angina pectoris, palpitations, tachycardia, bradycardia, arrhythmia, coronary heart disease, arteriosclerosis, aphasia
Complexion	Red face, itchy skin, carbuncles, boils
Digestion	Hiccoughs, nausea, vomiting, epigastic distress
Muscular problems	Stiffness and pain in the neck, scapula and shoulder, chest, upper back, hypochondrium and axillary fossa
	Joint pain, especially in the temporomandibular joint (TMJ)
Ears, eyes and throat	Red eyes, tinnitus, deafness, yellow sclera, mouth sores, tongue ulcerations, dry throat and thirst
Urogenital	Yellow urine, urine retention and frequent urination
Chest and lung	Cough, asthma and shortness of breath (SOB)
Lymphatic system	Lymph inflammation, immune deficiency, autoimmune diseases like lupus, multiple sclerosis (MS), Crohn's disease
Menstrual disorders	Irregular menses, fibroids and ovarian cysts, reproductive issues, infertility and impotence

Recommended Constitutional Treatment Protocol

Open the Du Mai contralaterally with the Eight Extraordinary meridians; SI-3 Houxi Back Ravine and Bl-62 Shenmai Extending Vessel.

Root Treatment
Kid-2 Rangu Blazing Valley (Right Side)
Kid-3 Taixi Great Ravine(Left Side)
Kid-2 Rangu Blazing Valley
Ying Spring Fire Point
Meeting Point of Yin Qiao Mai

Location	Anterior and inferior to the medial malleolus in the depression inferior to the tuberosity of the navicular bone
Functions	Clears deficient heat
	Cools blood
	Tonifies Kidney
	Strengthens Yin Qiao Mai
	Treats lower Jiao
Indications	Night sweats, insomnia, mental restlessness, heat in the 5 palms, dry, painful throat
	Fear, fright, forboding
	Dyspnea, epistaxis, diabetes
	Stabbing Heart pains
	Genital itching, impotence, infertility, uterine prolapse, menstrual imbalances
	Difficult urination, diarrhea
	Painful lower legs, restless feet, swelling and pain in the dorsum of the foot
Psychospiritual	Use Kid-2 Rangu when the patient is frightened, anxious, or nervous in body/ mind/spirit. This fire point on the Water element transforms water, and enables the patient to remember, affirm and advance further on their path in life
Comments	Usually, Ying Spring points treat excess heat and febrile conditions. However, since the Kidney meridian and organ is never in a state of excess, Rangu excels in clearing heat by keeping Mingmen fire in check, effectively addressing and treating Yin deficiency. This is a unique attribute of Kid-2 Rangu as the fire point on the Kidney meridian, which is the root of Yin and Yang in the entire body

Kid-3 Taixi Great Ravine
Shu Stream, Yuan Source Point
Earth Point

Location	In the depression between the medial malleolus and the tendocalcaneus
Functions	Nourishes Kidney Yin
	Tonifies Kidney Yang
	Benefits Yuan Qi
	Tonifies Lung Qi
	Strengthens back
	Treats Bi syndrome
Indications	Tinnitus, deafness, sore throat, dry mouth, diabetes
	Cough, epistaxis, asthma
	Insomnia, stabbing pain in Heart, poor memory
	Impotence, infertility, miscarriage, menstruation imbalances
	Frequent urination, yellow urine, constipation
	Lower back pain
	Rebellious Qi; cold hands and feet
	Bi syndrome; numbness, pain and swelling in the legs, ankle and heel
Psychospiritual	This point is a rushing stream, which washes away fears and increases the vitality and will of the patient
Comments	Kid-3 Taixi is a Yuan Source point, and it directly treats the Kidney organ, in cases of either Yin or Yang deficiency. It is the primary point employed to treat Kidney Yin deficiency, and for nourishing the Kidney. Taixi is also one of the Shu Stream points, which address intermittent diseases such as malaria. It also treats the other Zang organs, and, in this case, Heart not Communicating with Kidney, Heart Yang, Heart Yin and Heart Fire patterns. This is an excellent point for supporting and harmonizing the Heart function

SI-6 Yang Lao Nursing the Aged
Xi Cleft Point
Empirical Point for Longevity

A longevity treatment featuring either or both of the TCM points SI-6 Yang Lao Nursing the Aged and TH-2 Yemen Humor Gate, with its distinctive moistening qualities, is one of my personal favorites.

Location	When the palm faces the chest, the point is in the bony cleft on the radial side of the styloid process of the ulna
Functions	Benefits sinews
	Treats Wei atrophy of shoulder and arm
	Invigorates meridians and muscles, and alleviates pain
	Benefits eyes
	Acute conditions
Indications	Blurry, dim vision, eye pain
	Arthritis, muscular and joint pain
	Stiffness in neck, shoulder and arm numbness and swelling
	Contraction of sinews
	Hyperpigmentation, skin rashes
Psychospiritual	This point is used not only for older patients, but also for those who obsess over the past, have old habit patterns, addictions, past injuries, or childhood memories that debilitate and confuse them. Yang Lao aids the Small Intestine's function of sorting the pure from the impure, which helps these individuals to clarify and transcend old memories, assimilate and incorporate the new, and embrace the present moment
Comments	This Xi Cleft point treats acute conditions, such as severe shoulder pain. It is also good for joints, arthritis and contracted sinews. Deficient eye disorders that relate to aging, like blurred vision, dim vision and eye pain can also be addressed. It strengthens the Small Intestine function, and also effectively treats any chronic physical imbalances like general toxicity in the body and digestive complaints, fatigue, exhaustion, numbness and paralysis. When indicated, use SI-6 Yang Lao as a longevity tonic for all your patients, no matter what their age. This point has the ability to treat hyperpigmentation and skin rashes, as well. For patients who are dry, blood-deficient, or who have arthritis, joint, muscle pain and stiffness, I recommend a Chinese medicine decoction of vodka or brandy, mixed with Long Yan Rou, *Arillus euphoriae Longanae*, longan berries. Combine ⅓ longan berries with ⅔ vodka or brandy, in a beautiful decanter and let in marinate for at least 2 weeks. When it is ready, instruct the patient to drink only a single shot glass per evening before bed. This combination not only tastes good, it also tonifies blood, calms Shen and treats Heart and Spleen Qi deficiency patterns with symptoms of insomnia, palpitations, poor memory and melancholy. This preparation is contraindicated for alcoholics and for patients with excess heat, phlegm or dampness in the middle Jiao

TH-2 Yemen Humor Gate
Ying Spring, Water Point

Location	When the fist is clenched, the point is in the depression at the web margin between the 4th and 5th fingers
Functions	Moistens mucous membranes, and regulates fluids in the upper body
	Clears heat
	Benefits the ears
	Alleviates pain along the meridian
	Calms Shen
Indications	Tinnitus, earache, deafness, headache
	Red eyes and face, dry eyes
	Sore throat, toothache, bleeding gums
	Palpations, fright, mania, epilepsy, shortness of breath (SOB)
	Malaria
	Arm pain, Depuytren's contracture (contraction of five fingers)
Psychospiritual	Water circulates fluids and allows for movement and the Triple Heater controls fluids in the three Jiaos. TH-2 Yemen treats a patient who is unable to go with the flow, and lacks fluidity in their lives
Comments	This Ying Spring point clears heat in the body. Since the Triple Heater meridian ascends to the head and face, TH-2 Yemen clears and moistens this area of the body. Choose this point when treating patients who have red faces and eyes, are agitated and dry, nervous with palpitations and who have problems opening the chest and breathing freely. The Triple Heater's exterior/interior relationship with the Pericardium, which wraps around and protects the Heart, contributes to mental and emotional imbalances

Japanese Acupuncture Treatments

The Fire element patient is often a Type A personality, and is usually under a great deal of stress, which causes anxiety, restlessness, nervousness, insomnia and disturbed sleep. There may be a history of heart disease in the family, with symptoms of tachycardia, bradycardia, arrhythmia, angina pectoris and arteriosclerosis.

On the hara, there is tension under the sternum; pain on the left side of the chest at Kid-23 Shenfeng Spirit Seal, Kid-24 Lingxu Spirit Ruins and Kid-25 Shencang Spirit Storehouse, as well as under the nipple at St-18 Rugen Breast Root; a puffy area, especially at the left, SI-11 Tianzhong Celestial Gathering, which could be a harbinger of future heart attacks; pain at CV-17 Danzhong Chest Center and tenderness, especially at the left, Bl-14 Jueyinshu, in the area of the rhomboid muscles, also indicates heart-related stress issues.

If there is a history of rheumatic fever, pericarditis, a valvular disease, or the patient has an inherited mitral valve prolapse, he or she may have immune-related heart issues or autonomic nervous system imbalances, if under inordinate stress. Rheumatic arthritis is an inflammatory disease that relates to a Heart patient with fast pulses.

Most cardiac patients have an excess condition, unless they are recovering from a heart attack. In the case of excess conditions, use distal points and bring the energy down from the Heart, for symptoms like palpitations, shortness of breath, and blood pressure imbalances.

Insomnia

Treatment points	Nagano-sensei's Sp-3.2 Taibai Great White and Japanese PC-4 (JPC4)
Locations	Japanese Sp-3.2 is 0.5 cun distal to the TCM Sp-3 Taibai Supreme White; JPC4 is 3 cun below JPC3, which is at the location of the TCM Lu-5 Chize Cubit Marsh, on the radial side of the biceps brachii muscle
Palpation and needling protocol	Palpate for hyperdiaphragm tension below the sternum in the area of Ren-15 Jiuwei Turtle Dove Tail. This is the Luo Connecting point of the Ren Mai, located below the xiphoid process, 7 cun above the navel. Locate the point on the abdomen with the patient's arms lifted above their head. Needle the two points bilaterally as follows: Sp-3.2 45 degrees toward Sp-4 Gongsun and JPC4 45 degrees in the direction of the meridian flow
Indications	Insomnia
	Palpitations
	Sensations of pressure in the chest and Heart
	Nausea, indigestion, worse when sleeping, lying down or when experiencing stress, shock or anger
	Difficulty taking a deep breath
Comments:	Hyperdiaphragm can cause chest distress below the sternum and insomnia. In extreme cases, patients complain of symptoms that mimic a heart attack, even though, when tested by a cardiologist, there are no problems with the physical heart. Often there is pressure pain at St-11 Qishe Qi Abode, a tense sternocleidomastoideus muscle (SCM), and tightness under the xiphoid process. There may also be a lump or tightness at the left SI-11 Tianzhong Celestial Gathering, which is considered the cardiac reflex in Japanese acupuncture. A patient who is suffering from a hyperdiaphragm cannot hold their breath for 40 seconds

Mood Swings and Depression Due to Heart Imbalances

Treatment points	The Huatos of Bl-15 Xinshu Heart Shu and Ht-7 Shenmen Spirit Gate
Locations	The Huatos are located directly next to the spine. Bl-15 Xinshu is 1.5 cun lateral to Du-11, below the spinous process of the 5th thoracic vertebrae. Ht-7 Shenmen Spirit Gate is at the ulnar end of the transverse wrist crease, in the depression on the radial side of the tendon of the flexor carpi ulnaris muscle
Needling protocol	Angle the Bl-15 Xinshu Huatos toward the spine, bilaterally. Do needle deeply, only 0.5 cun. Insert the needle into Ht-7 Shenmen perpendicularly, about 0.3–0.5 cun, at the most
Indications	Shen disturbances
	Depression
	Sadness
	Mood swings
	Melancholy
Comments	Ht-7 Shenmen and the Huatos of Bl-15 Xinshu have similar functions, and, when used together, augment this Heart-related psychoemotional treatment. They both calm Shen, tonify and nourish the Heart, regulate Heart Qi and treat insomnia, poor memory, fear, palpitations, and excess and deficiency Heart conditions. Ht-7 Shenmen, in particular, treats sadness and melancholy due to Heart Qi deficiency, and Bl-15 Xinshu Huatos encourage the brain's function and alleviates depression, while lifting the spirits

Stroke and Speech Problems

Treatment points	Kawai-sensei's Special Speech point
Locations	The point is $\frac{1}{4}$ of the distance from GB-1 Tongziliao Pupil Bone Hole to Du-20 Baihui Hundred Convergences. It is found closer to GB-1 Tongziliao inside the hairline
Palpation and needling protocol	It treats aphasia, which can manifest as one of the sequelae following a stroke. First, palpate the St-9 Renying Man's Prognosis area bilaterally to see if your patient has pain there. Ask them to make a sound or speak, if they can, and feel the vibration in their larynx. Then, needle this scalp point bilaterally and transversely away from the face toward Du-20 Baihui. Use a thicker needle, such as a 32 gauge (Japanese #5), 40 mm. After the treatment, check St-9 Renying again to see if the pain has lessened or subsided in the throat. Once again, ask the patient to make a sound or speak, if possible, to discern if there has been any significant change in their situation. Please integrate this scalp treatment into your constitutional protocol

Continued

Indications	Stuttering
	Slurring of speech
	Difficulty speaking
	Inability to speak
	Aphasia
	Stiffness in the tongue
Comments	Distally, include Ht-5 Tongli Connecting Li, the Luo Connecting point of the Heart meridian, as a part of this treatment. It calms the Shen, addresses arrhythmia, a pounding heart, and is indicated for sudden loss of voice, stuttering, tongue stiffness, and an inability to speak, resulting from psychoemotional disorders and sequelae from windstroke

Blood Pressure Imbalances, Palpitations, Shortness of Breath (SOB)

Treatment points	Behind the 2nd toe for palpations; behind the 3rd toe for shortness or breath and/or blood pressure imbalances
Locations	Behind the 2nd toe is in the middle of the crease where the sole of the foot meets the toe. Behind the 3rd toe is in the middle of the crease where the sole of the foot meets the toe
Needling protocol	Needle behind the 2nd toe for palpitations, with a small gauge needle (40 gauge, 15 or 30 mm, #1 Japanese). You can also use an intradermal needle, a magnet, or a rice grain taped to this point behind the toe. You can leave the rice grain or magnet in place when they leave the clinic; instruct them to remove them in a few days, or earlier if they feel uncomfortable or have skin irritation. Contraindications: do not treat this point if the patient has a pacemaker, or a slow pulse. Needle behind the 3rd toe for blood pressure imbalances or for shortness of breath. If the patient has blood pressure issues, especially hypotension, and the feet are cold, it is appropriate to moxa this point
Indications	Behind the 3rd toe:
	Regulates both high and low blood pressure
	Treats shortness of breath, and 'White Coat' syndrome
	Behind the 2nd toe:
	Calms palpitations and anxiety

Comments	If the patient has cardiac issues, it is important not to treat the area around the Heart, but, rather, to bring the Qi down to the feet, or at least below the navel. It will exacerbate their condition to needle locally. Behind the 2nd toe calms anxiety, slows down the pulse and soothes Heart heat. Once again, do not treat this point, if the patient has a pacemaker or a slow pulse. Behind the 3rd toe is an excellent point for balancing not only low, but also high, blood pressure, and for patients with shortness of breath (SOB). I find that this point is good for patients who have a fear of the doctor or 'White Coat' syndrome. When patients reach a certain age, they are usually diagnosed with high blood pressure and given medication. They may or may not have this condition, but anxiety and dread of the physician's diagnosis causes them to react adversely. This stress, naturally, quickens their breathing and causes their pulse to race. I usually treat these patients prior to their doctor's visit, and teach them how to relax their breath, and to access deeper breathing in the Dan Tien. If they actually do require medication, they will receive it. Behind the 3rd toe also aids patients with low blood pressure, lethargy and cold sensations. This point homeostatically regulates blood pressure, and opens the chest. In this case, moxa can be applied to the point to alleviate cold, allowing the patient to breathe more easily and freely

CONSTITUTIONAL TREATMENT SUMMARY
FIRE ELEMENT: HEART, SMALL INTESTINE, PERICARDIUM, TRIPLE HEATER

Syndromes	Treatment Points	Indications
Longevity treatment	SI-6 Yang Lao Nursing the Old	Blurry vision, arthritis, hyperpigmentation, skin rashes
Moistening, calming treatment	TH-2 Yemen Humor Gate	Red face and eyes, dry skin, palpitations and emotional imbalances
Insomnia	(J) Sp-3.2, (J) PC-4	Hyperdiaphragm, palpitations, inability to sleep or breathe easily
Mood swings and depression	Huatos Bl-15 Xinshu Heart Shu, Ht-7 Shenmen Spirit Gate	Sadness, melancholy, Shen disturbances
Stroke and speech problems, stuttering, slurred speech	Kawai-sensei's special Speech Point Ht-5 Tongli Connecting Li	Stroke sequelae, aphasia, inability to speak, sudden loss of voice, calms Shen
Blood pressure imbalances, palpitations, shortness of breath	Behind 2nd toe, behind 3rd toe	Palpitations, SOB, blood pressure imbalances

(J), Japanese point.

The Water Element: Bladder, Foot Taiyang, and Kidney, Foot Shaoyin, Meridian

The Bladder Meridian Pathway: Foot Taiyang

- The Bladder Meridian starts at the inner canthus of the eye Bl-1 Jingming Bright Eyes, ascends to the forehead and joins the Du Mai at Du-20 Baihui Hundred Convergences, at the vertex.

- From the vertex, a branch descends to the temples above the ear, intersecting GB-7 Qubin Temporal Curve, through GB-12 Wangu Completion Bone.

- Another branch from the vertex enters, and communicates with, the brain, emerges and descends to the nape of the neck, where the meridian split into two branches.

- Branch A descends the neck posteriorly, and travels downward 1.5 cun later to the spine to the lumbar area.

- From the lower back, it enters the body cavity via the paravertebral muscles, connects with the Kidney and links to the Bladder.

- The lumbar branch continues to descend along the sacrum, through the gluteal region to the popliteal fossa of the knee.

- Branch B separates at the nape of the neck, descends along the medial aspect of the scapula parallel to the spine, 3 cun lateral to the midline, down to the gluteal area.

- It passes through the buttocks at GB-30 Huantiao Jumping Round, then descends along the lateral aspect of the thigh, where it meets the previous branch in the popliteal fossa.

- Both branches join and travel down the leg through the gastrocnemius muscle to Bl-60 Kunlun Kunlun Mountains to end at Bl-67 Zhiyin Reaching Yin, at the lateral side of the tip of the fifth toe, where it connects with the Kidney.

Symptoms of Bladder Foot Taiyang Meridian

- Headaches, nape of neck stiffness, chills, fever, runny nose, body aches.

- Yellow sclera, painful eyes with tearing, epistaxis, sinusitis.

- Pain and stiffness along spine, hip, knee, leg, foot, small toe.

- Nosebleed, head cold, clogged sinuses.

Internal Branch Disorders

- Urine retention, distention/pain in lower abdomen.

- Dysmenorrhea, leucorrhea.

- Worry, phobias, fears.

The Kidney Meridian Pathway: Foot Shaoyin

- The Kidney Meridian starts at the underside of the small toe, and travels to the sole of the foot, at Kid-1 Yongquan Gushing Spring.

- It emerges at Kid-2 Rangu Blazing Balley at the tuberosity of the navicular bone, curves around the medial malleolus, enters the heel, and ascends to Kid-6 Shaohai Shining Sea below the medial malleolus.

- Ascending along the medial aspect of the lower leg, it meets the Spleen Meridian at Sp-6 Sanyinjiao Three Yin Intersection.

- It continues up the leg to the popliteal fossa, along the posteromedial thigh to the tip of the coccyx, where it meets Du Mai at Du-1 Changqiang Long Strong.

- A branch travels from the pubic bone, lateral to the midline of the lower abdomen, and another branch intersects Ren Mai at Ren-3 Zhongji Central Pole, Ren-4 Guanyuan, Origin Pass and Ren-7 Yinjiao Yin Intersection.

- The main pathway continues up the abdomen to the chest, 2 cun lateral to the midline, and ends at Kid-27 Shufu Shu Mansion.

- From the coccyx, it goes internally into the spine, and enters the Kidney and the Bladder.

- A branch re-emerges from the Kidney, ascends and penetrates the Liver and diaphragm, enters the Lung, runs along the throat, and terminates at the root of the tongue.

- Another branch separates from the Lung, joins the Heart and links with the Pericardium at Ren-17 Danzhong Chest Center.

Symptoms of Kidney Foot Shaoyin Meridian

- Wei syndrome.

- Degenerative bone and joint disorders.

- Dry mouth, tongue and chronic sore throat.

- Pain and weakness in lower back, back of knees, spine, hip, lower extremities.

Internal Branch Disorders

- Infertility, impotence, poor memory.

- Edema, puffy face, dark circles and puffiness under the eyes.

- Blurred vision, dizziness.

- Chronic diarrhea/constipation, vomiting, nausea, hunger, but no desire to eat.

- Insomnia, somnolence, palpitations, shortness of breath.

- Fear, anxiety.

The Water Element: Wisdom

The Water element is represented by the Kidney Meridian, Foot Shaoyin, and its Yang companion, the Bladder Meridian, Foot Taiyang.

Water becomes every container, and over time wears away anything in its path, from a pebble to a rock or a boulder, or a large sequoia tree. It is fluid, and flows either gently and peacefully, or violently and powerfully.

It is paramount for life. The adult body is comprised of 70–78% water which includes lymphatic fluid, saliva, and synovial fluid, among other bodily fluids. In the womb, we are housed in amniotic fluid until our birth. We could not survive without water.

The Kidneys are the Official of Cleverness and Ingenuity; functionally, they store essence, produce bone marrow, dominate reproduction, and regulate water metabolism. The Bladder eliminates fluid waste, and stores and excretes urine.

A balanced Water element person has determination, will power, resourcefulness, stamina, ingenuity, adaptability, and the capacity to easily embrace change. When imbalanced, they are insecure, lethargic, fearful, phobic, overwhelmed, depressed and rigid.

The Spirit of the Water element is the Zhi or will power. An individual with a healthy Water element has the ability to realize their creative inspirations, dreams and ambitions in life. A weak-willed person may be overshadowed by others' personal power and will have difficulty accomplishing their own goals.

The wisdom to rest, balance and conserve one's water Qi and essence, especially during the winter months, revitalizes the Water element and recharges the Zhi.

WATER ELEMENT PATHOLOGY

Kidney Qi, essence and adrenal deficiency	Exhaustion, lower back and neck pain, general muscular aches and pains, poor memory, hair loss, tinnitus, deafness, blurry vision, vertigo
Bone and joint problems	Osteoarthritis, osteoporosis, arthritis in the knee joint
Gynecological and reproductive systems	Infertility, impotence, irregular menses, dysmenorrhea, leucorrhea, inflammation of the ovaries and fallopian tubes, prostatitis
Endocrine system	Hyper and hypothyroid, estrogen and progesterone and natural steroid hormonal imbalances
Urogenital system	Edema, frequent urination, retention of urine, incontinence, urinary tract infections (UTI), interstitial cystitis, kidney stones
Digestive system	Cock's crow diarrhea (at 5 am), constipation, abdominal distention
Addictions	Steroid hormones, heroin, morphine, codeine, also stimulants like coffee
Upper Jiao disturbances	Asthmatic breathing with difficulty inhaling, chronic cough, chest pain, palpitations
Complexion	Dark and withered skin, with dark, puffy circles under the eyes
Emotions	Fear, anxiety, depression, lack of will power

Recommended Constitutional Treatment Protocol

Open the Du Mai contralaterally with the Eight Extraordinary meridians.

Bl-62 Shenmai Extending Vessel as the master point and SI-3 Houxi Back Ravine as the couple point, if indicated for your patient.

Root Treatment

Kid-2 Rangu Blazing Valley (Right Side)
Kid-10 Yingu Yin Valley (Left Side)

The functions, indications, and psychospiritual qualities of Kid-2 Rangu Blazing Valley, Ying Spring Fire point, and the Meeting point of Yin Qiao Mai, were discussed in the Fire element Root Treatment section of this chapter.

Kid-10 Yingu Yin Valley
He-Sea Water Point
Horary Point

Location	On the medial side of the popliteal fossa, between the tendons of semitendinosus and semimembranosus muscles
Functions	Tonifies Kidney
	Expels damp heat from the lower Jiao
	Supports digestion
	Alleviates pain in the meridians
Indications	Infertility, impotence, genital pain
	Painful and difficult urination, frequent urination
	Uterine bleeding, leucorrhea
	Hypogastric pain, abdominal distention, diarrhea
	Knee pain
	Psychoemotional disturbances; manic depression, depression
	Hernia, kidney stones
Psychospiritual	As a horary Water point on the Kidney meridian, it restores, revitalizes, calms and cools damp heat in the system, which includes the treatment of Shen disturbances, as well as Kidney Qi deficiency, with symptoms of excessive urination, arthritis, and low back and knee pain
Comments	Use Kid-10 Yingu, and Kid-2 Rangu, the Water and Fire points of the Kidney, to support the root of Yin and Yang Qi in the Kidneys. This Vietnamese treatment addresses Kidney pulses when both pulses are deficient, but one is weaker than the other. It balances and harmonizes both Kidney pulses, and enlivens the Kidney Qi. It is rare that a patient's pulses are not more balanced and vital after this root treatment

Bac-si Truong Thin's Vietnamese Back Treatment

This is an effective lower back treatment for warming and tonifying Kidney Yang deficiency.

Treatment points	Bl-23 Shenshu Kidney Shu, Bl-52 Zhishi Will Chamber, and Essence Palace
Locations	Bl-23 Shenshu is 1.5 cun lateral to Du-4, below the spinous process of the second lumbar vertebrae. Bl-52 Zhi Shi is 3 cun lateral to Du-4, below the spinous process of the 2nd lumbar vertebrae. Essence Palace is a special Vietnamese treatment involving four points, with two points, respectively, on either side of the spine. One point is located $\frac{1}{2}$ cun outside of Bl-52 Zhishi, and another is $\frac{1}{2}$ cun below that point
Needling protocol	Needle Bl-23 Shenshu, Bl-52 Zhishi and the Essence Palace points bilaterally, angling the needles slightly toward the spine to consolidate Kidney Qi and essence, and to activate Du-4 Mingmen Life Gate Fire
Indications	Kidney Yang deficiency
	Cold, tight, aching back
	Low libido and poor sexual function
	Strengthens Zhi, will power
	Impotence, infertility
Comments	This Vietnamese lower back treatment is effective, practical and unconventional. After needling the lower back points indicated, and completing the constitutional treatment, apply liquid moxa to the entire lower back area. Warm the liquid moxa slightly to prevent shocking an already cold Kidney Yang deficient patient. Then warm the lower back with a hair dryer. Ask your patient to tell you when they feel completely warm; do not burn them by holding the hair dryer too close to the skin. Keep track of the amount of time necessary for them to experience the general warming effect. Every time that you treat them with this protocol, the duration will become shorter. Always first ask permission before employing this technique. A TDP lamp can be used in lieu of the hair dryer/liquid moxa combination, but, in my experience, the results are not as immediate or effective. If the patient is basically healthy, but is experiencing fatigue and a slight adrenal deficiency, this treatment should work well in one or two sessions. It is also effective for warming the uterus, and treating infertility due to Kidney Yang deficiency. I recommend covering the patient during and after the treatment with a light mylar, 'space,' blanket or parachute silk, to warm the entire body

Japanese Acupuncture Treatments

The Water element is indicated in issues of osteoarthritis, osteoporosis, adrenal insufficiency, natural hormone imbalances, and also imbalances due to synthetic steroid hormones, in addition to addictions to opiates like morphine, codeine and heroin.

There is also lower back pain plus cold in the quadratus lumborum muscle, which can cause infertility and impotence, as well as frigidity. Kidney/adrenal deficient patients have muscle aches and pains due to calcium insufficiency, arthritis in the knee joint, and neck pain that radiates to the entire trapezius muscle.

It is difficult for these patients to fall asleep, and consequently they experience fatigue and lower energy, which motivates them to drink between 5–10 cups of coffee daily in order to maintain their customary energy level. They may have thyroid imbalances due to hormone fluctuations, especially when peri-menopausal or menopausal.

Kidney problems develop from shock, trauma and stress over a long period of time. Lymph exhaustion from synthetic hormones, medications and drug addictions, taxes and toxifies the Kidneys. On the hara, the area below the navel represents the Kidneys, and when the Kidneys are out of balance, this part of the abdomen becomes hard and inflexible. Should the condition be more chronic, the Water element hara manifests a cold, loose, and 'cottony' consistency, which means that the treatment will take longer time to effect a change in the patient's condition.

Kidney Adrenal Treatment

Treatment points	Japanese Kid-6 Zhohai Shining Sea and Kid-27 Shufu Shu Mansion, or Kid-7 Fuliu Recover Flow and Kid-27 Shufu Shu Mansion

Kid-6 Zhaohai and Kid-27 Shufu

Indications	Adrenal gland exhaustion
	Trauma, shock, fright, depression
	Severe allergies
	A life-threatening experience
	Kid-6 Zhoahai can increase steroid hormone production

Kid-7 Fuliu and Kid-27 Shufu

Indications	Bone spurs
	Osteoarthritis and osteoporosis
	Shoulder pain and stiffness
	General muscle pain in the body

Continued   117

Both Locations

Palpation and needling protocol	Bilaterally palpate Kid-16 Huangshu or Kid-15 ½ Zhongshu Central Flow, just below the navel, for hard or painful tight tender points. If the hara were likened to a large pocket watch, these points would be observed at the 4:00/8:00 o'clock positions. This is a diagnostic reflex only, unless indicated. In review, Japanese Kid-6 Zhaohai is on a line drawn from the posterior and inferior edges of the medial malleolus and is at the point of the angle where they meet. Treat Japanese Kid-6 Zhaohai by needling obliquely, then transversely, toward the Achilles tendon. Kid-27 Shufu is needled in the same manner, toward the sternum to gather Kidney essence back to the Ren Mai. Kid-7 Fuliu is used in the treatment of post-menopausal patients, and is needled upward in the direction of the meridian flow. All points are treated bilaterally
Comments	This adrenal protocol is very effective when integrated into a Constitutional Facial Acupuncture treatment. Needle the adrenal points immediately after the Eight Extraordinary Meridians, and leave these needles in the body longer if there is a red, histamine reaction around the sites of insertion. Intradermals can be employed for these points if the patient is sensitive, and hypervigilant. Adrenal patients tend to manifest a variety of changing symptoms; therefore, apply 2500–3000 gauss magnets to support their Kidneys and adrenals before they leave the clinic. Normally, the north node of these magnets has a lip that protrudes, and disperses pain. The south node is flat and tonifies the point. In this case, the north node is placed on the lower numbered point of the meridian, and the south node on the higher numbered point. More specifically, the north node is applied to Japanese Kid-6 Zhaohai or Kid-7 Fuliu, and the south node to Kid-27 Shufu. Teach the patient how to locate these points, and instruct them to leave the magnets in place for 3 days, unless they experience a skin irritation or they do not feel comfortable. If the patient has a thyroid imbalance due to adrenal insufficiency, affecting the parathyroid gland, which regulates the amount of calcium in the blood and the bones, add Japanese Kid-3 Taixi Great Ravine. Angle the needles toward the Achilles tendon, and couple it with Kid-27 Shufu, bilaterally. After the treatment, apply 2500–3000 gauss magnets to Japanese Kid-3 Taixi, the north node, and Kid-27 Shufu, the south node. If there are also gynecological symptoms accompanying the adrenal deficiency, needle and moxa the 2nd and 3rd liaos of the sacrum

Kidney Detoxification Treatment

Treatment points	Japanese Kid-9 Zhubin Guest House is discussed in the Wood element portion of this chapter under Drug and Alcohol Detoxification, and is coupled with Liv-5 Ligou for Liver/Gall Bladder-related toxicity. For the Kidney Detoxification Treatment, it is paired with Kid-27 Shufu Shu Mansion for patients addicted to opiates
Needling protocol	In review, Japanese Kid-9 Zhubin is 3 cun below Kid-10 Yingu for chemical toxicity. Needle Japanese Kid-9 Zhubin perpendicularly or use moxibustion. Kid-27 Shufu is needled transversely toward the Ren Mai

Continued

Indications	Long-term drug addictions which damage the Kidneys
	Overuse of steroid hormones
	Anti-inflammatory drugs
	Opiate addictions: heroin, morphine, codeine
	Shen disturbances
Comments	This treatment was originally designated for opiate abuse and addictions, which toxify and damage the Kidneys. Japanese Kid-9 Zhubin and Liv-5 Ligou are more effective in the treatment of alcohol addictions. Kid-27 is the Kidney Transporting Shu point, where the Qi of the Kidney meridian is collected. It is a storehouse or mansion that abundantly contains Kidney Qi and essence. Japanese Kid-9 Zhubin addresses addictions and the attendant fear, fright and mania involved in being possessed by opiates or other toxic drugs

Hormone Imbalances and the 'Healthy Aging' Points

Treatment points	Huatos of Bl-25 Dachong Shu Large Intestine Shu, plus Japanese adrenal treatment, Japanese Kid-6 Zhaohai and Japanese Kid-27 Shufu
Needling protocol	Needle the Huatos of Bl-25 Dachong Shu and angle them toward Du 3. Follow the adrenal treatment cited earlier in this chapter for needling Japanese Kid-6 Zhaohai and Japanese Kid-27 Shufu
Indications	Balances female hormones
	Deficient steroid hormones
	Estrogen/progesterone imbalances
	Gynecological issues such as premenstrual syndrome (PMS)
	Menopause, morning sickness
Comments	Nagano-sensei created this treatment after many years of clinical practice. He discovered that hormone imbalances are caused by the side effects of birth control pills, patients who took steroid hormone injections, or used a steroid ointment or cream for a long time, which impacted the body's ability to manufacture natural steroid hormones in the adrenal cortex
'Healthy Aging' points	This is another protocol that supports healthy aging, and is effective in the treatment of prostatitis, the symptoms of menopause, urinary problems, low sexual energy, and indigestion. The point is located 1 cun lateral to Du-4 Mingmen Life Gate. Needle it bilaterally, or burn moxa on the point to warm the Mingmen Fire area

119

Impotence

Treatment points	Dr. Hukaya's Lu-10 Yuji Fish Border, Ying Spring Fire point
Needling protocol	Dr. Hukaya's Lu-10 Yuji is halfway between the Pericardium Fire point, PC-8 Laogong Palace of Labor, and the Lung Fire point, Lu-10 Yuji. Burn direct moxa on this point 7 times. The patient should feel heat from each individual moxa cone. Shiunko ointment can be applied as a barrier for the protection of the skin.
Indications	Low sexual function and energy
	Impotence
	Relaxes tension in the lower back due to Kidney deficiency
	Tonifies Kidneys
Comments	This is an excellent point that can be integrated into your constitutional treatment when there is chronic Kidney deficiency

Interstitial Cystitis

Treatment points	Bl-67 Zhiyin Reaching Yin, Jing Well, Metal, Tonification ppint, and Bl-66 Tonggu Valley Passage, Ying Spring Water and Horary point on the Bladder meridian
Needling protocol	First, palpate Bl-60 Kunlun Mountain for tight tender areas, puffiness or nodules. Kunlun Mountain clears heat from the Bladder meridian, invigorates blood and alleviates burning irritation. This is a diagnostic reflex for this treatment protocol, to be used along with your other diagnostic tools. Needle-Bl-67 Zhiyin bilaterally with a small, 40-gauge or Japanese #1 needle. This point is not only the Empirical point for Malposition of the Fetus, but it also relieves obstructions in the Bladder meridian, clears heat and invigorates blood. Bl-66 Tonggu is needled in a similar fashion to clear Bladder heat, address acute cystitis and to calm the Shen
Indications	Burning urination
	Obstructional pain in the Bladder meridian
	Shen disturbance
	Occipital and/or vertex headache
Comments	Interstitial cystitis is a painful Bladder syndrome with symptoms of urinary frequency and urgency, painful sexual intercourse and nocturia. Other symptoms may accompany this syndrome, such as: irritable bowel syndrome (IBS), fibromyalgia, chronic fatigue, lupus, endometriosis, chemical sensitivities and allergies, Sjogren's disease, chronic prostatitis and psychoemotional imbalances. Most patients suffer from a damaged Bladder lining due to frequent urinary tract infections (UTI), excessive coffee, tea and soda consumption, traumatic injury and high levels of stress and anxiety

CONSTITUTIONAL TREATMENT SUMMARY
WATER ELEMENT: BLADDER AND KIDNEY

Syndromes	Treatment Points	Indications
Bac-si Truong Thin's Vietnamese Back Treatment	Bl-23 Shenshu Kidney Shu BL-52 Zhishi Will Chamber Essence Palace Points	Impotence, infertility, frigidity, cold, tight, aching lower back, weak will power
Kidney Adrenal treatment	(J) Kid-6 Zhaohai Shining Sea Kid-27 Shufu Shu Mansion; or Kid-7 Fuliu Recover Flow Kid-27 Shufu Shu Mansion	Adrenal exhaustion, severe, allergies, low production of steroid hormones Osteoarthritis, osteoporosis
Kidney Detoxification treatment	(J) Kid-9 Zhubin Guest House Kid-27 Shufu Shu Mansion	Drug addictions; prescription drugs or opiates like heroin
The 'Healthy Aging' treatment	Huatos Bl-25 Dachong Large Intestine Shu and Kidney Adrenal treatment Lateral to Du-4 Mingmen Life Gate	Deficient steroid hormones, premenstrual syndrome (PMS), menopause, morning sickness, prostatitis, low libido, indigestion, urinary problems, menopause
Impotence	(J) Lu-10 Yuji Fish Border	Low sexual function, tense, cold lower back
Interstitial cystitis	Bl-67 Zhiyin Reaching Yin Bl-66 Tonggu Valley Passage	Burning urination and pain, emotional imbalances, headache

(J), Japanese point.

In this chapter, I have maintained the order of Qi flow through the three main circuits of the Twelve Regular Meridians. Therefore, you will find pathology, protocols and treatments for Pericardium, Hand Jueyin, and Triple Heater, Hand Shaoyang, included in the relevant Five Element section with Heart, Hand Shaoyin, and Small Intestine, Hand Shaoyang.

The Pericardium Meridian Pathway: Hand Jueyin

- The Pericardium Meridian originates from the chest, connects with the Pericardium, and descends through the diaphragm and abdomen to link with the upper, middle and lower Jiaos.

- A branch inside the chest emerges at PC-1 Tianchi Celestial Pool 3 cun below the axillary fold, and ascends to the axilla.

- The main pathway follows the medial aspect of the upper arm, travels down between the Lung and Heart Meridians to the cubital fossa, and further down to the forearm, between the tendons of the palmaris longus and flexor carpi radialis muscles to the palm, where it ends.

- From there, it passes to the tip of the middle finger PC-9 Zhongchong Central Hub.
- Another branch arises from the palm at PC-8 Laogong Palace of Toil, and follows the ring finger to its tip at TH-1 Guanchong Passage Hub, and links to the Triple Heater.

Symptoms of Pericardium Hand Jueyin Meridian

- Swollen, painful axillary fold.
- Yellow sclera, aphasia, red eyes.
- Spasms of elbow and forearm, hands, feet; fullness in chest and hypochondrium.

Internal Branch Disorders

- Palpitations, cardiac pain, restlessness, stuffy chest.
- Mental issues; depression, anxiety, syncope, manic depression.

The Triple Heater Meridian: Hand Shaoyang

- The Triple Heater Meridian originates at the ulnar side of the ring finger at TH-1 Guanchong Passage Hub, travels upward between the 4th and 5th metacarpal bones to the center of the wrist, and to the lateral aspect of the forearm, between the radius and the ulna.
- It continues on to the olecranon along the lateral aspect of the upper arm to the shoulder region, where it meets SI-12 Bingfeng Grasping the Wind and Du-14 Dazhui Great Hammer.
- From Du-14 Dazhui Great Hammer, it goes to the top of the shoulder, meets GB-21 Jianjing Shoulder Well, and enters the body cavity at the supraclavicular fossa.
- From the supraclavicular fossa, it spreads into the chest at Ren-17 Danzhong Chest Center, connects with the Pericardium, descends through the diaphragm down to the abdomen, and connects with the upper, middle and lower Jiaos.
- A branch from the chest emerges at the suprclavicular fossa, ascends to the neck, curves around the posterior border of the the ears to the temples where it meets GB-6 Xuanli Suspended Tuft, GB-5 Xuanlu Suspended Skull, and GB-14 Yangbai Yang White.
- From there, it travels down to the cheek and meets SI-18 Quanliao Cheek Bone Hole, then ascends to the infraorbital ridge under the eye.
- The auricular branch separates behind the ear, enters the ear, and re-emerges in front of the ear to meet SI-19 Tinggong Auditory Palace and GB-3 Shangguan Upper Gate.

- It crosses the previous branch at the cheek, reaches the lateral aspect of the eyebrow at TH-23 Sizhukong Silk Bamboo Hole, and ends at the outer canthus of the eye at GB-1 Tongziliao Pupil Bone Hole, where it links with the Gall Bladder Meridian.

Symptoms of Triple Heater Hand Shaoyang Meridian

- Migraines, ear pain, deafness.

- Pain in front of the ear, in the outer canthus, cheek and face; temporomandibular joint syndrome (TMJ), blocked ears.

- Pain in ears and shoulder.

- Pain and stiffness along arm and wrist and neck and shoulder.

- Red, painful eyes, toothache, swollen glands, and sore throat.

- Alternating chills and fever, hypochondriac pain, bitter taste in mouth, poor appetite.

Internal Branch Disorders

- Edema, puffiness, urine retention.

- Chest pain, cough, palpitations.

- Epigastic pain, vomiting, nausea.

- Abdominal distention and bloat, constipation and diarrhea.

- Hypothyroidism, swollen glands, diabetes, hyperthyroidism.

- Tumors, fibroids, cysts.

The Wood Element: Gall Bladder, Foot Shaoyang and Liver, Foot Jueyin

The Gall Bladder Meridian Pathway: Foot Shaoyang

- The Gall Bladder Meridian starts from the outer canthus of the eye at GB-1 Tongziliao Pupil Bone Hole, crosses in front of the ear to the upper border of the zygoma at GB-3 Shangguan Upper Gate, ascends to the corner of the forehead, and descends to TH-22 Heliao Harmony Bone Hole, just above the root of the ear.

- It curves behind the ear to the mastoid process and meets Th-20 Jiaosun Angle Vertex.

- It circles upward to the corner of the forehead at St-8 Touwei Head Corner, and descends to GB-14 Yangbai Yang White, above the eye orbit.

- It then travels along the side of the head to GB-20 Fengchi Wind Pool, below the occiput, and down to the shoulder via GB-21 Jianying Shoulder Well and TH-15, Tianliao Celestial Bone Hole to meet Du-14 Dazhui Great Hammer, then it passes laterally and anteriorly to enter the supraclavicular fossa at St-12 Quepen Empty Basin.

- A branch runs behind the ear, enters it at TH-17 Yifeng Wind Screen, comes out in front of the ear, meets SI-19 Tinggong Auditory Palace and St-7 Xiaguan Below the Joint and ends at the outer canthus.

- Another branch starts at the outer canthus, descends to the jaw to meet St-5 Daying Great Reception, joins the main pathway, rises to the infraorbital area Bl-1 Jinging Bright Eyes, descends to the jaw to meet St-6 Jiache Jawbone, then to the neck where it rejoins the main pathway in the supraclavicular fossa.

- It descends into the chest, meets with PC-1 Tianchi Celestial Pool, crosses the diaphragm, connects with the Liver, and unites with the Gall Bladder.

- Then, it penetrates the hypochondriac area, and emerges at the inguinal groove, curves around the genitals, travels along the pubic area to the hip joint, and emerges at GB-30 Huantiao Jumping Round.

- The external pathway descends from the supraclavicular fossa to the area below the axilla, to the lateral side of the chest and hypochondriac region, to meet Liv-13 Zhangmen Camphorwood Gate.

- It descends to the hip joint to meet GB-30 Huantiao Jumping Round from the previous branch, and continues down the lateral thigh and knee to the lower leg, the external malleolus and the foot, between the 4th and 5th metatarsals.

- It ends at the lateral side of the 4th toe at GB-44 Zuqiaoyin Foot Portal Yin.

- A branch from GB-41 Zulinqi Foot Overlooking Tears, goes to the lateral side of the big toe, where it connects with the Liver Meridian at Liv-1 Dadun Large Pile.

Symptoms of Gall Bladder Foot Shaoyang Meridian

- Pain in eyes, side of cheeks, ear, jaw, headache, deafness, tinnitus.

- Pain and swelling in the neck, glands, axillary fossa.

- Spasms along the side of the body, hip, knee, leg, ankle, foot.

- Shaoyang syndrome, alternating chills and fever, bitter taste in mouth, hypochondriac pain and distention, malaria.

Internal Branch Disorders

- Vomiting, nausea, belching, poor appetite.

- Dark complexion.

- Pain in scrotum, hernia, leucorrhea, pain in external genitalia, difficult urination.
- Deep sighing, depression, anger, indecision, insomnia, frustration.

The Liver Meridian Pathway: Foot Jueyin

- The Liver Meridian originates at the lateral aspect of the big toe at Liv-1 Dadun Large Pile, and follows the dorsum of the foot to Liv-4 Zhongfeng Mound Center, anterior to the medial malleolus.
- It ascends the lower leg medially to meet Sp-6 Sanyinjiao Three Yin Intersection, then continues to ascend anterior to the Spleen Meridian to an area 8 cun above the medial malleolus, where it crosses and runs posterior to the Spleen Meridian, up to the knee and medial aspect of the thigh.
- It continues to the pubic area via Sp-12 Chongmen Surging Gate and Sp-13 Fushe Bowel Abode, circles the genitalia, ascends to enter the lower abdomen meeting Ren-2 Qugu Curved Bone, Ren-3 Zhongqi Central Pole and Ren-4 Guanuyan Origin Pass, then travels up to curve around the Stomach, before entering the Liver and connecting with the Gall Bladder.
- It penetrates the diaphragm, spreads into the chest and hypochondriac region, ascends the neck, the posterior aspect of the throat, nasopharynx and connects with the tissues surrounding the eyes.
- It ascends across the forehead to meet Du-20 Baihui Hundred Convergences at the vertex, where it ends.
- A branch from the eyes descends through the cheek and encircles the inner surface of the lips.
- Another branch separates from the Liver, enters the diaphragm and the Lung, and connects with the Lung Meridian.

Symptoms of Liver Foot Jueyin Meridian

- Spasms in hands, feet, lower back, joints.
- Headache, lumbar pain referring to scrotum, hernia, swelling in lateral abdomen.

Internal Branch Disorders

- Hypochondriac pain, distention, dizziness, blurred vision, tinnitus.
- Dry throat, flushed face, fever, jaundice, bitter taste in mouth.
- Mood swings, nervousness, depression, anger.

- Irregular menses, infertility, leucorrhea, impotence, itching, burning genitalia, urine retention, enuresis, yellow urination.

- Stuffy chest, cough with blood-tinged sputum.

- Epigastric distention, belching, flatulence, eating disorders, nausea, vomiting.

- Palpitations, dream disturbed sleep.

- Masses, nodules, fibroids, cysts, Plum Pit Qi.

The Wood Element: Creativity

The Liver Meridian, Foot Jueyin, and the Gall Bladder Meridian, Foot Shaoyang, represent the Wood element. The life and growth of a tree can be compared to the life cycles of the human body, in that both incorporate structurally and dynamically the Three Treasures, Jing-Earth, Qi-Humanity and Shen Spirit-Heaven. Both tree and human root themselves downwards toward Earth, extend upward to Heaven, and stretch their Qi outward toward the wide open spaces to flourish and blossom.

When the Wood element is balanced, the person is flexible and strong, creative, motivated, adaptable, organized and easy going. When imbalanced, they are ungrounded, frustrated, angry and compulsive, and have difficulty making a decision or carrying any plans through to fruition. The Liver excels in strategic planning and functionally stores and regulates Blood, harmonizes emotions, and rules the patency of Qi throughout the body. The Gall Bladder excels in decision-making and judgments; functionally, it stores and excretes bile to aid in digestion.

The Hun, Ethereal, Soul represents the Spirit of the Liver. In the flow of the Twelve Regular Meridians, the Lung, Hand Taiyin, begins the cycle with our first breath, and the Liver, Foot Jueyin, ends the life cycle with our last gasp. According to the ancient Chinese, we shed our corporeal husk when we die, and the Hun Spirit lives on, is reborn, and we once again begin the experiential journey of life.

WOOD ELEMENT PATHOLOGY

Tendinomuscular	Spasms and tics
Bone and joint problems	Arthritis, osteoarthritis, spondylitis
Allergic landscape	Cosmetics, topical medications, seasonal allergies, pollen, insect bites, photosensitivity
Organ dysfunction	Hepatitis, cirrhosis, fatty liver
Addictions	Alcohol and drugs

Continued

Cancer	Chemotherapy and radiation treatments
Headaches	Migraines; triggered by alcohol, stress, rich foods, wind, and menstruation
Sleep disorders	Insomnia
Masses	Fibroids, cysts, nodules, cystic breasts
Gynecological and reproductive imbalances	Metorrhagia, dysmenorrhea, irregular menses, infertility, impotence, leucorrhea
Weight issues	Obesity, fat metabolism, high cholesterol
Eyes	Blurry vision, myopia/hyperopia, red, painful eyes, twitch in the eyes (wind)
Emotions	Depression; Liver; anger, frustration; Gall Bladder

Recommended Constitutional Treatment Protocol

Open the Dai Mai contralaterally with the Eight Extraordinary Meridians; GB-41 Zulinqi Foot Overlooking Tears and TH-5 Waiguan Outer Gate.

Root Treatment

Liv-2 Xingjian Moving Between (Right Side)

Liv-3 Taichong Great Surge (Left Side)

Liv-2 Xingjian Moving Between

Ying Spring Fire Point

Sedation Point

Location	On the dorsum of the foot between the first and second toes, proximal to the margin of the web
Functions	Clears Liver Fire and sedates Liver Yang Rising
	Regulates free flow of Liver Qi
	Cools the blood and stops bleeding
	Calms Liver wind
	Benefits the lower Jiao

Indications	Migraine headache, dizziness, dry throat, painful, inflamed eyes, epistaxis, tinnitus, red, flushed face
	Windstroke, Bell's palsy, epilepsy
	Emotions: anger, frustration, irritability
	Shortness of breath (SOB), sighing, insomnia, palpitations, mania
	Uterine bleeding, menorrhagia
	Masses; fibroids, cysts
	Constipation, painful urination, leucorrhea
	Empirical point for low back pain, contraction and inflexibility
Psychospiritual	Excess Fire: Wood, the Mother of Fire, is dry, irritated, agitated and inflexible
	Deficient Fire: Little joy or passion; no excitement about planning the future
Comments	I have selected Liv-2 Xianjiang as the active, fiery Yang point of the constitutional root treatment. It is the best point on the Liver meridian for resolving heat, febrile conditions, external pathogenic factors, sudden emotional shifts, such as rage, or for acute changes in the complexion. Not only can excess heat and Liver Yang Rising be sedated to address the symptom of a red, flushed face, but also, in heat deficient conditions, this point can be tonified. This approach is rarely used, but treatment with Liv-2 Xianjiang can cause a pale complexion to radiate a healthy color and glow

Liv-3 Taichong Great Surge
Shu Stream, Yuan Source Point

Location	On the dorsum of the foot, in the depression distal to the junction of the first and second metatarsal bones
Functions	Promotes free flow of Liver Qi
	Sedates Liver Yang and Liver Wind
	Clears damp heat
	Calms the Shen and emotions
	Tonifies Liver Yin and Liver Blood
	Expels cold in the Liver organ and meridian
	Calms spasms and tics
Indications	Treats anger, frustration and depression, pre-menstrual syndrome (PMS), mood swings, or fear
	Vertex headache, dizziness, deviated mouth, fright, epilepsy

Continued

	Both blurred and failing vision or swollen, painful eyes
	Menstrual cycle: amenorrhea, irregular menses or uterine bleeding, early menses
	Both difficult painful urination or incontinence, edema, enuresis
	Either constipation or diarrhea
Psychospiritual	This point addresses frustration, agitation and anxiety. The Earth quality of this Wood element point directly grounds and calms the Liver organ
Comments	The Shu Stream points are indicated for joint pain and arthritis in the Ling Shu, and the Source points treat the Zang, which directly impact the organs. Taichong is equally effective in treating both excess and deficiency patterns. For example: when Liver Yin is deficient, Liver Yang rises and disturbs the head, or, conversely, Liver Blood Deficiency contributes to the development of Liver Wind issues, such as epilepsy, Bell's palsy and windstroke

Suggested Body Points

My frequently used and recommended points for the Gall Bladder, Foot Shaoyang, and Liver, Foot Jueyin, meridians are GB-34 Yanglingquan Yang Mountain Spring, for tendinomuscular issues, GB-37 Guanming Bright Light for Liver-related eye disorders, Liv-8 Quguam Spring at the Bend for fibroids and masses in the abdomen, plus protocols for migraine headaches and seasonal allergies.

GB-37 Guanming Bright Light
Luo Connecting Point
An Empirical Eye Point

Location	5 cun directly above the tip of the lateral malleolus, on the anterior border of the fibula
Functions	Brightens eyes and clears vision
	Expels wind and moves dampness throughout the meridians
	Clears heat and pain
	Treats bruxism
Indications	Poor vision; night blindness, blurring vision, myopia and hyperopia
	Red, painful, itchy eyes
	Knee pain and atrophy of the muscles

	Breast fullness and infection
	Temporomandibular joint dysfunction (TMJ)
Psychospiritual	This point gives clarity of vision to bodymindspirit. It invests a person with courage and an ability to be flexible and see through challenges in life, while simultaneously gaining wisdom in the process
Comments	The transverse Luos are connecting branches that link the Yin and Yang points. These vessels are effective in treating blood issues; Liver stores blood, and GB-37 Guanming is an excellent distal point for spider veins or varicose veins, cysts or nodules in the body. In my experience, GB-37 Guanming is particularly effective in the treatment of unresolved anger issues. The Wood element rules the free flow of Qi in the body, and balances emotions; therefore, this point can support the release of latent anger, frustration or rage, and can illuminate Ming, the authentic life path. It is especially useful when treating a patient who has a long, deep, suspended sword line between the eyebrows, which is indicative of a past pattern of suppressing and internalizing anger

GB-34 Yanglingquan Yang Mound Spring
Lower He-Sea; Earth Point
Influential Point of Tendons and Sinews

Location	In the depression anterior and inferior to the head of the fibula
Functions	Promotes the smooth flow of Liver/Gall Bladder Qi
	Clears damp heat
	Supports sinews and joints
	Alleviates pain in the meridian
	Calms Shen
	Shaoyang syndromes
Indications	Hypochondriac pain, frequent sighing
	Stiff, tight muscles and joints, arthritis, osteoporosis
	Weakness, atrophy and numbness of lower extremities, hemiplegia, windstroke
	Bitter taste, vomit, jaundice, malaria
	For fear and shyness use GB-34 Yanglingquan with Liv-2 Xingjian, chills and fever, constipation

Continued

Psychospiritual	It calms frustrations, aids in decision-making, fosters hope and dispels negativity
Comments	Use GB-34 Yanglingquan for tendinomuscular issues, contractions, pain, and tightness in the muscles and tendons of the leg such as the gastrocnemius muscle, in the calf. It is also effective in treating sciatica, with numbness and pain radiating down the Gall Bladder channel. It alleviates the distress of inflamed joints, arthritis and spondylitis characterized by inflammation of the joints between the spinal bones

Liv-8 Quguan Spring at the Bend
He-Sea; Water Point
Tonification Point

Location	When the knee is flexed, the point is above the medial end of the transverse popliteal crease, in the depression anterior to the tendons of the semitendinosus and semimembranosus muscles
Functions	Tonifies Liver Yin and Liver blood
	Resolves damp heat in the lower Jiao
	Benefits the Bladder
	Relaxes the muscles and sinews
	Moves blood and benefits veins
Indications	Inflamed, dry eyes, poor vision, tinnitus, hearing loss
	Itchy skin and itching genitalia
	Menstrual cramps, uterine prolapse, leucorrhea
	Hernia, difficult urination and urine retention
	Fibroids and masses
	Coldness and pain along the Liver channel
Psychospiritual	When the Water element isn't balanced and there is too little water in the Wood element, the patient is fearful, rigid and cannot flow or let go. When there is a deficiency of water, they are overwhelmed, angry, depressed, even suicidal, and can't see any purpose in life

Comments	I have been successful treating fibroids and abdominal masses due to damp heat and blood stagnation with Liv-8 Yanglingquan. Needle this point and moxa it 21 times, then surround the masses or fibroids locally with intradermal needles, or, alternatively, with calibrated tuning forks. Certain intervallic combinations resonate through the fibroidal mass. These vibrations enliven circulation and subsequently diminish it in size. Tuning forks will be discussed in brief in Chapter 9. I also recommend dietary changes: non-greasy foods, the elimination of alcohol, coffee and other stimulants, accompanied by creative pursuits and an exercise regimen, as well as Chinese herbs and a homeopathic drainage technique. If the fibroids are too large, homeopathy works better than Chinese herbs

Migraine Headaches

Treatment points	GB-40 Qiuxu Ruin Hill; and Liv-5 Ligou Woodworm Canal

GB-40 Qiuxu Ruin Hill

Location	GB-40, a Yuan Source point, is located anterior and inferior to the lateral malleolus, in the depression on the lateral side of the tendon of the extensor digitorum longus muscle
Functions	Promotes the smooth flow of the Liver and Gall Bladder
	Cools fire, damp heat and hot phlegm
	Tonifies the Gall Bladder and supports decision-making
Indications	Pain in the neck and hypchondrium
	Acid reflux, vomiting, malaria
	Eye pain, headache, tinnitus, insomnia
Psychospiritual	This point allows people to gain perspective and clarity, gives them stability and alleviates a feeling of isolation

Liv-5 Ligou Woodworm Canal

Location	Liv-5 Ligou Woodworm Canal, is a Luo Connecting point, and is 5 cun above the tip of the medial malleolus on the medial aspect, and near the medial border of the tibia
Functions	Promotes smooth flow of Liver Qi
	Clears heat
	Resolves damp, as in vaginal discharge and cloudy urine
	Relieves wind heat
	Cold in the genitals

Continued

Indications	Hernia, urine retention, menstrual imbalances, headaches, leucorrhea, leg atrophy, skin irritation
Psychospiritual	This is a good spirit point for clearing out irritations, frustration, confusion, and for calming the patient. It can also manifest as either skin or mental irritation

Both Locations

Needling protocol	Needle only on the side of the migraine headache. First, needle the source point, which grounds the Gall Bladder, and then the Liver Luo Connecting point to drain the pathogenic heat from the Gall Bladder
Comments	If the migraine headache is not showing signs of improvement with this approach, resonating 2 Low Ohm Unison calibrated tuning forks on both of these points effects a quicker resolution. As a reminder, do not treat migraine patients with facial acupuncture until they are migraine-free for at least 3 months. Treat them constitutionally for the migraine prior to any facial needling. If, for some reason, after the 3-month period, facial acupuncture causes an incipient migraine, tuning forks, in addition to the needles, work very quickly and effectively

Seasonal Allergies and Sudden Weather Changes

Treatment points	Liv-14 Qimen Cycle Gate, and;
	Lu-1 Zhongfu Central Treasury

Liv-14 Qimen Cycle Gate

Location	Liv-14 Qimen, Front Mu, Liver Crossing Point of Yin Wei Mai, Exit point is located directly below the nipple in the 6th intercostal space
Functions	Promotes Liver Qi flow
	Clears heat and fire
	Cools the blood
	Benefits the Stomach
	Relieves obstruction in the chest
Indications	Hypchondriac pain, depression, problems with lactation, mastitis, nausea, acid reflux, belching, fever and unconsciousness
Psychospiritual	This point gives the patient hope for the future, and is an Exit point, which is a gate that needs to open and close freely to be balanced. If this gate is shut, the patient is frustrated, angry and intolerant. When the gate is stuck, the patient feels alone, hopeless and resigned to their fate

Continued

Lu-1 Zhongfu Central Treasury

Location	Lu-1 Zhongfu Front Mu Lung, Entry point is located 1 cun below the lateral end of the clavicle at the lateral side of the 1st intercostal space, 6 cun lateral to the Ren Mai
Functions	Regulates Lung Qi
	Stimulates the descent of the Lung Qi
	Disperses fullness in the chest
	Treats both acute and excess conditions
	Treats Lung Yin Deficiency
Indications	Cough, asthma, chest pain, lethargy
Psychospiritual	This Lung entry point rules inspiration, higher purpose and beauty. When the patient cannot enter, they feel isolated, lonely, separate, sad and stuck in the chest; they cannot take in the breath from Heaven, Tian. Liv-14 Qimen needs to be open to the Qi of Lu-1 Zhongfu, and *vice versa*, in order for the patient to be receptive to the divine wisdom. Heaven is represented by Lu-1 Zhongfu, which relates to inspiration; the Liver relates to aspiration

Both Locations

Comments	The Entry/Exit points of the Lung and Liver help in the treatment of pollen and seasonal allergies; the ingestion of medical grade pearl powder is an additional component that can alleviate these symptoms. Inserting a paste of pearl powder, Zhen Zhu, plus water into the navel every day makes a big difference for Wood element patients. In TCM, Zhen Zhu *Margarita* pearl powder anchors, settles and calms the Spirit, clears the eyes, promotes healing, generates flesh and sedates the Heart. It renews connective tissue, softens and naturally lightens the complexion, reduces blotchiness, irritation and inflammation
Treatment	For seasonal allergies that manifest as Liver Wind and Liver Heat, causing irritability, allergies and itchy skin: internally, ingest 1 vial medical grade pearl powder, Zhen Zhu, in 8 oz. of water every day for 3 weeks. Externally, apply pearl powder, Zhen Zhu to your navel; add water to the powder and make a paste, place it your navel and change it every day. Patients have reported release from seasonal allergies, skin rashes and itching from this treatment. The pearl powder treatment can also be used for Liver Yang Rising and Yin deficient patterns, seen in menopausal, perimenopausal or andropausal patients. It cools deficient heat, purifies the blood and balances the Liver. Insomnia due to Heart fire, with palpitations and anxiety, can be effectively treated, both internally and externally. However, drink the pearl powder, Zhen Zhu, decoction before bed for one month only. Stop the treatment for one month, and then resume it bi-monthly. Continue to use pearl powder, Zhen Zhu, in the navel daily. A Japanese acupuncture treatment for dermatological issues, such as inflamed, itchy skin caused by allergies or wind issues, as in urticaria, combines LI-5 Jianju Shoulder Bone with Kid-9 Zhubin Guest House. LI-5 Jianju is located in the upper portion of the deltoid muscle, antero-inferior to the acromian. When the arm is abducted, the point is found in the depression on the anterior border of the shoulder. LI-5 Jianju expels wind damp, stops pain, harmonizes Qi and blood, and locally treats the shoulder joint. In tandem with Kid-9 Zhubin, it expels organic toxins from the body and the skin. Use the TCM location for Kid-9 Zhubin, not the Japanese location, as outlined in the Drug and Alcohol Detoxification section of this chapter

Japanese Acupuncture Treatments

The Liver and Gall Bladder signs and symptoms usually are more pronounced on the right side of the body. The patient may have hepatitis, cirrhosis, or a fatty liver, and additionally manifest addictions to alcohol and drugs, including prescription drugs.

They may have undergone intensive chemotherapy and radiation treatments for cancer. Hormonal headaches involving the pituitary gland originate at Bl-2 Zanzhu Collecting Bamboo, with complaints of intense pain behind the eyeballs. With the involvement of the Gall Bladder, one-sided migraine headaches may ensue. There may also be tendinomuscular spasms, tics and temporomandibular joint dysfunction (TMJ). Shoulder pain is reported at Bl-43 Gaohuangshu Fatty Vital Hollow, which is the outer Pericardium Shu.

According to the Ling Shu, the emotional state of depression belongs to the Liver. Therefore, in Japanese acupuncture Gaohuangshu lifts the spirits, and also treats depression. Patients with insomnia awaken just after falling asleep. Liver rules the menstrual and reproductive cycles plus hormonal imbalances in the body.

Due to Liver Qi and blood stagnation, *oketsu*, masses, fibroids and cystic breasts can form. Obesity, fat metabolism and high cholesterol, in particular, are attributed to the Liver/Gall Bladder.

The Wood element patient presents an allergic landscape; patients have problems with any topical cosmetics, and insect bites persist longer than with the other elemental types. They are also photosensitive, and experience seasonal allergies to pollen, especially in the springtime. Their skin is easily irritated, and may develop red dots, which are not considered peticchiae.

Japanese Oketsu: Stagnant Blood

Treatment points	Japanese Liv-4 Zhongfeng Mound Center, and;
	Dr. Hukaya's Lu-5 Chize Cubit Marsh
Locations	Japanese Liv-4 Zhongfeng, Jing River, Metal point: 1 cun lateral to the medial malleolus, midway between Sp-5 Shangqiu Shang Hill, and St-41 Jiexi Ravine Divide, in the depression on the medial side of the tibialis anterior tendon
	Lu-5 Chize, He-Sea, Water, sedation point: the TCM location is in the cubital crease, in the depression on the lateral side of the tendon of the biceps brachii muscle
	The Japanese Lu-5 Chize is more lateral to the TCM Lu-5 Chize, and is located on the cubital crease midway between the TCM Lu-5 Chize, and Lu-11 Shaoshang Lesser Yang. The point can be found 1 cun above or below this area by palpating for tightness, small nodules or tenderness and pain in the area

135

Continued

Needling protocol	Needle only on the left side of the body, with the flow of the meridians. Therefore, Japanese Liv-4 Zhongfeng would be needled upwards toward the head, and Lu-5 Chize would be needled downward toward the feet, with the palm of the hand turned upward. To reinforce the effects of the treatment, 2500–3000 gauss magnets can be placed on Liv-4 (north node) and Lu-5 (south node)
Indications	Blood transfusions after surgery
	Scars, when the scar is different colors
	Right-sided occipital pain
	Premenstrual syndrome (PMS)
	Cystic breasts
	Dark circles under the eyes relating to the Wood element
Comments	This combination of points is used in Japanese hara treatments. In this system, the hara is palpated from St-25 Tianshu Celestial Root to St-27 Daju Great Gigantic on the patient's left side to discern where there is tight tenderness or tension in this area. Liver hara is only palpated on the left side, because the mesenteric and hepatic portal veins flow through the left side of the hara and up to the Liver organ, to cleanse toxic and stagnant blood. This may be why the Liver pulse is palpated on the left side of the wrist. Japanese hara protocols are elegant and simple, yet simultaneously complex and intricate. If you are not conversant with Japanese hara palpation, I recommend that you use the tongue and pulse, or other diagnostic tools. I have found that using this *oketsu* needling protocol with the indications that I have provided is very effective. I have had success treating premenstrual syndrome (PMS) with abdominal pain, tender, cystic breasts, and irritability. As the circulation of Qi and blood in the Wood hara begins to flow, the symptoms are alleviated, and Liver-related dark circles under the eyes begin to diminish, as well. There is customarily a noticeable difference with a single treatment

The Five Shu Transporting Points and the Corresponding Elements

The Five Shu Transporting points are sometimes referred to as the antique points, and are considered some of the most important points of the Twelve Regular Meridians. The qualities of these points, their indications, and the elements involved enhance their interrelationship. The Classic of Difficulties documented their indications, and the Spiritual Pivot expanded upon when to needle the points, plus the associated musical sounds, tastes and seasons involved. Japanese Liv-4 Zhongfeng is a Jing River point that traditionally relates to dyspnea, cough, asthma and alternating chills and fever. However, according to Peter Deadman in his book, *A Manual of Acupuncture*, Liv-4

Zhongfeng can be used to address changes in the patient's voice and frequent sighing.[1]

It is also a Five Phase Metal point on the Liver meridian, and one of its indications is a distended hypochondrium. This means that the qualities of the Metal/Lung and the hypochondriac restriction of Wood/Liver could give rise to breathing problems. The associated sighing may be interpreted as the patient's endeavor to alleviate the restriction in this area due to stagnation of Qi or blood and/or constrained emotions.

Lu-5 is a He-Sea point, which traditionally relates to rebellious Qi, and diarrhea due to Stomach imbalances and irregular eating and drinking habits.

Lu-5 Chize, in particular, indicates abdominal distention, diarrhea and vomiting, and is reinforced by the Lung meridians' internal pathway, which originates at Ren-12 Zhongmen Central Vertex, and travels downward to connect with the Large Intestine and then the Stomach.

The indications for this point include blood stagnation due to heat, and Lung heat and phlegm. It is a Water point on the Lung meridian and a sedation point, which strengthens its ability to quiet heat pathology, and also to treat *oketsu* blood stasis.

On the Five Phase Generation cycle, Metal is the Mother of Water. When Metal isn't balanced, it can cause pathological manifestations within the Water element, such as heat or mucus in the Lung, dry cough, grief or depression, and a rigid, dry attitude that lacks fluidity or flexibility.

Nagano-sensei's Obesity Treatment

Treatment points	Liv-14 Qimen Cycle Gate, St-27 Daju Great Gigantic, Ren-6 Qihai Sea of Qi and GB-26 Daimai Girdling Vessel
Locations	Liv-14 Qimen is 4 cun lateral to the midline in the 6th intercostal space
	St-27 Daju is located 2 cun below the navel, 2 cun lateral to Ren-5 Shimen Stone Gate
	Ren-6 Qihai is on the abdominal midline, 1.5 cun below the navel
	GB-26 Daimai is located directly below the end of the 11th rib where Liv-13 Zhongmen Camphorwood Gate is located, at the level of the navel
Needling protocol	All points are needled bilaterally except for GB-26 Daimai, and Liv-14 Qimen. Needle Liv-14 Qimen on the right side, pointed laterally between the ribs, with a 10-15 degree insertion, and GB-26 Daimai on the left side, angled toward the back. St-27 Daju and Ren-6 Qihai are needled at a 90-degree angle. Use direct moxa after needling

Continued

Indications	Abdominal obesity
	High cholesterol
	Fat metabolism imbalances
	Abdominal and hypochondriac distention and pain
	Damp heat
	Constitutional toxins in the Dai Mai
Comments	GB-26 Dai Mai is discussed in Chapter 5 on the Tendinomuscular Meridians, under 'Wandering Skirt' syndrome. Indications include abdominal bloat, obesity, anger, frustration, and an inability to make a decision. The patient is 'sitting on the fence,' and manifests phlegm, or lack of clarity in bodymindspirit. TCM describes an imbalance in Daimai as a feeling of sitting in cold water. Therefore, direct moxa is highly recommended. This Japanese acupuncture protocol indicates that only the left GB-26 Daimai is to be treated. This is most likely due to the Wood Element hara reflex, which is palpated only on the left side of the abdomen. Only the right Liv-14 Qimen is indicated because the Liver organ is on the right side of the body. The indications for Liv-14 Qimen were discussed under the Seasonal Allergies Treatment in this chapter. When Qimen's Exit Gate is closed, imbalances of anger, frustration, short temper and possible addictions and binge eating can arise. Obese patients also have imbalances in their fat metabolism. St-27 Daju is an Earth point which frees the Intestines, and when out of balance, manifests as an inability to let go of depression and co-dependence. It indicates problems with digesting not only food, but also thoughts and emotions. Ren-6 Qihai treats exhaustion, fatigue, depression, Spleen-related abdominal distention and weight issues. A person with weight problems often cannot digest fats. In this case, the patient could have developed a buffalo hump at the 7th cervical vertebra (C7), and problems with the pancreas manufacturing or secreting digestive enzymes. This treatment protocol is also effective with for patients with high cholesterol issues. In Sensei Nagano's experience, patients lost weight after they were treated with direct moxa every day. Patients with a fast pulse lost 10 lb a month without regaining the original weight

Drug and Alcohol Detoxification

Treatment points	Japanese Kid-9 Zhubin Guest House, Xi Cleft point of the Yin Wei Mai; and Japanese Liv-5 Ligou Woodworm Canal, Luo Connecting point
Locations	Kid-9 Zhubin's TCM location is 5 cun directly above Kid-3 Taixi Great Ravine, at the lower end of the belly of gastrocnemius muscle, on the line connecting Kid-3 Taixi to Kid-10 Yingu Yin Valley. The Japanese location for Kid-9 Zhubin is 3 cun below Kid-10 Yingu. Please note: Liv-5 Ligou was discussed in the Migraine Headache portion of this chapter. Japanese Liv-5 Ligou is found halfway between the external malleolus and Liv-8 Ququam
Palpation and needling protocol	Palpate Japanese Liv-5 Ligou for puffiness or pressure pain. Needle both Japanese Kid-9 Zhubin and Japanese Liv-5 Ligou at a 90-degree angle. Use direct moxa if there is edema present
Indications	Drug and alcohol addictions
	Toxicity from antibiotics and medications
	Neurosis and fright, mania, Shen disturbance
	Heavy metal poisoning
	Food poisoning
Comments	Kid-9 Zhubin is translated as 'Guest House' in most acupuncture manuals. In ancient Chinese texts, according to Grasping the Wind, the radical for Zhu means 'to attack' and the radical for Bin 'to expel.'2 To simultaneously expel and attack implies that this point could expel pathogenic Qi from the Kidney meridian. This description is in alignment with the overall function of detoxing the entire body from chemicals. It is a Xi Cleft point, which addresses emergency conditions and pain. In the case of Kid-9 Zhubin, because it is a Yin point, it also treats blood issues. Blood rules the Shen, which makes Kid-9 Zhubin a perfect point for the treatment of acute mental imbalances, such as mania and manic depression. As the Xi Cleft point of the Yin Wei Mai, it also opens the chest, and addresses Heart pain, not only on the physical level, but also spiritually and psychoemotionally. In Japanese acupuncture protocols, Kid-9 Zhubin is also designated the 'Happy Baby' point, because it nourishes the uterus. This point is needled following the conclusion of the 1st and 2nd trimesters to support the fetus; this can dispel the impact of any negative imbalances inherited from the parents. There are several ways to treat this point; use a stainless steel or a gold needle, or direct moxa 9 times. Utilize the TCM location for Kid-9 Zhubin; this is not a chemical detox. We have already discussed Japanese Liv-5 Ligou in the section on Migraine Headaches this chapter. In Japanese acupuncture, Liv-5 Ligou detoxifies and cleanses the Liver, but does not treat the withdrawal symptoms or severe addictions. The Japanese Kid-9 Zhubin is a good detoxification point because of its diuretic properties. Liv-5 Ligou is a transverse Luo point, and it uses blood and fluids to keep pathogens latent, so that they do not penetrate or harm the Twelve Regular Meridians. Ligou does not treat pathogenic Qi, but forms a safe container for Kid-9 Zhubin to expel pathogens from the body

CONSTITUTIONAL TREATMENT SUMMARY
WOOD ELEMENT: GALL BLADDER AND LIVER

Syndromes	Treatment Points	Indications
Empirical eye point	GB-37 Guanming Bright Light	Night blindness, blurry vision, painful, red, itchy eyes, psychospiritual vision and perspective
Tendinomuscular and joint problems	GB-34 Yanglingquan Yang Mound Spring	Stiff, tight muscles, arthritis, osteoarthritis, atrophy of the lower limbs (windstroke)
Abdominal masses	Liv-8 Ququan Spring at the Bend	Fibroids, pain in the Liver meridian, menstrual cramps, leucorrhea, difficult urination
One-sided headaches	GB-40 Qiuxu Ruin Hill Liv-5 Ligou Woodworm Canal	Migraine headaches
Seasonal Allergies	Liv-14 Qimen Cycle Gate Lu-1 Zhongfu Central Treasury	Se asonal allergies due to pollen, with cough, sneezing, irritability, itchy skin
Oketsu Stagnant Blood	(J) Liv-4 Zhongfeng Mound Center (J) Lu-5 Chize Cubit Marsh	All right-sided occipital pain, premenstrual syndrome (PMS), cystic breasts, dark circles under the eyes, irritability
Nagano-sensei's Obesity Treatment	Liv-14 Qimen Cycle Gate St-27 Daju Great Gigantic Ren-6 Qihai Sea of Qi GB-26 Daimai Girdling Vessel	Abdominal obesity, high cholesterol, fat metabolism imbalances
Drug and Alcohol Detoxification treatment	(J) Kid-9 Zhubin Guest House (J) Liv-5 Ligou Woodworm Canal	Addictions to drugs, alcohol, antibiotics, heavy metal poisoning, food poisoning, Shen disturbances

(J), Japanese point.

REFERENCES

1. Deadman P, Al-Khafaji M. A Manual of Acupuncture, Journal of Chinese Medicine Publications, 2nd ed. East Sussex, UK: Hove; 2007.

2. Ellis A, Wiseman N, Boss K. Grasping the Wind: An Exploration into the Meaning of Chinese Acupuncture Point Names. St. Paul, MN: Paradigm Publications; 1989.

CHAPTER 5

The Twelve
Tendinomuscular Meridians

"He who knows others is wise; he who knows himself is enlightened."
— Lao Tzu

The Tendinomuscular Meridians (TMM) are discussed in chapter 13 of the *Nei Jing* and *Ling Shu*, and are considered conduits of Wei Qi. While they protect the body from damp, wind, heat, cold and trauma, there are no indicated exterior signs and symptoms, such as aversion to cold, fever, or sore throat.

Even though they circulate deeper than the Cutaneous Regions, they are still located on the superficial aspect of the body. They overlap each other, involve more than one channel, are nourished by the Regular Channels, circulate Qi and blood on the exterior of the body, and treat imbalances of the muscles, joints, ligaments and tendons.

- They do not connect with internal organs; however, the internal organs influence the TMMs.

- All of them begin at the extremities and travel up to the head and face, or to the trunk.

- Structurally, they are wide band-like areas that follow the Twelve Regular Meridians.

- They have no points of their own, but borrow points from the Twelve Regular Meridians.

- Their symptomatology includes sprains, spasms, stiffness, restricted movement of the joints, and muscle weakness, due to overuse, injuries or muscle tension caused by stress or trauma.

Qi and blood knot, bind or converge in specific areas, such as large muscles and joints, and are more reactive in these particular locations. These groups

TABLE 5.1	MEETING POINTS OF THE TENDINOMUSCULAR MERIDIANS		
Yin/Yang Meeting	Area	Points	Meridians
Three Leg Yang	Face/zygoma	SI-18 Quanliao Cheekbone Hole	Bl/GB/St
		St-3 Juliao Great Bone Hole	
Three Leg Yin	External genitalia	Ren-3 Zhongji Central Bone Hole	Sp/Liv/Kid
Three Arm Yang	Corner of the head	GB-13 Benshen Root Spirit	SI/TH/LI
		St-8 Touwei Head Corner	
Three Arm Yin	Diaphragm	GB-22 Yuanye Armpit Abyss	Lu/PC/Ht

each have meeting points that can effectively treat signs and symptoms of nearby TMMs. For example, low back pain can be treated distally by using Three Leg Meridian meeting points; SI-18 Qianliao Cheekbone Hole; or St-3 Juliao Great Bone Hole. The three affected meridians are Bladder, Gall Bladder and Stomach.

In Table 5.1 we see that the Tendinomuscular Meridians areas have their respective points and meridian involvement, plus a strong relationship and mutual influence upon these channels.

Applications for the Tendinomuscular Meridians

1. Ashi tight tender points are palpated and treated locally, distally and on adjacent meridians. Use distal points first to treat acute pain.

   The painful areas of the body can be moved by the patient while the practitioner manipulates the needle distally. For example: for rotator cuff injuries, deconstrain St-38 Tiaokou Ribbon Opening on the same side, as the patient moves the shoulder in various directions. This point removes meridian obstruction, and is an empirical point for shoulder pain and stiffness.

   The meeting point of the Three Arm Yang Meridians could also be needled; either GB-13 Benshen Root Spirit or St-8 Touwei Head Corner, can effectively influence the Small Intestine, Triple Heater or Large Intestine Tendinomuscular Meridians.

2. Depending upon which meridian has pain or strain, treat the corresponding area on the opposite side of the injury.

   For example: if there is left-sided hip pain at GB-29 Juliao Squatting Bone Hole, treat the right GB-21 Jiangjing Shoulder Well, or use the right TH-15 Tianliao Celestial Bone Hole, which is on the Shaoyang Channel. If the

TABLE 5.2   THE SIX ENERGIES/DIVISIONS, THE THREE YANGS AND THE THREE YINS

Level	Meridian/Organ	Polarity
Taiyang ('Greater Yang')	Small Intestine (fire)	The Three Yangs
	Urinary Bladder (water)	
Shaoyang ('Lesser Yang')	Triple Heater (fire)	
	Gall Bladder (wood)	
Yangming ('Yang Brightness')	Large Intestine (metal)	
	Stomach (earth)	
Taiyin ('Greater Yin')	Lung (metal)	The Three Yins
	Spleen (earth)	
Shaoyin ('Lesser Yin')	Heart (fire)	
	Kidney (water)	
Jueyin ('Terminal Yin')	Pericardium (fire)	
	Liver (wood)	

elbow is painful, treat the knee, or, with the wrist, address and treat the ankle; both treatment points should be on the opposite side from the injury.

3. For Bi syndromes: heat a thick needle and insert and remove it immediately from the affected area; this is especially effective with cold or damp Bi syndromes. You may also employ moxa on the handle of the needle to warm the area. Many of these needling methods have been described in the *Nei Jing*.

4. Other treatment methods use direct or indirect moxa, such as moxa stick, tiger warmer, and also TDP lamps, cupping, electrostimulation and bleeding techniques. The Vietnamese often apply liquid moxa, and then warm the area with a hair dryer.

I also recommend using trigger and Ashi points. At a deeper level, integrate the needling of motor points to alleviate symptoms of Bi sydromes, muscle strain and overuse, contraction from stress and possible emotional imbalances.

Table 5.2 describes how the Twelve Tendinomuscular Meridians follow the areas associated with the Six Divisions or Energies, which delineate specific pathological factors derived from climatic changes, such as cold, wind, heat, damp, dryness and fire. In other words, they are the first line of defense and circulate Wei Qi throughout the muscles and joints.

In addition, they also control the flow of Qi from the exterior of the body to the interior, and from the Yang to the Yin pairs.

Taiyang flows to Shaoyin

Shaoyang flows to Jueyin

Yangming flows to Taiyin

Therefore, I have grouped the Tendinomuscular Meridians according to the Six Stages of the *Shang Han Lun*, starting with the most Yang and ending with the most Yin. The following summary of the tendinomuscular pathways will enable you to visualize them when you are applying the Wei Qi treatments to release the exterior, or for tension and tightness at the superficial level in the shoulders, neck or waist. The individual summaries and the accompanying charts will help you to needle these areas more effectively.

The Taiyang is used to treat the TMM area of the Bladder and Small Intestine meridians, and because it is the most superficial, it is the first part of the body to be exposed to external pathogens. The neck, shoulders, back, buttocks, hamstrings, calves, ankles, outer malleolus and foot are especially vulnerable to muscle imbalances, pain, strain and sprains.

Taiyang: Greater Yang

Bladder and Small Intestine TMM

The Bladder TMM Pathway

Starts: little toe

Ends: nose

1. It originates at the little toe and ascends past the lateral malleolus, and up to the lateral aspect of the knee where it binds.

2. A lower branch travels along the external malleolus to bind at the heel, and then up to the lateral popliteal fossa.

3. Another branch separates from the branch in the calf at the two heads of the gastrocnemius muscle, and travels up to the medial popliteal fossa.

4. Both branches unite and travel up the hamstrings to the gluteal area where they bind at the buttocks, and then ascend along the side of the spine to the nape of the neck. From there, another branch penetrates and binds the root of the tongue.

5. The main branch continues to ascend and binds at the occipital bone, passes over the head and binds at the bridge of the nose, circles around the eyes and sends capillary branches to the upper eyelids; it then binds at the zygomatic bone.

6. Another branch separates at the back, ascends the posterior axillary fold and binds at LI-15 Jianyu Shoulder Bone.

7. Yet another branch travels through the axilla up to the chest, emerges at the supraclavicular fossa and binds at GB-12 Wangu Completion Bone, behind the ear.

8. Finally, one more branch emerges from the supraclavicular fossa to rise to the cheekbone, and ends at the side of the nose.

SUMMARY: BLADDER TMM

- Starts at the little toe; travels up the lateral ankle to the lateral knee (binds)
- Lower branch travels along the ankle to the heel (binds), then up to the lateral popliteal fossa
- Separates at the calf and ascends to the medial popliteal fossa
- Both branches ascend the hamstrings to (bind) at the buttocks, up along the spine to the back of the neck, to penetrate the root of the tongue (binds)
- Ascends to the occipital bone (binds), up over the head to the bridge of the nose (binds), circles around the eye to the upper eyelid and (binds) at the zygoma
- Separates at the back, ascends to the posterior axilla to LI-15 Jianyu (binds)
- Another branch travels through the axilla to the chest, emerges at the supraclavicular fossa, and (binds) at GB-12 Wangu
- Emerges from the supraclavicular fossa, rises to the cheekbone and ends at the side of the nose

---

Signs and Symptoms

- Numb, tingling little toe.
- Swollen painful heel.
- Popliteal fossa spasms (knee).
- Spasm and pain in the erector spinae muscles (Bladder meridian).
- Sore and painful back of the neck.
- Inability to raise the shoulder.
- Pain in the axilla radiating to the supraclavicular fossa.
- Tight, tense painful shoulder.

The Small Intestine TMM Pathway

Starts: ulnar side of the little finger

Ends: corner of the forehead

1. The main branch starts at the ulnar side of the little finger and travels up to bind at the wrist, then along the forearm to bind at the elbow.

2. From the elbow, it ascends the back of the arm, along the triceps muscles to bind at the axilla, the posterior deltoid muscle.

3. From the axilla, it circles around the scapula and rises to the neck, just anterior to the Bladder TMM, and binds at the mastoid process.

4. It then travels and binds behind the ear, and enters the ear.

5. It continues to ascend behind and above the ear, then descends to bind at the mandible, and travels upward to bind at the outer canthus of the eye.

6. It ends and binds at the corner of the forehead where it meets the Three Arm Yang TMM.

SUMMARY: SMALL INTESTINE TMM

- Starts at the little finger (ulnar side), travels to (bind) at both the wrist and the elbow
- Ascends the back of the arm, (binds) at the axilla
- Circles the scapula, ascends to the neck and (binds) at the mastoid process
- (Binds) behind the ear and enters it
- Ascends above the ear, descends to the mandible (binds), and to the outer canthus of the eye
- Ends at the corner of the forehead (binds)

Signs and Symptoms

- Painful, stiff little finger.

- Pain in elbow (medial epicondyle of the humerus).

- Pain and tightness below the axilla, in the triceps and posterior deltoid muscles.

- Scapular and neck pain.

- Tinnitus.

- Ear pain; refers to the mandible.

- Delayed vision/vision impairment.

- Neck spasms, swelling and muscle atrophy.

- Neck stiffness due to external pathogens, like cold and heat.

Shaoyang: Lesser Yang

Gall Bladder and Triple Heater TMM

The Gall Bladder TMM Pathway

Starts: lateral side of the fourth toe

Ends: outer canthus

1. It begins at the fourth toe and binds at the lateral malleolus.

2. It ascends to the lateral aspect of the leg and binds at the lateral side of the knee.

3. A branch begins with the upper portion of the fibula and ascends along the later thigh.

4. Another branch travels anteriorly to bind just above St-32 Futu Crouching Rabbit, along the rectus femoris muscle, and then moves posteriorly to bind at the sacrum.

5. A branch ascends across the ribs, travels anteriorly to the axilla, then links with the breast. It then travels up the pectoral muscle to bind the supraclavicular fossa, St-12 Quepen Empty Basin.

6. Another branch ascends from the axilla, passes through St-12 Quepen Empty Basin, anterior to the Bladder Channel, passing behind the ear to the corner of the forehead; it then continues upward to the vertex of the head where it meets its bilateral pathway.

7. A branch descends from the forehead, crosses the cheek and binds at the side of the nose.

8. The meridian ends and binds at the outer canthus of the eye.

SUMMARY: GALL BLADDER TMM

- Begins at the fourth toe and (binds) at the lateral ankle
- Ascends the lateral part of the leg to the knee (binds)
- Begins in the upper portion of the fibula and ascends laterally along the thigh
- Travels anteriorly just above St-32 Futu (binds) and moves to the sacrum (binds)
- Crosses the ribs to the axilla, links with the breast, to the supraclavicular fossa, St-12 Quepen (binds)
- Ascends from the axilla, through St-12 Quepen, anterior to the Bladder Channel, and passes behind the ear to reach the corner of the forehead; it then travels to the vertex to meet the bilateral pathway
- Descends from the forehead, across the cheek, to the side of the nose (binds)
- Ends at the outer canthus of the eye (binds)

Signs and Symptoms

- Spasms and pulling sensation at the fourth toe.

- Stiffness and cramps at the lateral side of the knee, with an inability to bend the knee.

- Spasms at the popliteal fossa, referring to the upper thigh and the sacrum.

- Pain in the hypochondriac area and spasms in the supraclavicular fossa, breast and neck areas.

- Paralysis on the left side of the body, from an injury in the right temporal area, and *vice versa.*

CLINICAL NOTE

The *Nei Jing* explains that a traumatic injury to the head area can cause internal bleeding and paralysis to the opposite side of the body; this includes cardiovascular accidents (CVA).

The Triple Heater TMM Pathway

Starts: ulnar side of the ring finger

Ends: corner of the forehead

1. The main branch starts at the ulnar side of the ring finger and travels up to the lateral aspect of the wrist, where it binds and continues up the arm to bind at the tip of the elbow.

2. It continues laterally up the arm, over the shoulder to the neck, where it connects with the Small Intestine TMM.

3. One branch separates at the angle of the mandible, and internally enters the root of the tongue.

4. Another branch ascends anterior to the ear, then to the outer canthus and ends and binds at the corner of the forehead, where it meets the Three Hand Yang TMM.

SUMMARY: TRIPLE HEATER TMM

- Begins at the ulnar side of the ring finger, (binds) at the wrist, ascends the arm laterally and (binds) at the elbow tip
- Continues up the lateral arm, the shoulder and the neck
- Separates at the angle of the jaw and enters the root of the tongue
- Ascends anterior to the ear, passing to the outer canthus, and ends at the corner of the forehead (binds)

Signs and Symptoms

- Spasms, swelling and pain along the meridian.
- Curled or contracted tongue.

Yangming: Yang Brightness

Stomach and Large Intestine TMM

The Stomach TMM Pathway

Starts: middle three toes

Ends: in front of the ear

1. It begins at the three middle toes and binds on the dorsum of the foot.

2. It then ascends the lateral aspect of the leg and binds at the lateral knee, where it connects with the Gall Bladder TMM, and binds at the hip joint.

3. Continuing on, it passes through the hypochondriac and connects to the spinal column.

4. A branch separates on the lower leg, follows the tibialis anterior muscle to bind at the knee, then ascends to the thigh to bind in the pelvic area just above the genitals.

5. From there, it ascends the abdomen and chest, and binds at St-12 Quepen Empty Basin.

6. It continues to ascend the neck to the jaw, mouth, and the side of the nose, and binds below the nose.

7. From the nose, it joins the Bladder TMM to form a circular network around the eye. The Stomach TMM forms the lower network, below the eye, and the Bladder TMM forms the upper network, above the eye.

8. Another branch separates from the jaw and binds, ending at the anterior aspect of the ear.

SUMMARY: STOMACH TMM

- Begins at the three middle toes and (binds) at the dorsum of the foot
- Ascends the lateral leg to the knee (binds) and to the hip joint (binds)
- Passes through the hypochondriac to the spinal column
- Separates from the lower leg, travels to the knee (binds), and up the thigh to the pelvis above the genitals (binds)
- Continues up the abdomen and chest to St-12 Quepen (binds), and ascends the neck, jaw, mouth and side of the nose, (binds) below the nose
- Forms a net around the lower portion of the eye
- Separates from the jaw and ends in front of the ear (binds)

Signs and Symptoms

- Stiffness and spasms of the third toe and cramping in the tibialis anterior muscle.

- Jumping, spasms and hardness in the muscles of the dorsum of the foot.

- Spasms of the thigh (rectus femoris muscle).

- Swelling and distention in the inguinal groove.

- Hernia.

- Abdominal muscle spasms traveling up to the supraclavicular fossa and to the face.

- Sudden deviation of the mouth (wry mouth), i.e., Bell's palsy, neuropathies, windstroke.

CLINICAL NOTE

If a contraction is caused by heat, there will be paralysis, loss of muscle tone, and an inability to open the eye. Cold causes a spasm that deviates the mouth to the opposite side (wry mouth).

The Large Intestine TMM Pathway

Starts: index finger

Ends: mandible

1. It begins at the end of the index finger and binds at the wrist, then continues up the forearm to bind at the lateral aspect of the elbow.

2. It ascends the upper arm to bind at the shoulder, LI-15 Jianyu Shoulder Bone.

3. From there, a branch winds around the scapula and attaches to the upper thoracic spine between the shoulder blades.

4. From the shoulder, the main channel ascends to the neck, where a branch crosses the cheeks to bind at the side of the nose.

5. It continues to ascend anterior to the Small Intestine TMM, binds at the corner of the forehead, crosses over the head, and ends at the mandible on the opposite side of the face.

SUMMARY: LARGE INTESTINE TMM

- Begins at the index finger, (binds) at the wrist, and also at the lateral elbow
- Travels up the arm, (binds) at the shoulder, LI-15 Jianyu
- Circles the scapula, and connects to the thoracic spine between the shoulder blades
- Ascends to the neck, crosses the cheeks, and travels to the side of the nose (binds)
- Continues to the corner of the forehead (binds), and ends at the mandible on the opposite side of the face

Signs and Symptoms

- Pain and spasms along the pathway.

- Difficulty raising the shoulder (frozen shoulder).

- Restricted neck rotation.

Taiyin: Greater Yin

Spleen and Lung TMM

The Spleen TMM Pathway

Starts: medial side of the big toe

Ends: the spinal column

1. It begins at the medial side of the big toe and ascends the foot to bind at the medial malleolus.

2. It continues up the medial aspect of the leg to bind at the medial knee area.

3. It ascends the medial thigh area to bind at the inguinal groove, where it meets the external genitalia.

4. Traveling up the abdomen, it binds at the umbilicus, enters internally and binds at the ribs, dispersing in the chest.

5. It loops backward and connects with the spinal column.

SUMMARY: SPLEEN TMM

- Begins at the medial big toe, and (binds) at the medial ankle
- Continues up the leg and (binds) at the medial knee
- Ascends the medial thigh to the inguinal groove (binds), and meets the external gentialia
- Ascends the abdomen to the navel (binds), enters internally, (binds) at the ribs, and disperses in the chest
- From the ribs, it loops backward and connects with the spine

---

Signs and Symptoms

- Pain in the big toe spreading to the medial malleolus.

- Pain and cramping along the pathway.

- Medial knee, thigh and inguinal groove pain.

- A gripping and pulling feeling in the genitals, reaching the umbilicus, hypochondrium, chest and spinal column.

The Lung TMM Pathway

Starts: At Lu-11 Shaoshang Lesser Shang

Ends: hypochondriac region

1. It begins at Lu-11 Shaoshang Lesser Shang on the thumb, and ascends to bind at the thenar eminence.

2. It travels up the forearm and binds at the center of the elbow.

3. It continues to climb the upper arm and enters the chest below the axilla, emerging at the supraclavicular fossa, St-12 Quepen Empty Basin area, and travels to the shoulder, LI-15 Jianyu Shoulder Bone, where it descends into the chest.

4. Here it spreads over the diaphragm and branches out into small blood vessels in the hypochondriac region (floating rib area).

SUMMARY: LUNG TMM

- Starts at Lu-11 Shaoshang and (binds) at the thenar eminence
- Ascends the forearm to the elbow (binds)
- Continuing up the arm, it enters the chest below the axilla, emerges at the supraclavicular fossa and travels to the shoulder, and descends into the chest
- Spreads over the diaphragm and meets in the hypochondriac region

---

Signs and Symptoms

- Cramping and pain along the channel.

- Spasms and pain in the chest and hypochondriac region. When the pain is severe, there can be hematemesis (spitting up blood).

Shaoyin: Lesser Yin

Kidney and Heart TMM

The Kidney TMM Pathway

Starts: beneath the little toe

Ends: nape of the neck/occiput

1. It begins under the little toe and meets the Spleen TMM below the medial malleolus.

2. It then binds in the heel and meets the Bladder TMM, and ascends the leg to bind at the medial aspect of the knee, where it again meets the Spleen TMM, and travels further up the medial thigh to bind at the genitals.

3. An internal branch travels into the spine, ascends to the nape of the neck and binds to the occipital bone, where it converges with the Bladder TMM.

> **SUMMARY: KIDNEY TMM**
>
> - Begins under the small toe and meets Spleen TMM below the ankle
> - (Binds) in the heel, meets Bladder TMM, ascends the leg to the medial knee (binds), meets the Spleen TMM, continues to the medial thigh to the genitals (binds)
> - Travels internally through the spine, ascends to the nape of the neck and occiput (binds) and meets Bladder TMM

Signs and Symptoms

- Spasm and cramping in the plantar area of the foot, i.e., plantar fasciitis and bone spurs.

- Cramping and pain along the pathway. All chronic Bi syndromes.

- Because the Kidney TMM goes to the nape of the neck and to the brain, it can be used to treat epilepsy, convulsions, trembling, twitching and shivering.

- Difficulty bending forward and backward; this includes the neck, back and lumbar spine.

> **CLINICAL NOTE**
>
> If Kidney Yang is imbalanced, the patient cannot bend forward. With Kidney Yin imbalances, they cannot bend backwards.

The Heart TMM Pathway

Starts: at the radial side of the little finger

Ends: umbilicus

1. It begins at the radial side of the little finger and binds at the pisiform bone of the wrist.

2. It ascends to bind at the medial aspect of the elbow.

3. It continues to ascend the arm where it enters the axilla and meets the Lung TMM.

4. From there, it travels to the breast and binds in the center of the chest, passes through the diaphragm and ends at the navel.

> **SUMMARY: HEART TMM**
>
> - Begins at the little finger and (binds) at the wrist bone
> - Binds at the medial elbow
> - Enters the axilla, and meets the Lung TMM
> - Travels to the breast, the center of the chest (binds), the diaphragm, and ends at the navel

Signs and Symptoms

- Stiffness, pulling pain and spasms along the channel.

- Internal cramping below the Heart, which can produce symptoms, such as anxiety, hiatal hernia and Stomach disorders.

Jueyin: Terminal Yin

Liver and Pericardium TMM

The Liver TMM Pathway

Starts: at the dorsum of the big toe

Ends: external genitalia

1. Beginning at the dorsum of the big toe, it ascends the foot to bind in front of the medial malleolus.

2. It ascends along the medial tibia to bind at the medial aspect of the knee.

3. Then it travels up the medial thigh to the external genitalia and connects with other TMM channels.

> **SUMMARY: LIVER TMM**
>
> - Begins at the big toe, and (binds) in front of the inner ankle
> - Ascends the medial leg, to the medial knee (binds)
> - Travels up the thigh to the genitalia, and connects with other TMMs

Signs and Symptoms

- Pain in the big toe to the medial malleolus.

- Pain and spasms in the medial aspect of the knee and thigh.

- Dysfunctions of the genitalia:

  1. Internal injury; inability to get an erection.

  2. Cold injury; genital contraction.

  3. Heat injury; persistent erection.

The Percardium TMM Pathway

Starts: tip of the middle finger

Ends: diaphragm

1. It starts from the tip of the middle finger and joins together with the Lung TMM to bind at the medial aspect of the elbow.

2. Ascending the antero-medial aspect of the upper arm, it binds at the area below the axilla, then descends to spread over the anterior and posterior rib cage.

3. A branch internally penetrates the chest below the axilla and binds at the diaphragm.

SUMMARY: PERICARDIUM TMM

- Begins at the tip of the middle finger, joins the Lung TMM, and (binds) at the medial elbow
- Ascends the upper arm below the axilla (binds), and spreads over the rib cage
- Penetrates the chest area under the axilla and (binds) at the diaphragm

---

Signs and Symptoms

- Cramps and pain along the pathway.

- Pain in the chest, labored breathing and panting in the diaphragm, cardiac orifice area.

- Xufen syndrome, an 'inverted cup' sensation below the lower right ribs.

CLINICAL NOTE

Xufen is an accumulation disorder due to Lung Qi stagnation, combined with phlegm and heat symptoms, which includes a mass below the right hypochondrium. This mass resembles a cup with a cover on it, and it could be a tumor, lung abscess, tuberculosis or possibly pleurisy.

Specific Constitutional Facial Acupuncture Wei Treatments

Releasing the Wei Qi, whether it be a tight tender Ashi point, a trigger point or a motor point, is very effective in Constitutional Facial Acupuncture treatments. While I do present seminars in which I treat both constitution and face with these points, these applications are not within the purview of this book. (See the Bibliography for book recommendations on this topic.)

However, I will offer you three syndromes that continually appear in Constitutional Facial Acupuncture treatments.

1. 'Coat Hanger' Syndrome

This syndrome involves the upper trapezius muscle. The patient resembles a coat hanger, because their shoulders are elevated to their ears, and they appear to have no neck. The character of Maggie in the American playwright

Tennessee Williams' play, *Cat on a Hot Tin Roof*, would refer to these patients as 'no-neck monsters.' Obviously, these individuals are very tense, tight, frustrated, stressed, and feel as if they are carrying the weight of the world on their shoulders.

In describing the treatment strategy for this syndrome, I will give both a local and a distal approach, based upon your patient's diagnosis of either excess or deficiency.

2. 'Wandering Skirt' Syndrome

This syndrome relates to the Belt Meridian, the internal oblique muscles and issues of bloat, obesity and other imbalances, manifesting around the waist. The patient has the attendant Shaoyang emotions of frustration, anger, with an inability to make a decision, and a tendency to stuff these damp viscous feelings under their belt. Since one of the TCM indications for the Dai Mai is a subjective feeling of sitting in cold water, the patient may also have a Kidney imbalance, and will lack courage.

I have named this syndrome after one of my patients, who always wore slimming, A-line, skirts with a bias or seam down the middle, so that she appeared thinner. She was a lawyer in a large multinational company, and secretly desired to leave this job to work for a non-profit corporation that supported the arts.

Being a frustrated artist herself, she longed to be connected with that world. However, the fear of abandoning her high salary was palpable, and she never did act upon her dream, but continued to vacillate. She literally was sitting on the fence, half-in/half-out, and couldn't make any sort of decision.

I always knew when she had experienced a particularly frustrating day, because her A-line skirt would always list to one or the other side of her waist, just off the centerline. Even though I always checked for any hip imbalances, it was usually the Belt area that was the culprit. In releasing her internal oblique muscles at the waist, I was able to give her temporary relief. Afterwards, her skirt would line up beautifully!

Other benefits of this treatment include weight loss, resolution of bloatedness and damp, and an easing of pain in the lower back, quadratus lumborum area.

3. 'The Wakefield Point'

I was flattered and honored to have this point named after me by my Japanese students in Tokyo. 'The Wakefield Point' is accessed by needling the nuchal notch of the occipitalis muscle. This point is not only effective in the treatment of neck issues; it also addresses tension in the frontalis muscle or forehead area. 'The Wakefield Point' became the everything point to them because it alleviated neck pain, whiplash, disturbed Shen, fright and surprise, manifesting in horizontal lines on the forehead, and relaxed the entire galea aponeurotica, the scalp.

In Table 5.3, the local treatment for 'Coat Hanger' syndrome is outlined, along with the muscle involved, the acupuncture points, indications, palpation and needling techniques for both trigger and motor points.

Motor points are neuromuscular junctions. The stimulation of this area causes the muscle spindles to fire and reset, which allows the muscle to grab the needle, and simultaneously balances the muscle. This action relays a message to the patient's central nervous system (CNS), which causes a tense muscle to relax and a flaccid muscle to strengthen. When needling a motor point, the muscle rarely jumps, as is the case with trigger point needling.

While motor points may be more comfortable for a patient than trigger points, both of these treatments are local and may be quite strong in their response.

Some patients are hypervigilant, adrenal or Spleen-deficient, and they are frightened by the body's involuntary response to the needling of trigger points. The sudden jumping of the muscles is not really painful, but it can evoke the uncomfortable feeling of being out of control, and this can bring up emotional responses. The motor points may also twitch when needled, which could be disconcerting for a deficient patient. With these patients, a distal treatment may be more effective and less disturbing.

When a patient has a deficient Spleen pulse, and the Kidney pulses are also deficient, the tongue appears scalloped and puffy, and with a red tip, I recommend a distal treatment to gently release the 'Coat Hanger' syndrome. With this Spleen deficiency, there is insufficient blood to fill the vessels, and the Kidney pulses are also weak. Palpation of the GB-21 Jianjing Shoulder Well area may reveal a deficiency tightness. There may also be tightening and pain around the navel and also at Sp-15 Daheng Great Horizontal, which is located 4 cun from the navel, lateral to the rectus abdominis muscle.

In examining the Five Element Destructive Cycle, we can observe that the Wood element is overacting on Earth.

'Coat Hanger' syndrome, a Five Element Japanese distal treatment is shown in Table 5.4. The GB-21 Jianjing Shoulder Well area presents a deficiency tightness, because the Spleen is hypoactive and the Gall Bladder oversteps its boundaries and invades the Spleen.

TABLE 5.3 'COAT HANGER' SYNDROME

Muscle	The upper trapezius muscle elevates the shoulder, bends the neck and head to the same side, and aids in the rotation of the head to the opposite side. GB-21 Jianjing Shoulder Well treats the anterior muscle fibers
Treatment point (1)	GB-21 Jianjing Shoulder Well is located midway between Du-14 Dazhui Great Hammer, and the acromium at the highest point of the shoulder
Indications (1)	The crossing point of the Yang Wei Mai, Triple Heater and Stomach meridians
	It relaxes the muscles, treats shoulder pain and tension
	Promotes lactation
	The patient senses a great weight and responsibility on their shoulders
	Contraindicated for pregnancy
Treatment point (2)	TH-15 Tianliao Celestial Bone Hole is located on the superior angle of the scapula, midway between GB-21 Jianjing Shoulder Well, and SI-13 Quyuan Crooked Wall. TH-15 Tianliao Celestial Bone Hole treats the posterior muscle fibers
Indications (2)	The crossing point of the Gall Bladder and Yang Wei Mai meridians
	Neck and shoulder stiffness and pain
	Temporal headache
	An alternative name for this point is Tianting Celestial Hearing, and it can be used to treat patients who neither take time to listen to their inner voice, nor to process events that occur within their lives
Signs and symptoms	The indications for the trigger and motor point are similar to GB-21 Jianjing: shoulder and neck pain, a tension headache referring pain to the temple and behind the eye, and emotional stress and frustration
Trigger point palpation	Pincer grasp the upper trapezius muscle between your thumb and fingers, so that it is safely lifted off the top of the lung, to prevent pneumothorax
	Palpate it by rolling the muscle bands between your fingers; this action may elicit a twitch or jump response in the muscle, which will help you locate the trigger point area prior to needling. The patient will report referred pain in the neck, occiput, temple or behind the eye as you palpate. Needling this point bilaterally will relieve 'Coat Hanger' syndrome

Continued

TABLE 5.3 'COAT HANGER' SYNDROME—cont'd

Trigger point needling techniques	Needle transversely into the muscle with a 38 or 36 gauge, 30–40 mm needle
	Do not use a thinner needle. Insert the needle for both the anterior fibers of the trapezius muscle, GB-21 Jianjing Shoulder Well toward TH-15 Tianliao Celestial Bone Hole, and the posterior fibers of the muscle, TH-15 Tianliao Celestial Bone Hole toward GB-21 Jianjing Shoulder Well, directly into the trapezius muscle
	When treating the back, needle the posterior fibers; when treating the front of the body, treat the anterior fibers
	Once the trigger point is located, continue the pincer grasp with your non-dominant hand, and needle transversely 0.5 cun directly into the muscle
	Utilize a pecking, thrusting technique, which positively irritates the muscle sufficiently, until it releases, jumps or twitches
	Peck directly into the muscle, only stopping for a second to allow the muscle a moment's rest, then begin again. This tricks the muscle, and allows old holding, tightening patterns to release, not only physically, but also emotionally
	If there is any discomfort for the patient, please stop after the next release, and do not persist. Massage arnica into the area, and inform them that they may feel a bit sore, similar to the achiness felt after a workout session
	Do not needle downward toward the lung, but transversely down toward the massage table. If this treatment is new to you, do ask a teacher who is conversant with trigger points to help you with the techniques
Motor point needling techniques	The motor point is needled in the same way, and in the same area as the trigger point, but it has a different needling technique
	Needle the point 0.5 cun transversely down toward the massage table, using a 36 or 38 gauge, 30–40 mm needle
	Make sure that you hold the trapezius muscle in a pincer grip as you needle, to prevent pneumothorax. When you insert the needle, it will grab. There is no thrusting or pecking technique involved
	Leave the motor point needle in for the entire treatment

TABLE 5.4 'COAT HANGER' SYNDROME; A FIVE ELEMENT JAPANESE DISTAL TREATMENT

Treatment point	Sp-9 Yinlingquan Yin Mound Spring is located on the inferior border of the medial aspect of the knee, in the depression on the medial border of the tibia
Indications	Resolves damp accumulation; heavy body, joint pain, cloudy urine, vaginal discharge, diarrhea
	Regulates blood production
	Treats dizziness and palpitations
	Strain and stress
Needling techniques	Needle Sp-9 Yinlingquan Yin Mound Spring bilaterally and perpendicularly 0.5 cun, then transversely up toward the trapezius muscle, GB-21 Jianjing Shoulder Well area
	Use a 40 mm, 36 or 34 gauge needle to traverse this area
	Integrate this protocol into a Constitutional Facial Acupuncture treatment

This is not a trigger, motor or Ashi tender point treatment, but a Japanese Five Element protocol for Spleen-deficient patients. The shoulders will be considerably released and softer after this treatment, and the patient will feel refreshed and unstressed.

'Wandering Skirt' syndrome treatment given in Table 5.5 can be used with patients who have been in an automobile accident and complain of low back pain, with difficulty rotating their spine to one side of the body. This technique also temporarily ameliorates lower back pain due to kidney stones.

Remember, that once you have needled the motor point, you do not need to continue with the trigger point needling, if your patient is particularly sensitive. I always ask permission to needle the trigger point, and first explain to them what they might expect to feel.

'The Wakefield Point' in Table 5.6 relaxes the entire scalp, as well as the forehead and the back of the neck. This point addresses a wide range of symptoms, and since it is located near GB-19 Naokong Brain Hollow, it can be used to treat brain imbalances, such as epilepsy and convulsions, and also psychospiritual issues.

All these constitutional Wei syndromes, as outlined in Table 5.7, not only manifest as physical symptoms; they are also connected to stress and emotional imbalances seen as furrows and lines on the face.

TABLE 5.5 'WANDERING SKIRT' SYNDROME

Muscle	The internal obliques are a fan-shaped abdominal muscle, whose fibers range from vertical to diagonal to horizontal. All the muscle fibers meet at the inguinal ligament, and the iliac crest of the lower spine. They flex and rotate the spine and trunk to the same side of the body
Treatment point	GB-26 Daimai, Girdling Vessel is directly below the free end of the 11th rib where Liv-13 Zhangmen Camphorwood Gate is located, at the level of the navel
Indications	It regulates the uterus; irregular menses, dysmenorrhea, uterine prolapse and cramps
	Resolves damp heat issues, such as leucorrhea
	Treats abdominal pain and hernia
	Pain in the lumbar area and hypochondria
Signs and symptoms	The indications for both trigger and motor points are similar. Imbalances include fibrocystic nodules or tightness near GB-26 Daimai Girdling Vessel and the pubic bone, difficulty flexing and bending the spine to the same side, lower back pain, an imbalance of the right and left sides of the body when standing for long periods of time or walking for hours. It also increases the intra-abdominal pressure for urination and defecation
Trigger and motor point palpation	The motor point will grab the needle, and the trigger point, when needled with the pecking technique, may elicit a jump or twitch within the muscle
	Pincer grasp the waist at GB-26 Daimai Girdling Vessel, between your thumb and fingers, with your non-dominant hand
	Locate the internal obliques muscle, which feels like a tight band next to the waist area
	Palpate it by rolling the bands between your fingers. This will make your patient aware of the tightness of this long, fan-like muscle. They may feel a local twitch, or a jump referring up the muscle, but not necessarily
Trigger and motor point needling technique	Continue to hold the internal oblique muscle and needle transversely downward, 0.5–1 cun, toward the massage table, with a 36–34 gauge, 40 mm or longer, needle. Needling in this fashion will not puncture the peritoneum. Do not needle toward the waist, but downward through the muscle
	The motor point will grab and the skin will pucker at the site of the needle insertion. If you use the pecking technique after the muscle has grabbed, you will activate the trigger point
	When the trigger point releases, the patient usually experiences a wave-like release, flowing up and down the entire muscle
	If the muscle is very tight on one side of the body, first needle the other side; this will release the tense side
	Massage arnica gel or cream into the area, and inform your patient that they may experience muscle soreness, such as they would after a strenuous workout

TABLE 5.6 'THE WAKEFIELD POINT'

Muscle	The occipitalis muscle moves the scalp backwards and forwards, and assists the frontalis muscle in raising the eyebrows and horizontally wrinkling the forehead, as in the expression of fright and surprise
Treatment point	The points are 2 cun above GB-20 Fengchi Wind Pool and also 2 cun above Bl-10 Tianzhu Celestial Pillar. The point is located by palpation up from GB-20 Fengchi Wind Pool, in the indentation of the nuchal notch of the occipital bone
Indications	GB-20 Fengchi Wind Pool, when pressed, refers to, and is felt in the ear. It resembles a pool in the back of the neck, which is a receptacle for pathogenic wind factors
	Treats:
	Wind heat
	Benefits eyes and hearing
	Headaches, pain and stiffness in the neck
	Vertigo, tinnitus, insomnia
	Convulsion, epilepsy
	Sinus obstruction
	Bl-10 Tianzhu Celestial Pillar resembles two pillars supporting the head, which, according to the ancient Chinese, was considered the heavenly part of the body
	Treats:
	Headache, sinusitis
	Sore throat
	Neck rigidity and pain in the shoulder and back
Signs and symptoms	Both motor and trigger points can be treated with 'The Wakefield Point,' because the occipitalis and frontalis muscle function as a single unit. The galea aponeurotica or scalp is involved, and affected by the action of these muscles, and must also be taken into consideration
	Neck pain, headache

Continued

TABLE 5.6 'THE WAKEFIELD POINT'—cont'd

	Decreased vision, glaucoma
	Occipitalis: cervical neck tension and tightness; contracts the forehead and scalp muscles
	Frontalis: habitually wrinkling the forehead causes lines and wrinkles in the skin around the eyes, as well as neck pain and tightness at the back of the neck and scalp muscles
	Whiplash and trauma
	Sinusitis
	Pain behind the eye
	Disturbed Shen; fright and surprise
	Emotional tension
Motor/ trigger point palpation and needling technique	'The Wakefield Point' is 2 cun above GB-20 Fengchi Wind Pool in the indentation of the nuchal notch of the occipital bone
	Locate GB-20 Fengchi Wind Pool and trace your thumb directly above it until you find the indentation in the skull
	Use a 36 or 34 gauge, 30–40 mm needle
	Needle transversely 0.2–0.3 cun from 'The Wakefield Point' above GB-20, toward a location above Bl-10 Tianzhu Celestial Pillar
	The needle will grab when pulled backward, or it may twitch slightly. You do not need to use the trigger point pecking technique
	Needling bilaterally; the patient will be comfortable with this transverse needling and it will not adversely affect them while they are lying on their back
	If 'The Wakefield Point' elicits too strong a response, slightly retract the needle

TABLE 5.7 A SUMMARY OF WEI SYNDROME TREATMENTS

Syndrome	Muscle/Area	Motor/Trigger Points	Signs/Symptoms
'Coat Hanger' syndrome	Trapezius muscle (excess condition; local treatment)	GB-21 Jianjing Shoulder Well TH-15 Tianliao Celestial Bone Hole	Shoulder/neck pain, tension headache (temporal and behind eye; emotional stress)
	Medial aspect of tibia (deficiency condition; distal treatment)	Sp-9 Yinlingquan Yin Mound Spring	Deficiency tight shoulders, dizziness, palpitations, damp issues, possible blood deficiency, stress and strain
'Wandering Skirt' syndrome	Internal oblique muscles	GB-26 Daimai Girdling Vessel	Pain in lower back, difficult flexion and bending of spine to same side, urination/defecation problems, imbalances in the gait (walking) cycle
'The Wakefield Point'	Occipitalis/frontalis muscles (occipito-frontalis)	2 cun above GB-20 Fengchi Windpool and Bl-10 Tianzhu Celestial Pillar	Whiplash, headache, neck pain, pain behind the eye, sinusitis, disturbed Shen

CHAPTER 6

Practical Specifics

"Teachers open the door, but you must enter by yourself."
— Chinese Proverb

This chapter will focus on all the practical guidelines and necessary technical information for Constitutional Facial Acupuncture treatments, including benefits and contraindications, the definition of facial acupuncture, recommended supplies, the 'Wrinkle Rule,' treatment length and timelines, the short and long-term effects, maintenance treatments, a complete treatment protocol with Chinese topical herbs and poultices, and soothing botanicals. Also provided are explanatory pages summarizing the details of treatments, which can be given to your patients before a treatment session, or made available as an informational pamphlet in your clinic.

A Definition of Constitutional Facial Acupuncture: The 'Elevator Speech'

Even though you may not have an elevator in your building, it is important to define, and educate your patients about Constitutional Facial Acupuncture. If you find yourself in the position of having to answer questions about this modality and you take too much time, or are somewhat vague about explaining what you do, your audience will lose interest, walk away, or get out of the elevator. If this happens, it will make it impossible for you to offer them one of your business cards.

This is advice born of experience, because I encountered this situation when I was just beginning to establish my own acupuncture practice.

There are several components to this concise and interesting definition of Constitutional Facial Acupuncture:

1. Constitutional Facial Acupuncture uses a constitutional approach to the facial landscape, which treats the body, as well as the face.

   New patients may be under the impression that facial acupuncturists are like estheticians or cosmetologists, and that we only address the face in our treatments. This is obviously not the case, and it is important to educate prospective patients about the constitutional aspects of this modality.

2. When the face is needled, blood and Qi flow to the area transporting nutrients to the cells. Making reference to both Oriental and Western medicine will help the patient to better understand what is involved.

3. Needling the face also creates a positive microtrauma, and activates the body's wound healing response. This stimulates the fibroblasts and can promote increased production of collagen/elastin.

   Make certain that you explain to the prospective patient that there are no scientific studies definitively linking facial acupuncture treatments with increased collagen/elastin production. However, I have observed that facial needling can plump up and flesh out sunken areas of the face.

If the patient is new and has never had acupuncture treatments, you may wish to omit the information about the microtrauma. Use your judgment and your discretion.

I have found that saying much more than that in a short period of time subjects new patients to information overload. Of course, they will eventually realize that these treatments can make a real difference with lines, wrinkles, sagging tendencies and puffiness, as well as more serious issues like Bell's palsy, windstroke and neuropathies. Facial acupuncture treatments also brighten the Shen, alleviate stress, promote increased self-esteem, and more.

Your prospective patients may ask you a few questions, which you can answer briefly during this first encounter. Finally, after you have successfully piqued their interest, make sure that you give them a card, and/or a brochure, both of which should refer them to your website.

Benefits of Constitutional Facial Acupuncture

The constitutional foundation of these treatment protocols insures that any conditions that can be addressed in a conventional acupuncture treatment can be incorporated into the constitutional component of a given facial acupuncture session. Consequently, a variety of constitutional, facial and psychospiritual benefits are provided.

The beauty of acupuncture is manifested in the connection, interrelationship and flow of the meridians throughout the body, head, neck and face. This constitutional connection benefits and balances both face and body. Patients not only look refreshed, but they also feel better.

Constitutional Benefits

In addition to acupuncture, the practitioner provides the patient with lifestyle counseling, dietary and nutritional recommendations, and a topical herbal treatment protocol that supports and enhances the results of the facial needling.

Constitutional benefits of these treatments include the following:

1. Issues of acne, rosacea, eczema and other skin conditions can be improved. This is accomplished not only with acupuncture, but also topical herbal poultices and suggestions regarding diet and nutrition. Chapter 9 provides information concerning the use of topical Chinese herbs for the treatment of certain skin issues.

2. The treatment of irregularities in reproductive cycles and other gynecological imbalances can be incorporated. Menarche, perimenopause, menopause, premenstrual syndrome (PMS), and andropause are just some of the conditions that may be positively impacted within a course of treatments. In particular, the Eight Extraordinary Meridians have a significant connection to the endocrine system, and are a powerful Jing treatment for hormonal imbalances (see the Jing level treatments: Chapter 2).

3. Treating the body distally can relieve sinus congestion and headache. Of course, your approach will depend upon what you discern from the patient's diagnostics, a consideration of external pathogens, and, with respect to headaches, the location of the symptoms, and what meridians or organ systems are involved.

4. Both hyper- and hypothyroid issues can be addressed. Each patient presents with a different pattern in these cases. For hyperthyroidism, clear heat and tonify Kidney Yin; with hypothyroidism issues, it is necessary to tonify Kidney Yang and expel cold in the body.

5. A wide range of gastrointestinal issues, such as diarrhea and constipation, are easily treated constitutionally. Heat in the Stomach manifests on the face as red eyes or red spots around Stomach points (St-1 Chengqi Tear Container, St-2 Sibai Four White, St-3 Juliao Great Bone Hole and St-4 Dicang Earth's Granary); gas, bloating and puffiness are not only apparent in the abdominal area, but also on the face.

6. Facial acupuncture benefits the sensory organs – eyes, ears, nose, mouth – and the brain. Imbalances in these systems can be treated locally, for example: GB-1 Tongziliao Pupil Bone Hole affects the vision and the

intrinsic muscles of the eye, and distally, GB-37 Guangming Bright Light improves and clears vision, and also regulates the Liver.

7. Facial acupuncture treatments help with insomnia, dizziness and vertigo; Anmian, N-HN-54, an extra point, can be used locally for insomnia, vertigo, palpitations and mental imbalances. In addition, GB-44 Zuqiaoyin Foot Portal Yin is effective as a distal treatment point for these issues, as well as Liv-3 Taichong Great Surge or Liv-2 Xingjian Moving Between.

8. Constitutional Facial Acupuncture eliminates global edema and puffiness. Ren-9 Shuifen Water Divide is a wonderful point for systemic edema, retention of urine and abdominal pain. Sp-9 Yinlinquan Yin Mound Spring is a classic treatment point for dispelling damp and stagnation from the lower burner, in the knees, legs and ankles.

9. Constitutionally, these treatments can help to retard hair loss and graying. The treatment, and support of the Kidneys, especially with the Eight Extraordinary Meridians, and the addition of the Yuan Source points, which support the organs, can gradually slow the rate of hair loss and foster hair regrowth. This is very difficult to accomplish simply with acupuncture; herbal remedies are recommended which conform to the patient's particular constitutional pattern and symptoms.

Further, graying hair can be successfully addressed over time, with the consumption of He Shou Wu *Polygonum multiflorium*; fleeceflower root herbal tea, taken both in the morning and evening. While this is a gradual process, it is usually effective, and, in my experience, with both patients and members of my family, there has been a noticeable change in the coloration of the hair. He Shou Wu tonifies the Liver, Kidneys and the blood, and augments essence. In addition to its effects as an anti-graying agent, it also treats blood deficiency and helps with vision.

Facial Benefits

1. Facial acupuncture can improve collagen/elastin production. There is a great deal of misinformation about this aspect of the modality, as many practitioners claim outright that these benefits are a matter of course. However, I am always careful to point out that a direct correlation between the act of facial needling and the regeneration of this vital component of the skin structure is still speculative, because no targeted research has yet been undertaken in this area. I can state categorically, that the microtrauma produced by the acupuncture needle activates a wound healing response, and mobilizes the flow of Qi and blood to the site of the insertion. The microtrauma appears to stimulate the fibroblasts, and this action can be the precursor to the production of collagen/elastin.

Facial acupuncture increases muscle tone. All of these points, whether they be related to origin and insertion, motor points, or the antagonist/

protagonist component of the muscle, serve to reharmonize the muscle structure, causing the relevant areas to be lifted and toned. This becomes quite noticeable after several treatments.

2. Issues of wind in syndromes such as Bell's palsy, windstroke and facial neuropathies may also be treated, especially with motor points. Trigeminal neuralgia and temporomandibular joint dysfunction (TMJ) syndromes can also be balanced and lessened with the use of acu-muscle points.

   Syndromes that are not purely cosmetic are easily addressed with these facial protocols. As a facial acupuncture practitioner, it is important for you to be knowledgeable in the treatment of all these facial syndromes.

3. Constitutional Facial Acupuncture helps to reduce under-eye bags and alleviate other sagging tendencies in the neck, jaw, nasolabial fold and upper eyelids. While bags under the eyes have specific correlations to imbalances in various organ systems and the associated Five Element disharmonies (see Chapter 7), the sagging muscles seen in turkey wattles, the two folds below the neck, jowls, the smile lines of the nasolabial fold and the upper eyelids, all will respond to treatments with acu-muscle points.

   Treatments that address these various drooping and sagging tendencies customarily begin to demonstrate their effectiveness after 5–7 sessions, when you will begin to notice a substantial difference. Naturally, this depends upon your patient's general health and the strength of their constitution.

   I have treated patients in the throes of extreme grief, those with emphysema, and individuals who consumed very little protein, either vegetable or animal, in their diets, which is necessary for muscle strength and flexibility. These patients have required two courses of 20 treatments each to support their constitution, address psychospiritual issues, and to have ample time to make beneficial changes to their diet and general lifestyle.

4. Sunken areas can be fleshed out with facial acupuncture. One particular problem area is the buccinator muscle (see Chapter 7) and the area across the lower cheek 1 cun lateral to St-4 Dicang Earth's Granary. Patients who are anorexic, chronically ill, Jing deficient, or those who have had certain types of dental work, or are missing teeth, those with malocclusions, bruxism, or individuals who are losing the collagen/elastin layer of their skin due to waning hormones, usually manifest a characteristic gauntness here.

   Needling the acu-muscle points for the buccinator muscle in a healthy person will usually plump up the cheek area in just 2–3 visits. Of course, the constitutional needling component is of utmost importance in all these treatments.

5. Puffiness, fine lines and larger wrinkles can be diminished. However, it is important to bear in mind that the majority of facial wrinkles have an

emotional component, and it is the habit of contorting the musculature of the forehead – to express, for example, fright and surprise – or furrowing the brows when frustrated or angry that over time makes its impact upon the skin.

Facial puffiness is usually constitutionally based, and Du-26 Shuigou Water Trough is an empirical local point which will address this problem.

6. The eyes are brightened, pores tightened and the skin looks more radiant. Even after an initial treatment with Constitutional Facial Acupuncture, the patient's face will appear more open and relaxed. The eyes are clear, sparkling and bright, due to the work with all the Shen points in the face, and the very fact that the patient has been compelled to rest during the treatment, and may have even had a little restorative nap.

After the facial needling, I apply a topical egg white poultice infused with Chinese herbs. This mask is astringent; it closes the pores and calms the redness from the needling (see Chapter 9).

When Qi and blood enlivens the face, and soothing creams and botanicals are administered, the skin takes on increased vitality – glowing, hydrated, and tranquil.

7. Facial needling increases local blood and lymph circulation, and improves facial color and tone. As we have previously indicated, needling the face causes a positive microtrauma, and mobilizes blood and Qi. The lymphatic system can also be drained into the brachial plexus in the clavicle by using jade rollers, rolling down from the forehead along the side of the face and cheeks. This is a rhythmic and very gentle massage using two rollers in parallel motion.

8. Facial acupuncture promotes total health and well-being. When working with the constitution as a springboard for facial transformation, the entire system is balanced and supported – promoting a sense of well-being and joy.

Psychospiritual Benefits

The face is a mirror of the constitution and the most emotive part of the body. Beyond this, it is the focal point for our sense of personal identity. Therefore, when we perceive life to be filled with happiness and satisfaction, it is only logical that we would experience an increased spiritual benefit. Moreover, as we incorporate treatment points into the protocols that specifically target Shen, it becomes possible to see changes in the person's outlook and philosophy.

1. One of the most common benefits is stress reduction. Patients will feel more relaxed, grounded and rested after even a single treatment session. When

both face and body are treated, stress levels are reduced and there is a release of beneficial endorphins.

2. Facial acupuncture encourages healthy Shen, and aids self-esteem, because it addresses the seven emotions: anger, fear, grief, worry, fright, melancholy and excess joy. In Chinese face reading, different parts of the face correspond to these emotional expressions. For example, when the risorius muscle, located at the corner of the mouth, is needled and lifted up, the patient who was previously sad may feel more positive and this confidence will be reflected in the Shen. Self-esteem is cultivated when they feel and look better.

3. Working with the facial acu-muscle points can alleviate depression. As the psychospiritual points are engaged on the face, scalp and body, feelings of depression may subside. A treatment that includes the Three Shens scalp points and the Kidney Spirit points, coupled with the muscle exercise for the levator labii superioris, is especially effective for depressed/angry patients.

Often issues of abuse, whether physical, emotional or spiritual, may be brought into consciousness and healthily released during a treatment series with Constitutional Facial Acupuncture. The Eight Extraordinary Meridians, particularly Chong Mai, coupled with facial needling, can release and transform cellular memory which informs the subconscious mind. It is important to remember that we, as facial acupuncturists, are not psychotherapists, but it is appropriate for us to incorporate these Shen and other psychospiritual points into a treatment.

Do not hesitate to refer your patients to other health care professionals who specialize in these types of psychospiritual imbalance. You can also address certain addictive behaviors in your treatments, if you have your patient's consent. For example, cigarette smoking responds well to auricular therapy points and herbs. I have also noticed that facial beauty, and the stimulus of what I refer to as 'healthy vanity' are often highly significant in motivating certain patients to abandon these self-destructive habits.

Bear in mind that patients who are in strong states of denial about their addictions to alcohol and drugs will not be amenable to your suggestions about lifestyle changes; be realistic as to what you think you can accomplish. I had a patient for a number of years who was addicted to cocaine, which they snorted in order to maintain their energy level while working long hours at night at a job that demanded all of their resources.

They were often very hyperactive when they arrived at my clinic, but repeatedly denied that they were taking any drugs. However, in all conscience, I could not continue my treatments with them, because it would not have been appropriate for me to give them facial acupuncture while they were high, despite the fact that they would not confirm my suspicions.

I was compelled to let them go, and recommended them to other professionals who I felt might be able to help them, if they would permit it.

4. These treatments can be used effectively to reduce anxiety and prevent the recurrence of panic attacks. Symptoms of this nature do not arise from logic; they are based in irrational fears. I had a patient who experienced frequent panic attacks, was always anxious and had taken anti-depressants for years. They attributed their condition to being abducted by aliens when they were very young; as is consistent with these experiences, they reported that the aliens subjected them to invasive sexual experimentation and poking and prodding.

I discovered only later that they had been repeatedly sexually violated by a relative, from age 5 to 12. This revelation, as it arose organically during the course of treatment, eased their anxiety, but they would never acknowledge that the alien abduction story was a mask for something more prosaic, closer to home and equally disturbing in its implications. There was only so much I could do to help them, even though they had repeatedly sought counseling and other remedies.

Once again, I must stress that our role in administering to our patients who have these psychoemotional disturbances is not that of a therapist, and there are limits to the kind of help that we can provide. Admittedly, I have had my successes, but there is no shame in directing these individuals elsewhere; wisdom lies in knowing our limitations as practitioners.

Contraindications

Despite the fact that there is increasing interest in facial acupuncture worldwide as a holistic alternative to cosmetic surgery and other procedures, it is important to recognize that these treatments are not for everyone. There are certain patients that should not receive facial acupuncture, and others with whom you should proceed very cautiously. Of course, the exercise of appropriate caution is at your own discretion, and whom you choose to work with as a patient very much dependent on your assessment of their general health through your diagnostics and your experience as a practitioner.

1. Do not treat hemophiliacs because they bleed and bruise easily; however, it should be noted that there are varying degrees of hemophilia. A student successfully treated her fiancé during one of my seminars, because she knew that his condition was mild, and she was, of course, accustomed to treating him as a patient. Ordinarily, I would not recommend this.

2. Exercise caution when treating patients who may be taking blood-thinning medications, and ensure that you are informed as to the precise dosage. Examples are: Coumadin, Plavix, warfarin, aspirin, supplements like omega 3s and 6s, vitamin E, *Gingko biloba*, and turmeric. This also includes

blood invigorating and moving herbs like Chuan Xiong, *Ligusticum chuanxiong* or *Ligusticum wallichii,* Szechuan lovage root, Dan Shen, *Salvia miltiorrhiza,* Salvia root, Yi Mu Cao, *Leonurus heterophyllus,* Chinese motherwort, and Tao Ren, *Prunus Persica,* peach kernel, among others.

3. Hypertension should be under control, so address that first constitutionally prior to any facial needling. Facial acupuncture causes the Yang Qi to rise to the head, and this may provoke blood pressure spikes, a fast pulse and a red face. It is imperative to thoroughly anchor the Yang and confirm that the patient is taking their medication. A Japanese distal treatment point that regulates both hypo- and hypertension is located beneath the 3rd toe of the foot in the crease where the toe intersects with the sole of the foot. Needle bilaterally in the middle of this crease, or use a magnet or some other means to activate the point.

4. Diabetics are similarly prone to bruise or bleed easily; it is imperative for you to ascertain that they are having regular injections of insulin, and not deviating from their dietary regimen.

5. Be particularly cautious when working with patients who have had cosmetic surgery. Wait until at least 6 months after any procedure to treat the scars behind the ears and in the scalp; scar treatment will break up and dissolve any adhesions in the area. I always have these patients sign a release form signifying their willingness to have facial acupuncture. Usually, these individuals will not be interested in exploring alternative methods immediately after a face lift, but 20 years later, they may seek help for the scar adhesions that are affecting muscles and tendons in their scalp and neck.

Face lifts, over time, can droop on one side and be tight on the other, because of the adhesions, and they will give rise to certain undesirable side effects, which may cause these individuals more than a little discomfort. Protect yourself, despite the vintage of their surgery, by having them sign a release form.

6. Avoid needling patients who have had injections of Botox or other facial fillers, as the insertion of acupuncture needles in close proximity to injection sites will enliven the facial muscle and the effects of the Botox will abate. Do not perform Constitutional Facial Acupuncture until 3 weeks after laser resurfacing, and a minimum of 2 weeks after microdermabrasion or chemical peels, or if the patient has a severe sunburn.

Laser resurfacing burns off the epidermis, the top layer of the skin, and leaves the patients red, vulnerable and prone to infection. Needling the face at that time would bring even more Qi and blood to the area, which could be potentially damaging.

Microdermabrasion is analogous to sandblasting, in that many tiny granules are used to exfoliate the face. Sometimes, these granules are not fine, and the patient exhibits facial redness and tenderness after the treatment. Harsh chemical peels can provoke an inflammatory reaction.

7. Avoid ulcerated, irritated, bruised areas, warts or any irregularly shaped or pigmented skin. This contraindication is self-explanatory. Please refer patients who present these conditions, or other suspicious looking skin lesions or unusual pigmentation to a dermatologist.

8. Do not treat a patient with migraine headaches until they are migraine-free for at least 3 months. You should first address the constitutional pattern. The patient should be made aware of the fact that unregulated migraines will predispose them to a negative reaction to the facial needling; an excess of Yang Qi will rise to the head, and will most likely trigger an episode. In my experience, three months is the magic number; however, it is still possible that a migraine-prone patient may experience a headache even after that period. Should this occur, immediately cease needling the face, and bring the energy down by needling distal points.

9. Do not perform Constitutional Facial Acupuncture on patients with compromised immune systems:

   a. For example, when a patient has the beginnings of a cold or flu, do not given them a full facial acupuncture treatment, so as to avoid driving the pathogen further into the body. The appropriate strategy here is to treat the Wei Qi, and release the surface, but this does not mean that you cannot use any points on the head. You may treat the sinuses, or use Yintang or auricular points.

   Do not treat pregnant women with facial acupuncture, but support them constitutionally. In Chinese medicine (TCM), pregnancy is defined as a phlegm ball, or Qi and blood stagnation. It is important to keep this Qi and blood in the womb to nourish the fetus. The mother's face is usually flushed with hormones, and she does not need facial acupuncture during the time that she is carrying the child. However, she will need the treatments later, particularly after a protracted labor.

   b. If a patient has had a recent herpes simplex I or II outbreak, simply treat their constitution, and especially the immune system.

   c. With any acute allergic reactions, tonify the immune system, and try to identify the allergen to the best of your ability. Do your best to insure that your clinic space is as clean and sterile as possible, with no extraneous scents, dust or other potential allergens.

10. Caution should be exercised with patients who have chronic immune deficiency conditions:

    a. Treat patients that have chronic fatigue syndrome with strong constitutional support. Depending upon the severity of their condition, it is possible for you to perform facial acupuncture; however, you should not overload the patient with too many needles in the face.

b. Fibromyalgia is characterized by a pronounced emotional component, and it is a very debilitating condition, which tends to affect women more than men. I have had good results giving Constitutional Facial Acupuncture treatments to these patients, but once again, I am careful not to subject their systems to undue stress by over-needling, and I monitor them very closely.

c. Hashimoto's disease affects the thyroid and is also a very debilitating syndrome, but there are varying degrees of severity. I had occasion to treat a student with moderate Hashimoto's in one of my seminars; she was very sensitive, and I was careful to use very few needles, while providing support for the immune system. Afterwards, she reported that she felt wonderful, had experienced a refreshing night's sleep, and woke the next day with more energy than usual.

11. Patients with Cushing's syndrome or Addison's disease should not be subjected to facial needling. Cushing's disease presents as an excess of adrenocorticotropic hormone (ACTH), adrenal function. These patients usually have a tumor in the pituitary gland, with thin skin that bruises and bleeds easily, and a high level of irritability. Their bodies are typically rounded, like a bumblebee or butterball, with thin arms and legs, and a noticeable buffalo hump in the C7 area at the back of the neck. They look a bit like Humpty Dumpty in the nursery rhyme.

Individuals who have Addison's disease also have marked tendencies to bruise and bleed, and they have deficient heat that rises to the head. This is a hereditary condition, and it presents as deficiency, with low-functioning adrenal glands. These patients are noticeably weak and the stress of facial needling might cause them to faint, and you might then need to rush them to the emergency room. This does not mean that you cannot treat them constitutionally.

12. Do not treat patients who are suffering from acute emotional or psycho-spiritual conditions. For example, someone in the throes of a panic attack or fright, extreme trauma or shock, or an acute Shen disturbance – ranting and raving, talking to themselves while pulling out their hair, and other symptoms of mania.

I think that all of these contraindicated conditions that I have outlined should be reasonably easy to detect and address within the context of facial acupuncture treatments. Please rely on your better judgment as to when to treat or not treat patients. If you have any questions about whether or not you should treat a given patient, do research to ensure that you are sufficiently informed about the precise nature of the syndrome or disease, trust your intuition and then make an informed decision.

Supplies

In Chapter 7, you are introduced to a facial acupuncture needling protocol that is both subtle in execution and profound in effect. However, even with these sophisticated needing techniques, you are going to require the appropriate tools in order to give the most effective treatments possible, and insure that you will have satisfied patients.

The most important component of your facial acupuncture supply kit in your clinic is the acupuncture needles. I always prefer to perform facial acupuncture treatments with Japanese acupuncture needles, especially Seirins. I am not averse to using other needles for constitutional points, but I find that Japanese needles are well-made, sterile and do not subject my patients to pain. It is not good business practice to shock or inflict discomfort on your patients, and drive them away.

I have taught several seminars in Japan, and was invited to tour the Seirin factory facility in Shimizu, where I witnessed at first hand how exacting and careful they are manufactured.

Needles

Here is a breakdown of the Seirin needles I customarily recommend for the Constitutional Facial Acupuncture needling protocols:

1.   Spinex Intradermal Needles (Spin.6, 6 mm x 0.14 mm):

Along with these small needles, you will require the following:

a. A small magnet.

b. Tweezers.

The magnet is extremely useful for locating any intradermals that may have gone astray, hiding in a patient's hair or on their clothing. Tweezers are my preferred method of insertion for intradermals in the face; I do not use my hand, because it not as accurate or as sterile.

2.   Seirin J Type Needles (Blue; 36 Gauge, 20 x 30 mm), with Tubes: These are of an appropriate size and thickness for men's faces, as they have thicker skin, and can also be used on the body.

3.   Seirin J Type Needles (Yellow; 38 Gauge, 18 x 30 mm), with Tubes: These needles work very well on women's faces, and also for needling body points.

4.   Seirin J Type Needles (Red; 40 Gauge, 16 x 30 mm), with Tubes: These needles are thinner, and, while they can be used for facial points, they are too thin to needle motor and trigger points, as the muscle can easily bend them. You can employ them in the origin and insertion technique, if you are working with someone whose face is sensitive.

5.   Seirin J-15 (Lime Green; 42 Gauge, 14 x 15 mm): Even though these needles have accompanying tubes, I prefer to insert them, without the tube, into lines on the forehead, neck, and other smaller facial wrinkles.

6.   Pyonex Individual Press Needles (Pyon.N.09, Green, 0.9 x 20 mm): I find these press needles are appropriate when needling the body of a sensitive patient. For example: when a patient does not have both the palmaris longus and brevis tendons, or PC-6 Neiguan Inner Gate is very sensitive, I will insert a press needle at that point. The Pyonex can also be used on certain facial points to fill in lines or wrinkles. Make sure that you insert them gently, so that it is easy to remove them without pulling on your patient's skin.

I recommend that you use Seirin D type needles without tubes for auricular therapy (1 gauge, 16 x 15 mm). However, I use ear needles sparingly when performing Constitutional Facial Acupuncture treatments. Too many needles in the face, coupled with ear points, can cause the Yang Qi to rise.

Other Supplies

Homeopathic Arnica Pellets (6C, for Acute Bruising; 12C, for Chronic Bruising): I recommend that you administer 1 pellet of arnica 6C to your patient prior to treatment, to prevent bruising. Another 3 pellets should be taken during the remainder of the day to insure that they don't develop a hematoma. The pellet should be taken sublingually by the patient and allowed to dissolve naturally.

Accu-Band 800 Gauss Magnets (Non-Gold Plated): If your patient has systemic blood stagnation, it is possible that they could bruise several days after the treatment. I always give new patients several of these magnets to apply to a hematoma, should one develop later. These non-gold plated ferrite magnets disperse the blood stagnation and the bruise will disappear.

Two Silver Spoons on Ice: If the patient manifests a hematoma after I remove a needle, I immediately press upon the site of the stagnation with cotton and arnica gel or cream or Wan Hua oil, until the swelling subsides. The next step is to apply one of two cold silver spoons, which has been kept on ice in a mug, on the area to prevent bruising. I roll the cold spoon over the point; when one spoon gets warm, I swap it for the other, and interchange them until the bruise dissipates.

I guarantee that, if you use this technique, you will find it extremely rare for a bruise to remain in the skin. The combination of the dispersing quality of silver with the cold temperature is very effective. I once bruised a patient's neck during a DVD taping and by using this technique, 'un-bruised' them right in front of the student audience. However, do ensure that you have access to ice and that your spoons are always on hand.

Two-Sided Magnifying Mirror: After the completion of a facial acupuncture, I always have the patient examine the results while they are still lying on the table. Invariably, they remark upon their open, relaxed look and the increase in Shen. There is a brightness in their eyes, the skin appears soft and smooth and there is a lovely, rosy, glow to the cheeks.

They usually cannot quite believe how their wrinkles have lessened, even in a single treatment; however, I ask them to sit up and take into account the effects of gravity, and then offer my assessment of their response to the facial needling and recommendations for a course of treatments. The transformation is always a source of great delight, even after gravity demonstrates its impact, and their enthusiasm for the process is quite noticeable. It is after this initial consultation session that they have a much greater appreciation for the organic nature of the work, and they are more amenable to committing to a treatment series.

Lavender Essential Oil: Lavender essential oil is wonderfully effective for healing scar tissue, because it has properties of cellular regeneration. It treats burns, acne, bug bites, jellyfish stings and calms wind and heat in the head. I always have it in my facial acupuncture kit. Sometimes, I apply lavender to Yintang or Ear Shenmen after I have needled them, to calm the Shen.

If either you or one of your patients should get burned, you can apply it neat to the affected area. It will have an immediate analgesic effect, and the wound will begin to heal. A few drops of lavender in a spray of distilled water is wonderfully effective for cooling heat that rises to the face, which can cause hot flashes and red faces that result from exposure to microwave radiation from cell phones or computers.

These recommended supplies will serve you well as the basis for your own facial acupuncture treatment kit, but do feel free to investigate other items that may be more specific to your patients' needs. Use your imagination, be inventive, but also practical!

General Rules for Facial Acupuncture

The 'Wrinkle Rule'

Facial wrinkles can be addressed in one of two ways: 1) by threading the needle superficially through a line, or 2) by treating the acu-muscle points.

In order to ascertain which method to use for a given wrinkle, you need to assess the line, and determine whether it is in the muscle or the skin.

How to assess facial wrinkles: simply spread the skin around the line. If the wrinkle disappears, it is still in the muscle. If it remains visible in the skin, treat the skin level by using the threading technique on the next page. Habitual contracture of facial muscles associated with emotional reactions will impact the skin, and, over time, cause the formation of a line or wrinkle.

Threading the needle through the line engenders a wound healing response, sends Qi and blood to the area, and stimulates fibroblasts, which are the precursor to collagen/elastin production.

Threading: Lines that remain in the skin should be treated by threading transversely and superficially under the skin. Do not thread across the line, but follow and pass the needle directly through it.

Muscle Treatment: Wrinkles that disappear during assessment have not progressed to the skin level, and can be treated using the origin/insertion or other techniques involving acu-muscle points. Re-harmonizing the muscle in this fashion will help to reverse the effects produced by a habitual emotional response, and will ameliorate sagging tendencies.

Do not treat both the muscle and skin level in the same treatment; it is not necessary, and there will be too many needles in the face. It is important not to overwhelm the patient, and overload them in a single session, when you have ample opportunity to work with their facial landscape over a scheduled series of treatments.

Do not treat heavily wrinkled areas all at once; focus on the area of the face that your patient would like you to target. Many patients will want you to treat every line and wrinkle in one session. For example, if you needle all the lines in the forehead simultaneously, you may disturb the patient's Shen. Heat and fire rise to the forehead, and in Western medicine this rising heat is associated with conditions of fright and surprise.

Have them choose a single wrinkle that they would like to see improved; there are three reasons for doing this:

1. Shen may be disturbed, and you may trigger a hot flash or a blood pressure spike, due to rising heat and fire.

2. Needling more than one line will be extremely time-consuming, and will not permit you to be on time for your other patients.

3. Your patient will not be able to see the difference in their face if you needle too many areas in one session.

The 'Anti-Wrinkle' Rule: An Exception

If you have a patient that has a sagging neck with many lines, and when they lie down to receive the treatment, the loose skin covers their ears, so that they cannot hear you, it will be inappropriate for you to treat the neck lines. Treat the muscle points instead. Once the neck is no longer sagging, which will take some time, you can then move on to thread the actual lines.

Treatment Protocol for Constitutional Facial Acupuncture

Prior to Treatment

1. Prescreen your patients prior to booking an appointment; ask them about any possible contraindications for treatment, including serious migraines, immune deficiency problems or pregnancy.

2. Have every new patient complete medical intake/release form, and e-mail or fax it to you prior to their first session.

3. Clarify expectations and inform them of the possible facial bruising in the treatment process. Review their medical history in depth – surgeries, accidents, medications they are taking, previous treatments, any history of cosmetic surgery, Botox injections, and fillers.

    It is fairly standard for most new patients to be less than forthright with you about Botox and other injectables. Inform them that the facial needling will enliven any muscles deadened by Botox and unfreeze the muscle. Usually when you advise them of this, they will tell you immediately. I am always surprised that these individuals are of the opinion that their facial work is undetectable.

4. Have the patient examine their face in the mirror and tell you what areas they would like you to address in your treatment. You can learn a great deal about people by observing how they react to seeing themselves in a mirror. Some of them pucker their lips, as if blowing themselves a kiss, others refuse to look at their reflection at all. Well-adjusted individuals will point out things that they like, and others may not find anything that particularly disturbs them.

    Whether your new patient has low self-esteem, is narcissistic, shy, inse- cure, or balanced, this engagement with the mirror will give you an instant insight into their emotions. A word of caution: please do not impose your own opinions on the patient, pointing out a large line between the brows or elsewhere that they have not brought to your attention. This may be quite difficult as you'll be mystified that they didn't notice it. Please try to refrain from offering this extraneous information.

5. Make a graphic record of the patient's wrinkles, and note the areas that they have singled out for your attention on a blank facial template. Use a pencil to make these notations, with the tacit understanding that all these lines and wrinkles will change, and may be erased on the chart.

    Beginning the Treatment: note that all products used in the herbal treat- ment protocol will be discussed in Chapter 9.

6. Have the patient go into the bathroom, change into a robe and don a headband. Instruct them how to wash their face using a combination of

Chevre Lait de Luxe goat's milk cleanser and *Oats 'Ooh-la-Laver'* exfoliating scrub.

7. Do your diagnostics: tongue, pulse, hara, Five Element, etc.

8. Prior to preparing the face for the needling protocol, ascertain what kind of skin your patient has: 1) if their skin is essentially normal and in need of hydration, you will dip a cotton mask into *The Nutritif*; 2) if their skin is characterized by damp heat conditions – acne, rosacea, or other heat signs – you will perform the same procedure using *The Calme* (see Figure 7.1).

   Heat a gel mask for 20 seconds in a microwave or in warm water, and place it on the patient's face, over the herb-infused cotton mask. Leave both masks in place for 5 minutes or less (see Figure 7.2).

9. Needle the three constitutional body levels: Jing, the Eight Extraordinary Meridians; Ying, the TCM points and Wei, the muscle origins and insertions, trigger or motor points. Also needle hara points and auricular therapy points if needed.

10. Remove the gel mask and Chinese herbal poultice, and give your patient a pellet of arnica 6C prior to the facial needling to prevent bruising.

11. Use jade rollers on the face to cool the skin, and further minimize the chance of bruising, then perform the Constitutional Facial Acupuncture needling protocol. Leave the needles in for 15–40 minutes, depending on what you have ascertained through your preliminary diagnostics and whether the patient is deficient or excess.

12. When the appropriate amount of time has passed, remove needles from the face.

13. With a fan brush, paint on a frothed egg white mask infused with Chinese herbs (see Figure 7.17); the frothing of the egg whites activates the protein in the egg, which feeds the facial muscles. It also permits the Chinese herbs to more fully penetrate the skin; this mask closes the pores after the facial needling and astringes the face.

14. Remove the remaining needles from the body as the mask dries.

15. When the mask is sufficiently dry, use a bar towel dipped in warm water to gently wipe it off the face (Figure 7.18). A bar towel is longer and thinner than most towels, and works beautifully at this stage of the protocol. Do not scrub the face, but hold the warm towel over it for a moment, and then gently cleanse the face. You can also add a few drops of essential oil to the water – rose, lavender, geranium, orange blossom.

16. Take a small amount of *Crème Vitale ESP* moisturizing cream, place it on the back of your hand, and then massage it into the skin (see Figures 7.19A and B). Follow with two jade rollers to further allow absorption of the

cream and to call forth the Yin moisture to the complexion. Jade is always cool, evens out the skin, and decreases hyperpigmentation and red spots (see Figure 7.20).

17. The final stage of the treatment protocol features the use of a hydrosol, spritz the face with organic Bulgarian rose, organic lavender or organic neroli (see Figure 7.21).

After you have finished this protocol, and the patient has had an opportunity to view the results, you will then estimate how many times they need to see you in order to achieve the desired goal of renewal.

The following Treatments page will provide you with a summary of everything you need to know about these treatments, and an encapsulation of the material previously touched upon in this chapter. It covers benefits, contraindications, treatment timeline and frequency, maintenance treatments, use of Chinese herbs and jade rollers and short and long-term effects of facial acupuncture. This information is not only for you as the practitioner; it can also be used to further your patients' education and understanding of the process of Constitutional Facial Acupuncture.

Treatment Summary

Constitutional Facial Acupuncture is a safe, painless and effective treatment for renewing the face, as well as the whole body. Fine lines may be entirely erased, deeper lines reduced and bags around neck and eyes firmed.

Fine needles are placed at a variety of acupuncture points on the face, neck and around the eyes to stimulate the body's natural energies, or Qi. Since muscle groups are addressed, as well the acupuncture points, the face lifts itself, via the acupuncture points, through the muscles' toning and tightening action. The needles also stimulate blood and circulation, which improves facial color.

Benefits
Constitutional

• Improves acne (caused by hormonal imbalance).

• Helps menopause, perimenopause, PMS and other GYN issues.

• Helps sinus congestion and headache.

• Improves hyper- and hypothyroidism.

• Reduces symptoms of toothache, TMJ, trigeminal neuralgia, and Bell's palsy.

- Helps headaches (except severe migraine).
- Treats diarrhea and constipation (most digestive issues).
- Helps to eliminate edema and puffiness.
- Benefits eyes, ears and brain.
- Can help insomnia and dizziness.
- Helps depression and aids self-esteem.

Facial

- Can improve collagen production and muscle tone.
- Helps reduce bags and sagging tendencies.
- Helps eliminate fine lines and diminish larger wrinkles.
- Helps reduce double chin and lift drooping eyelids.
- Improves metabolism.
- Tightens pores and brightens eyes.
- Increases local blood and lymph circulation.
- Improves facial color.
- Reduces stress and promotes total health and well-being.

Is Facial Acupuncture for Everyone?

It would probably be more instructive to list the few contraindications for facial acupuncture, because, for the vast majority of prospective clients, it is a safe and beneficial treatment, not only for prevention of wrinkles, but also the reversal of the customary signs of aging.

Contraindications

1. Severe high blood pressure (it is OK when the blood pressure is under control and the patient is seeing a medical doctor).

2. Severe migraines (if the patient is having a migraine only once every 3 months or so, they can receive facial acupuncture treatments).

3. Be aware that it takes a patient 3 weeks to recover from laser resurfacing on the face. Do not needle during that time; wait 2 weeks after microderm-abrasion or chemical peels.

Do not perform during:

- Pregnancy.
- Colds or flu.

Treatment summary

183

- Acute herpes outbreak.

- Acute allergic reactions.

In the latter three instances, once the condition has passed, the patient may receive a facial acupuncture treatment.

How Long is the Treatment?

Constitutional Facial Acupuncture involves the patient in an organic process, in which a series of treatments is necessary to achieve maximal effect. After an initial session, the practitioner evaluates the patient's response, and then can determine the number of follow-up visits that will be required.

After this evaluation, and taking into consideration other variables, such as stress, diet, lifestyle, genetic inheritance, proper digestion and elimination, sleep, emotional balance, and age, the following durations of treatment are customarily recommended:

- Usually 12–15 treatments.

- 20 treatments for smokers or people whose skin tends to sag, i.e., who manifest jowls, 'turkey wattles,' droopy eyes, etc.

It should be noted that age is not as crucial as might be estimated; an older patient with a healthy lifestyle and good genetics, may in fact have a better prognosis than a younger person who is prone to dissipate themselves.

Treatment Timeline

- 2 times a week (if possible), for 45 minutes to 1 hour.

- 1 treatment per week, 90 minutes.

Maintenance Treatments

Within the normal parameters of aging, the completion of a series of treatments should be effective. To ensure long-lasting results, ongoing maintenance treatments are recommended:

1. One treatment per month for basically healthy patients.

2. Two treatments per month for saggers, smokers or patients who need more care.

3. Of course, the patient can also embark upon a subsequent series after a week's respite.

The Use of Chinese Herbs

The Constitutional Facial Acupuncture treatment protocol incorporates Chinese herbal masks, poultices and moisturizers. Jade rollers, which enhance blood circulation, remove fine lines and age spots, and prevent premature aging, are used to massage moisturizer into the skin. The ancient empresses of China used jade as a precious stone to be worn, not only around their necks, but also to attract Yin and nourishment into their skin. The stone served a double purpose of promoting beauty and for magical protection.

Short and Long-Term Effects of Facial Acupuncture

After the first treatment, one usually observes an increased glow to the complexion, the result of increased Qi and blood flow to the face. The person's face appears more open, there is a clarity in the eyes ('clear Shen'), and the patient appears to be more rested; wrinkles start to lessen and the skin appears more toned.

A significant difference in their appearance can be ascertained following the 5th to 7th treatment; even more marked changes in wrinkles, skin tone, etc. The impression of relaxation and calm is more pronounced; they appear as if they have returned from vacation. Lifting of the jowls, neck and the eyes has begun and is usually noticeable. With continuing treatment, constitutional issues like gynecological, digestive and circulatory system complaints have been ameliorated or have subsided.

By the end of a series, the patient should look and feel 5–15 years younger. These results may vary slightly, depending upon how well the patient has taken care of themselves during the process, and afterward. At this stage, maintenance treatments provide ongoing support within the normal process of aging.

Constitutional Facial Acupuncture is non-invasive, less costly than surgical procedures, and draws upon the ancient Chinese wisdom related to longevity, beauty and balance.

CHAPTER 7

Constitutional Facial Acupuncture Protocol

"Whatever you can do, or dream you can do, begin it. Boldness has genius, power and magic in it."
— *William Hutchinson Murray, from* The Scottish Himalayan Expedition *(1951)*

The Face: The Most Emotive Part of the Body

The face is an organic calling card that allows us to communicate and connect with our fellow human beings. This non-verbal communication telegraphs to the world what we think, how we feel, and how we react to inner and outer stimuli. By interpreting our facial expressions, our friends, loved ones, acquaintances, and even strangers are alerted to the ebb and flow of our emotional states prior to the actual voicing of anger, frustration, sadness or joy.

Because our facial expressions are the first impression that other people have of us, they can have a strong positive or negative impact on our business and personal interactions. We can make a bad first impression if our facial expressions do not match the message we are trying to convey.

The emotional significance of the face assumes greater importance in a social environment increasingly dominated by video communications technology, such as webcams, which are found on virtually every PC and laptop, and hand-held devices, such as iPads, iPhones, Androids, cell phones, and Blackberrys. An ill-timed frown or winsome smile now possesses even more power to repel or attract the things and individuals that we wish to have in our lives. This is because the close proximity of the video screen subjects our faces to scrutiny that would ordinarily only occur under the most intimate of life circumstances, without the attendant level of trust that is fostered by authentic relationship.

"Face to face relationships create trust in a way that online interactions do not."
— Susan Cain, from Quiet[1]

No part of the body is more expressive than the face. Without its fluent, but mute, vocabulary, our inner emotional being would remain a mystery to all but ourselves. The beauty of Shen spirit emerges from the recesses of our being and reveals itself through the face, which reflects the wonders of the individual soul and the heart's compassion.

The Tibetan Buddhist lama, Tarthang Tulku, has said that 'the opening heart is the most beautiful flower of all. The greatest beauty in the world is compassion." Beauty does not exist in a vacuum, but unfolds from awareness, our inner resources, and the individual tapestry of our life experience.

Archetypal beauty originates in the spiritual realm. No expression is more beautiful than love or compassion, and the revelation of this inner blossoming, as described by Tarthang Tulku, can only be accomplished through the face. The individual who embodies this beauty, born of acceptance and self-love, possesses an authentic grace that has no age limit. The beauty of compassion is timeless and ageless, and does not have an expiration date.

Facial Lines are not Proof of Aging

Contrary to popular opinion, expression lines or wrinkles are not necessarily a sign of aging. Unlike other parts of the body, facial muscles do not form lines or droop, due to inadequate activity only. These muscles are subject to conscious or unconscious expression. Wrinkles form because of the habit of habitually contracting the facial muscles in a particular position.

For example, the frown line between the eyebrows is a product of the corrugator supercilii muscle – which pulls the eyebrows down and together to express anger, frustration, impatience or deep concentration – and can be seen in people of all ages.

The combination of a frozen emotion, muscle movement, and the habit of frowning, which shortens the tissue and muscle fibers in this area, can cause a line to develop between the eyebrows. However, the extent that these lines are etched in the skin depends on how long this particular muscle is held in a contracted state, the frozen emotion expressed, the moisture and elasticity of the skin, gravity, sun exposure, diet and one's age, among other factors.

In one of my facial acupuncture seminars, a fellow acupuncturist threaded a needle superficially through the 'suspended sword' between a colleague's eyebrows in a treatment session. This long, deep crease between the eyebrows became very red after the treatment and remained so throughout the class.

In my experience, redness that does not subside within a few hours, especially in this area of the face, usually indicates past emotional issues that have not been totally processed or resolved.

When he returned to class the next day, he shared with his colleagues that he had realized he still harbored anger over a difficult divorce that had taken place 20 years before. He was surprised that the turbulent emotions associated with that earlier phase in his life were still lodged in his cellular memory.

Even though the event had long passed, the process of voicing this anger to the class freed his throat of plum pit Qi and helped him claim Liver Qi that he had involuntarily surrendered years before.

In claiming Liver Qi, he accessed his life force and reclaimed his power. According to the precepts of Oriental face reading, the reclamation of Qi, such as was accomplished in this initial treatment, can lead to the manifestation of reconstituted Jing.

Jing essence and Yuan Qi are both experienced at the cellular level. However, according to Chinese medicine theory, Yuan Qi is pre-natal and cannot be replaced. Jing essence represents both pre- and post-natal Qi, and it can slowly be replaced, changed, supported, and enhanced by lifestyle changes, which include dietary modification, herbal therapy, Qi-gong, acupuncture, Tui-na, psychospiritual health and stress reduction.

Therefore, it is possible to reconstitute Jing, to restore Jing to its original state and create a new cellular structure that reflects the patient's present growth and psychospiritual evolution. Needling the glabellar crease can wake up patients who have been living as if in suspended animation.

In this case, revisiting this old wound and releasing ancient emotions shifted and changed the man's vital energy and gave him back the life force that had been etched as a line between his eyebrows.

I refer to this as 'emotional cryostasis,' because the unexpressed emotions leave these individuals frozen in time. This condition persists until they are resuscitated by the acupuncture needle, which triggers the memory of the anger and frustrations related to the specific life experience, the significance of which was not fully realized at the time.

Emotions that can't be expressed in a forthright manner are short-circuited and find their outlet in unconscious tension in the muscle that eventually leaves its mark embedded in the skin. The act of needling these areas can bring unconscious cellular memories to the fore; however, this only transpires when the patient is ready to re-visit the trapped emotions.

His suspended sword was still present, but it looked softer, less deep, and definitely not as angry red as it had been the previous day. He didn't totally lose this line, but he definitely accessed more of his natural Jing and Qi.

This true story is important for us as practitioners, because it makes us aware of the potential ramifications of a 'suspended sword' that may appear between your patients' eyebrows. We then can understand that thought and stuck emotions, specific muscle involvement and a particular Traditional Chinese Medicine (TCM) pattern can constitutionally affect our patients over time. All of this information is encoded in your patient's facial expression.

I have found this knowledge to be a very valuable tool in my own facial acupuncture practice. That is why I say that the face is the barometer of the health and well-being of the body. Nothing is separate in Chinese medicine; all Yang meridians travel to the face and the crown to Baihui, which is the convergence point of all six Yang channels.

The head is considered the most important part of the body because it is the meeting place of 100 Spirits, the Sea of Marrow point, and most importantly, because it houses the brain. These Yang meridians rise up the head to clear the mood and lift the spirit, and open the portals to the crown chakra, which makes the head and the face the seat of our divine connection to heaven, Tian.

When we are babies, we are masters of face reading. We know when our parents are pleased, angry, loving or impatient with us. Because our survival depends upon keeping these large beings happy, we smile, coo, and are delightful to encourage their natural protective instincts. Of course, the joy inherent in most babies is a spontaneous expression of being, but the primal instinct to read facial expressions is part of our cellular memory. It is an innate gift that we carry in our DNA. In Neolithic times, reading an antagonistic, violent neighbor's facial expressions correctly could not only save our lives, but also our family and tribe's lives, as well.

Despite esthetic trends to the contrary, such as Botox, which seek to immobilize the face and its muscles in a timeless and characterless present, more and more evidence has emerged in recent years to demonstrate the primacy of facial expression as the *sine qua non* of human communication. In his best-selling book, *Blink*, Malcolm Gladwell has documented the development of a scientific analogue to traditional physiognomy, the Facial Action Coding System (FACS). This modern attempt to decode the repertory of facial expression has its origin in an interesting experiment between Paul Ekman and his mentor, Silvan Tomkins.

While Ekman was studying psychology in graduate school, Professor Tomkins challenged him by claiming to be able to discern the subtleties of character of any individual or group, simply through an examination of their facial expressions. This assertion was completely at variance with the conventional wisdom of the time. Ekman was nonplussed at such an audacious hypothesis, and resolved that he would discover the truth for himself.

Some years later, he decided to subject Professor Tomkins to the ultimate test. He had procured and carefully edited film footage of two obscure aboriginal tribes from Papua New Guinea, polar opposites in their social structure and psychospiritual nature; one was inherently pacifistic and gentle, with harmonious family and societal relationships, and the other exhibited traits of aggression, dominance, violence and physical and sexual abuse of offspring and intimate partners.

Despite his lack of familiarity with these two disparate groups, the lack of any apparent social context, and his incomprehension of their language, Professor Tomkins quite accurately delineated the not-so-subtle differences between them simply by analyzing their facial expressions.

After this, Mr. Ekman could only conclude that facial expressions are universal, the result of untold eons of human evolution – the bedrock upon which all communication is founded – and building upon the results of their previous research, he and his partner, Wallace Friesen, thereafter developed FACS.[2]

Thus, changes in our facial appearance are not only dependent on bone structure, the collagen/elastin layer of the skin, genetics and hormones, but also on the movement and intensity of facial muscles, which are activated by our thoughts and emotions. A line etched in the facial landscape, facilitated by an unconscious habit of contracting the facial muscles when encountering a specific situation, can express a long-forgotten emotion.

This emotional palette was acknowledged centuries ago by Chinese medicine in Five Element theory with the Five Primary Emotions – anger, joy, worry, grief and fear – and their connection to the balances and imbalances of the internal organ systems. In the old Chinese axiom, "The Shen leads the Qi."

"The Shen Leads the Qi"

Since the face functions as a mirror of the health and well-being of the body, every blemish, mole, wrinkle, line, scar, or discoloration can indicate a constitutional imbalance. For this reason, I do not view facial acupuncture as a cosmetic, stand-alone treatment. My approach honors the face as an integral part of the meridian pathways that flow from the soles of the feet to the extremities, and up to the head, skull and brain.

The face can also indicate a healthy constitution and the emotional well-being of the patient. In my experience, in the ShenMind, a thought or feeling is the precursor to a facial line, wrinkle, mark or discoloration. Where these lines are formed depends upon Chinese physiognomy, the Five Element emotion, organ imbalances, and the movement and intensity of the facial muscles made to express these emotions.

First the thought arrives in the ShenMind, then the emotion propels the movement of Qi in the facial muscles to express a particular feeling. The Shen leads the Qi: over time, a repetitive movement of Qi becomes a pattern in the body. In times of trauma or intense stress, this process can happen very quickly.

As previously discussed, a long deep vertical line between the eyebrows is called a 'suspended sword' in Chinese physiognomy, and is indicative of a Wood or Liver Qi imbalance. We could liken it to the sword of Damocles, which features prominently in a famous Greek legend, later related by the Roman orator Cicero in his Tusculan Disputations:[3]

> Dionysius II was a fourth century B.C. tyrant of Syracuse, a city in Magna Graecia, the Greek colony in southern Italy, now located in modern Sicily. To all appearances, Dionysius was very rich and comfortable, with all the luxuries money could buy, tasteful clothing and jewelry and delectable food. As one might expect, his retinue was filled with envious courtiers who secretly coveted the privileged status of their ruler.
>
> The most notorious of these was Damocles. Having endured Damocles' obsequious behavior for a long time, the tyrant singled him out one day and made the following unanticipated proposition: 'If you think that I am indeed so fortunate, perhaps you would like to experience what my life is truly like?'
>
> Damocles, although thunderstruck by this unexpected notion, readily agreed to assume the place of his ruler, and so Dionysius ordered everything to be prepared so that Damocles' experience should be as authentic as possible. Everything was as he anticipated – the most sumptuous of garments, wonderful food and drink, his every whim catered to … until, as he was savoring a fantastic meal in the throne room, Damocles glanced up and was horrified to catch sight of a sharp sword hovering over his head, suspended from the ceiling by a single strand of hair from a horse's mane. This, Dionysius explained to Damocles with relish, was more specifically the nature of his exalted status.

Damocles clearly had no idea of the precarious nature of the power wielded by his tyrant overlord. While the legend does not inform us of his ultimate fate, we can presume that he quite readily realized the folly of coveting his ruler's creature comforts and contentedly lived out his own life in more modest circumstances.

It is simple to draw a parallel between the actual weapon which dangled above poor Damocles, threatening him with imminent physical harm, and the self-sabotage and emotional toxicity that accompanies the formation of that line between the brows, with its linkage to the Liver.

Lillian Bridges, in her book, *Face Reading in Chinese Medicine*, describes the 'suspended sword' as "a single line between the eyebrows that is very deep. It is a symbol that the Liver energy is cut in half, and that, at some point, the issues behind this marking will stop forward progress because the sword will drop and cut off the foot. This sign is also called 'estrangement'. It is considered a sign of estrangement from the father, estrangement from sons, or estrangement from the person's own male or Yang energy. It is correlated with a person using only half of the Liver Qi."[4]

Because this anger is turned inward and not expressed outwardly, many health problems can manifest. This individual does not claim their own power, and mollifies and placates other people. They do not want to be like the past violent Yang figure in their life, and they are afraid of finding their voice and speaking their own truth.

Over time, this 'suspended sword' becomes a facial fixture between the eyebrows, and with this emotion turned inward, Liver Qi Stagnation can develop. A woman with a 'suspended sword' may have signs and symptoms, such as premenstrual syndrome, painful periods, distended, painful breasts before menses, irritability and fibroids.

The Facial Landscape

The expressive muscles of the face communicate thoughts and emotions. They are layered in the superficial fascia and enervated by the seventh cranial nerve. The expressive muscles developed from the mesoderm, and thus represent the middle layer of the primary germ layers of the early embryo.

One of the jobs of the expressive muscle layer is to form connective tissue, and the crosswise and lengthwise partitions of the muscles *in utero*. On the head and the face, the expressive muscles include the areas of the scalp in front of and around the ears, the eyelids, the mouth, the corner of the nose, the forehead and both the back and front of the neck. The expressive muscles work synergistically with the sphincter muscles that surround the eye and the mouth.

For example, several muscles interlace with the orbicularis oris muscle, which encircles the mouth. The zygomaticus muscle draws the mouth upward as in laughing, and mingles with the depressor labii inferioris, which depresses the lower lip laterally to express irony, and the depressor anguli oris, which depresses the angle of the mouth to express deep-seated grief.

The connection between the depressor anguli oris and the expression of grief is generally acknowledged by scientists. Paul Ekman, creator of the Facial Action Coding System (FACS), believes this muscle can only be fully activated when the emotion is genuine, and that even the most skilled actor cannot feign the facial terrain of grief.[5] The transformation is involuntary and often instantaneous, pulling down the corners of the mouth in a way that is unmistakable.

Not only do emotions cause the facial muscles to move; the movement of muscles can also trigger emotions. One might argue that the movement of Qi similarly motivates Shen.

A Western consultant conducted a smile clinic in India, where public expression of emotion has historically been regarded as somewhat inappropriate. He assembled a very large group of people in an open field, and persuaded them all to emulate his smiling countenance; the emotions evoked by the smile became infectious, and soon everyone began laughing uproariously. The simple mechanics of activating the muscles involved in laughter caused neurotransmitters to be secreted in the brain, which allowed the uncustomary emotion to burst forth.

Additionally, compelling evidence has emerged documenting the impact of Botox injections on an individual's recognition and response to facial expressions. As recently reported in *Science News*, even a single Botox injection in the glabellar crease diminished study subjects' ability to identify negative emotional states in the faces of others for up to 2 weeks after the experiment.[6]

It seems apparent that immobilizing the corrugator supercilii, which is actively involved in the expression of the Wood element's anger and frustration, rendered the study subjects incapable of recognizing the characteristic muscular activity associated with those emotional states on another person's face. Not only did the Botox freeze the muscle involved with the emotion, it also severed the communication between the muscle and the brain, effectively lowering the test subjects' emotional intelligence. They could neither utilize the physical mechanisms involved in the expression of anger and related emotions themselves, nor respond to them neurochemically to recognize those emotions, and the possible danger to themselves from people who were noticeably angry. Thus, we cannot overemphasize the evolutionary linkage between the outward manifestation of emotional states and brain chemistry.

Other muscles, like the levator anguli oris, which elevates the angle of the mouth in smiling, counteract the depressor anguli oris, which lowers the corners of the mouth in grief. Both the orbicularis oris and the orbicularis oculi eye area are sphincter muscles with more than one muscle overlapping and intermingling with each other, which enables them to demonstrate several different emotions, and contributes to the formation of more lines, wrinkles, pouches and bags in these facial areas.

The facial muscles are also called cutaneous muscles because they are layered superficially over the bone, scalp, fat and skin. The cutaneous muscle fibers are very flexible, like a rubber band, to allow for mobile facial expressions. However, as we age, these rubber bands lose their elasticity and become too loose, flexible or hyper-mobile, causing areas of the face to sag, drop and droop, especially the platysma, or neck muscle.

Since the superficial platysma muscle is very thin, it is usually the first muscle to sag and droop. The two cords under the neck are sometimes called "turkey wattles." These wattles are loose cords or bands that extend up from the clavicle up to the underside of the chin. The platysma is so paper-thin that it is usually peeled away in a cadaver during dissection.

The good news is that the platysma can be worked on, toned and lifted, especially in facial acupuncture treatments.

The Origin and Insertion of Muscles

All of my facial protocols focus on muscle structure and acupuncture points because I've discovered that such an approach works faster and has a longer, much more lasting effect.

The protocol that we are introducing in this chapter uses the origin and insertion of the muscle. In a treatment, the acupuncture points are chosen based on the muscle function and the areas of the face involved. Combining Eastern and Western modalities makes for a very successful outcome, especially when treating sagging areas of the face. When there are deep lines etched in the face, I treat the skin by superficially threading the needle through the line (see Chapter 6). The movement of the muscles can produce drooping and sagging, plus bags and wrinkles at the muscle's insertion site, which is flexible and attaches to the skin.

The origin of the muscle is the beginning of the muscle, because it is usually attached to the bone. This origin anchors the muscle, and it is needled first in Constitutional Facial Acupuncture treatments. This fixed attachment permits the insertion of the muscle to move and make facial expressions.

The insertion of the muscle attaches to the skin or muscle fibers, and is needled after the muscle origin. The insertion attachment supports muscle movement in making facial expressions, and allows the face to be mobile and flexible. Without this ability to move the skin to express a feeling such as joy, sadness, anger or frustration, we would not be able to communicate these non-verbal emotional states to others.

The expressive movement of the facial muscles is an interplay between the origin and insertion of the muscles, which pulls the skin in the direction of a facial expression when a person laughs, smiles or frowns. This interplay is similar to the balance between Yin and Yang in Oriental medicine. Wrinkles are formed cross-fiber or transversely to the fiber direction of the muscle involved.

For example, the orbicularis oris is involved in the formation of vertical lines, parentheses, and larger 'marionette' lines around the mouth. The frontalis muscle fibers run vertically from the eyebrows to the forehead, but wrinkles in the forehead form horizontally, as in raising the eyebrows in fright or surprise.

Also be aware that skin growths or tumors tend to grow cross-fiber to the muscles involved in the lines and wrinkles. Understanding the origin and insertion of the muscles, the muscle fibers and the direction of wrinkle formation can aid you in your facial acupuncture treatments.

If you recognize the emotion held in the face by the lines appearing in the skin and can identify the specific muscles involved in facial expression, you can treat the origin/insertion of the muscles successfully with my Constitutional Facial Acupuncture protocol. This protocol provides a simple and effective way to work with your patients, in a clinical setting, to change the facial landscape of the patient.

Muscle Function, Emotions, Associated Wrinkles and Facial Acupuncture Treatment Protocols

Each muscle has a specific function, range and direction of motion, associated emotion and specific wrinkles formed by repetitive and habitual movements.

The following twelve areas of the face are used in expression and consequently are the places where wrinkles, lines, pouches, puffiness and sagging become more apparent as we age, or exhibit repetitive facial expressions.

Included in this chapter are: the origin and insertion of the muscles, the associated lines or wrinkles, the emotional reflection involved in muscle movements, needling techniques, depth and insertion, gauge of needles, examples and recommendations, diagrams of the facial muscles and the bones of the face, plus color photos of all the needling steps involved in the Constitutional Facial Acupuncture protocol.

The treatment photographs below represent a constitutionally based facial system. Please do not assume that you know and are able to successfully execute this protocol merely by examining the photos.

The information is comprehensive, and the techniques are unusual, such as 'wrapping around the bone.' Each area of the face is addressed with acu-muscle points to increase the efficacy of the treatments.

Protocol Treatment Photos

Figure 7.23 illustrates the facial muscles, which represent the most expressive part of the body. When the facial muscles are activated, the skin moves to express a particular emotion.

196

Text continued on p. 208

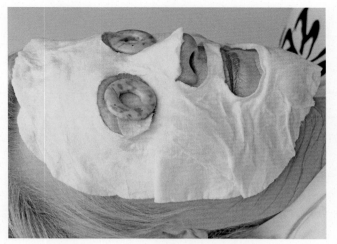

Figure 7.1 Cotton mask with gem discs. The cotton mask is saturated with a Chinese herbal tea to either hydrate, calm or cool the skin. Jade gem discs are placed over herb soaked cotton rounds to moisten the eye area and relax the patient.

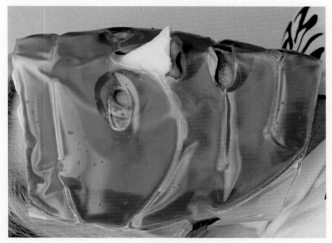

Figure 7.2 Green gel mask. A warm gel mask is placed over the cotton herb infused mask for 5–8 minutes to further allow absorption of the herbs into the skin.

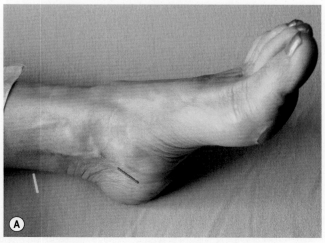

Figure 7.3A Kid-6-7, 2 needles in the foot. Kid-6 Shaohai and Kid-7 Fuliu nourish the Yin, tonify the Kidneys and support Yuan Source Qi.

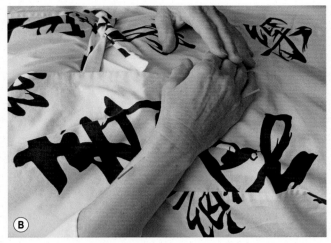

Figure 7.3B Lu-7-TH-2, 2 needles in the hand. Lu-7 Lieque is coupled with Kid-6 Shaohai to open the Ren Mai; TH-2 Yemen brings fluids up to the face to nourish dryness.

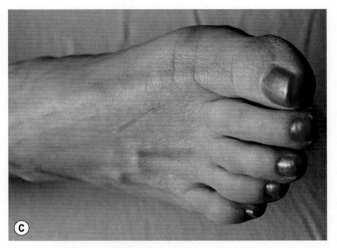

Figure 7.3C Liv-3, 1 needle in the foot. Liv-3 Taichong balances emotions and distally treats Liver related dark circles under the eyes.

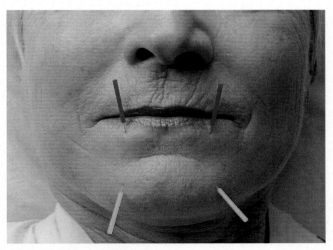

Figure 7.4 The Chin: 4 needles in the chin. This area of the face relates to the mentalis muscle, and emotionally expresses doubt or disdain.

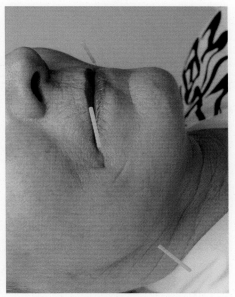

Figure 7.5 The Grin: 2 needles at both mouth corners and jaw (St-6–St 4). In ancient China, the Emperor prized concubines whose mouth corners turned up into a grin, because he knew that they were happy, cheerful, and more easily satisfied.

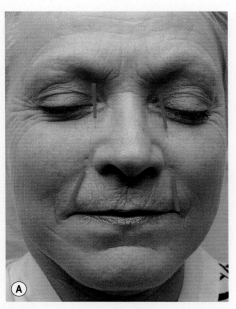

Figure 7.6A The Smile: Bitong-LI-20; 2 dark green needles on either side of the nose. This angular head of the levator labii superioris muscle lifts up the upper lips and dilates the nostrils, as in a sneer.

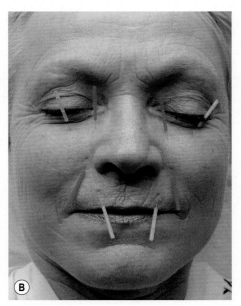

Figure 7.6B The Smile: St-2-LI-19; 2 lime green needles under the eyes and in the upper lip. The infraorbital muscle portion raises the corners of the mouth and confirms that this is a smile, not a sneer.

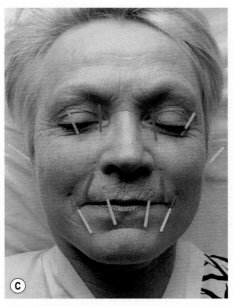

Figure 7.6C The Smile: SI-18-St-4; 2 yellow needles in the cheek and above the mouth corners. The zygomatic muscle elevates the upper lip laterally, and completes the smile.

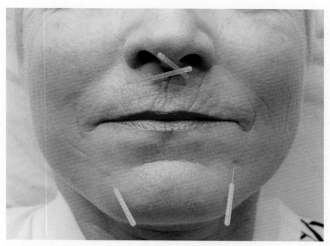

Figure 7.7 Lips: 4 needles around the mouth (upper and lower lips). Lines and wrinkles that form around the mouth can express a smile, sneer, a laugh or despair, anger or joy.

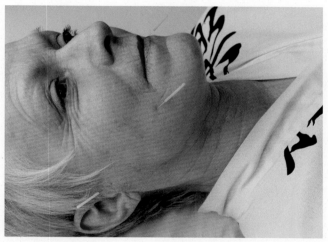

Figure 7.8 Sunken Cheeks: 2 needles in front of ears and the mouth corners. This area treats sunken, hollow cheeks, due to the loss of collagen/elastin Jing deficiency, anorexia or chronic illness.

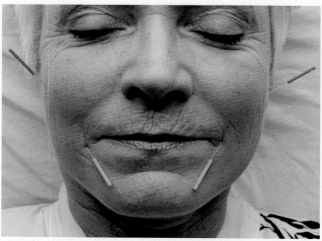

Figure 7.9 Laugh: 2 needles in the cheeks and at the corners of the mouth. A laugh is more than a smile; it is pure delight, which also highlights and lifts the cheekbones.

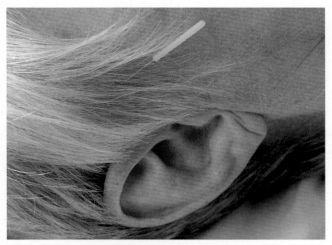

Figure 7.10 Crow's Feet: 1 needle in scalp above the ear. Wiggling the ears activates this small muscle under the temples and prevents lines at the corners of the eyes. It also alleviates headaches, frustration and anger.

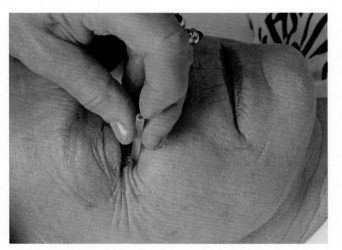

Figure 7.11 Eye Bags: 1 needle placed below the eye. This point treats dark circles and puffiness under the eye, and also relieves grief and stagnant emotions.

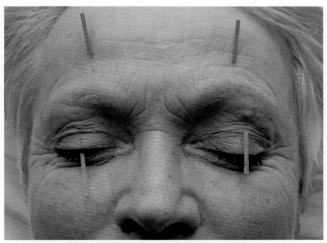

Figure 7.12 Droopy Eyelids/Sagging Brows: 2 needles under and above each eye. The extra point under the eyebrow is called Upper Brightness, because it lifts the upper eyelids, so that the patient can clearly see out of their eyes.

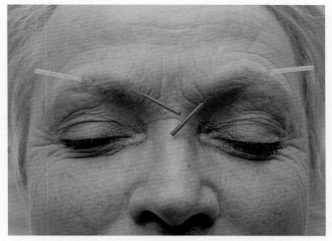

Figure 7.13 Frown: 2 bilateral needles in each eyebrow. Two gentle vertical lines are visible between the model's eyebrows, which means that she is comfortable voicing her anger and displeasure.

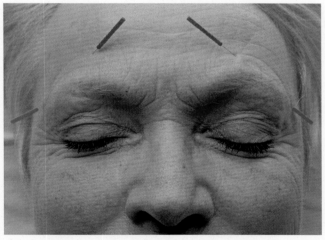

Figure 7.14 Forehead: 2 bilateral needles above the eyebrow. In Chinese medicine, horizontal forehead lines and raised eyebrows indicates disturbed Shen.

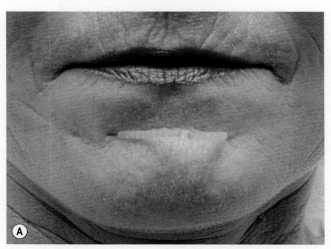

Figure 7.15A Sagging Neck: 2 lime green needles in the chin (Jiachengjiang). The chin area wrinkles horizontally, which runs cross-fiber to its related mentalis muscle.

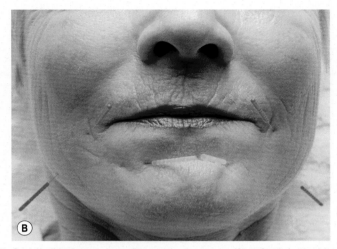

Figure 7.15B Sagging Neck: 4 red needles at mouth corners (St-5-St-4), both sides of the jaw plus lime green needles in the chin. The corners of the mouth pull down to express grief or disappointment.

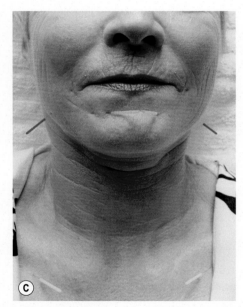

Figure 7.15C Sagging Neck: 2 yellow needles in chest (St-13 Qihu), lime green in chin, and reds in mouth corners and jaw. This area is responsible for sagging, horizontal lines on the neck, and the two cords that form below the chin called 'turkey wattles.'

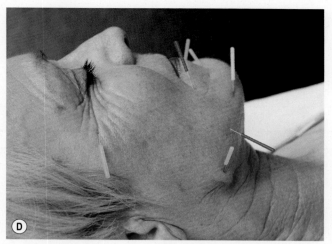

Figure 7.15D Sagging Neck: 2 blue needles under the jaw, 2 yellow needles under St-4, all face needles. 1 needle threaded at the side of the eye for crow's feet. Both SI-17 and St- 4¾ use one needle to "Wrap Around the Bone." This technique accesses the muscle ligaments and tendons above and below the jaw, which lifts and tones the neck.

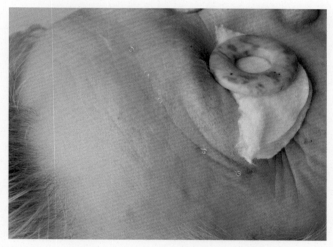

Figure 7.16 Intradermals: close-up forehead with small silver needles. These small needles inserted into facial lines encourage local Qi and blood circulation to the area and diminish wrinkles.

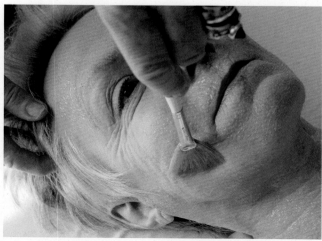

Figure 7.17 Mask with brush. After the facial needles are removed, a frothed egg white mask infused with Chinese herbs is brushed on the neck and face to astringe and close the pores.

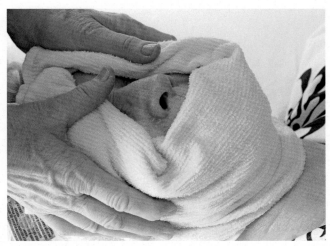

Figure 7.18 Towel. A towel soaked in warm water laced with essential oils gently cleanses the face.

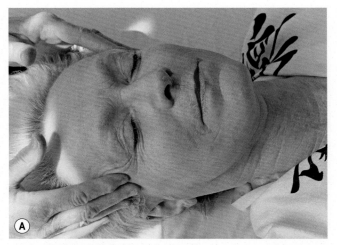

Figure 7.19A Facial massage: hands on temples. Organic cream is massaged into the Taiyang area of the face in a circular fashion.

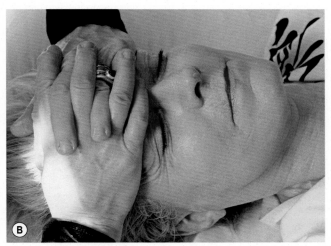

Figure 7.19B Facial massage: hands on forehead. This technique is called 'The Butterfly', because the fingers are interlaced like wings, and then massaged across the medial forehead to the lateral hairline.

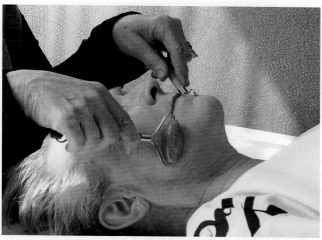

Figure 7.20 Jade rollers. 2 jade rollers further massage in the cream, even out the complexion, calm any redness and "call forth the Yin to the face."

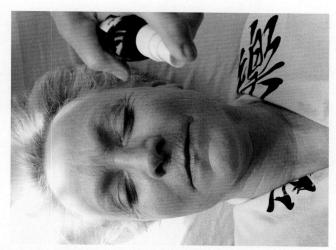

Figure 7.21 Hydrosol spritz. The practitioner selects a specific hydrosol – organic Bulgarian rose, lavender, or neroli hydrosol, which is then is spritzed over the face to hydrate, cool or calm the complexion.

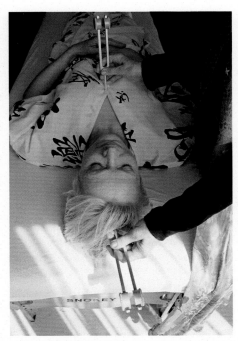

Figure 7.22 Tuning forks. 2 Ohm Unison tuning forks, one on Du-20 Baihui and the other on Ren-17 Danzhong, harmoniously balance, ground and complete the treatment.

Figure 7.24 not only includes the facial bones, but also depicts the head, which houses the brain, our seat of awareness and memory. The Chinese called the head Tian, because it is the most Yang point of the body, and relates to our connection with Heaven or the Divine.

1. The Chin

This area of the face relates to the mentalis muscle, which raises and protrudes the lower lip, as in pouting, and wrinkles the skin of the chin.

Emotion

The emotions expressed by the mentalis muscle are doubt or disdain. These expressions can be seen when a person is presented with a suggestion or idea with which they do not necessarily agree, or about which they are unsure.

Gustave Rodin's famous sculpture, The Thinker, comes to mind, with his chin resting in his large hand, pondering, perhaps doubting, or thinking about what's next. Of course, no one knows what he's thinking and that becomes part of the allure. However, we do know that being carved in solid marble, he is eternally Botoxed, and will not have a line on his chin. His muscle insertion is not flexible like ours, which could be both a curse and a blessing.

Since the chin area in Oriental medicine relates to the water element or the Kidney, your patient may be more Yang with a jutting jaw and the

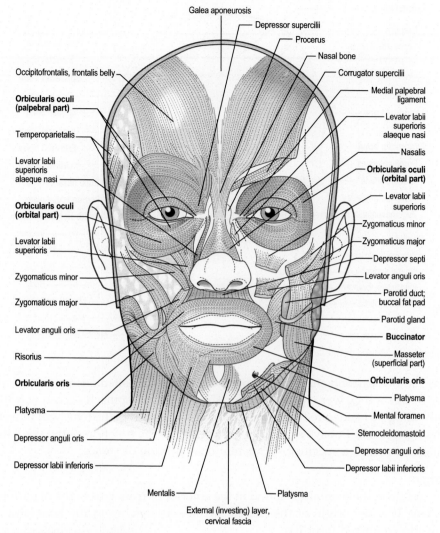

Galea aponeurosis
Depressor supercilii
Procerus
Nasal bone
Occipitofrontalis, frontalis belly
Corrugator supercilii
Orbicularis oculi (palpebral part)
Medial palpebral ligament
Temperoparietalis
Levator labii superioris alaeque nasi
Levator labii superioris alaeque nasi
Nasalis
Orbicularis oculi (orbital part)
Orbicularis oculi (orbital part)
Levator labii superioris
Levator labii superioris
Zygomaticus minor
Zygomaticus major
Zygomaticus minor
Depressor septi
Zygomaticus major
Levator anguli oris
Levator anguli oris
Parotid duct; buccal fat pad
Risorius
Parotid gland
Buccinator
Orbicularis oris
Masseter (superficial part)
Orbicularis oris
Platysma
Platysma
Mental foramen
Depressor anguli oris
Sternocleidomastoid
Depressor anguli oris
Depressor labii inferioris
Depressor labii inferioris
Mentalis
Platysma
External (investing) layer, cervical fascia

Figure 7.23 Muscles of the face.

accompanying stubbornness and strong will power, or they may be more Yin, with a receding chin, little will power and deficient Zhi.

The strong-willed person usually expresses disdain and disgust, while the Jing-deficient patient exhibits more doubt in everything they do and think they know. Use your diagnostics to discern between these two types, treat them constitutionally, and balance the chin area by using the origin and insertion of the muscle.

Lines and Wrinkles

Lines run transversely to the vertical fibers of the mentalis muscle. However, there may be no lines on the chin, but rather a very tight bilateral muscle that protrudes and flexes itself in obstinacy.

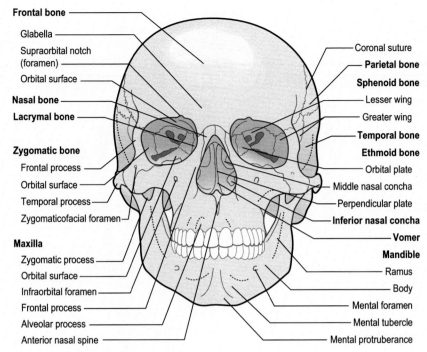

Figure 7.24 Bones of the face.

The famous cartoon character, Popeye the Sailor, exhibited such a chin. Popeye's chin and Qi were regularly nourished by eating spinach – a can was the only thing he needed to bolster his post-natal Qi and replenish his will power. The tightness of Popeye's chin not only reflected the function of the mentalis muscle, but also a specific psychoemotional attitude or stance.

Origin
The origin of the mentalis is found in the anterior or front part of the mandible, or jaw. It is the origin of the muscle because it attaches to the bone and is considered a fixed insertion.

Insertion
The insertion attaches to the skin of the lower lip and the chin; this allows for movement when a person makes a facial expression.

If you look at the anatomy of this bilateral muscle, you will see that it is closer to the center of the chin than the depressor labii inferioris muscle, which pulls the corner of the mouth downward as in an expression of irony. I chose acupuncture points that activate the origin and insertion by observing the muscle's anatomy, function and expression.

Needling Techniques
This small area only needs a single 15 mm, 40 gauge needle (Japanese #1). I always needle the origin of the muscle first, and then the insertion, so that the

fixed attachment to the bone is firmly grounded first to support the mobile insertion in the skin. Needle the mentalis bilaterally.

Origin: A special point 0.5 cun lateral to Ren-24 Chengjiang Sauce Receptacle, between Ren-24 and the extra point Jiachengjiang M-HN-18. Needle obliquely and then transversely upward toward the lower lip, 0.2–0.3 cun.

Insertion: This area is attached to the skin of the lower lip. Needle obliquely and then transversely downward toward the origin of the muscle in the chin, 0.2–0.3 cun.

Remember to needle the origin and insertion of this muscle bilaterally. This muscle has two parts and both sides must be balanced. If we, as practitioner needle this area simply and effectively, the patient's body will balance, tone, relax, tighten or release the muscle. Also, by needling the face, we can more effectively support the constitutional health and well-being of the patient.

Point Locations and Indications
Since the location of this point is so close to Ren-24 Chengjiang Sauce Receptacle, it shares similar indications. It expels both internal and external wind from the face, and treats facial paralysis, Bell's palsy, windstroke, epilepsy, sudden loss of voice, and toothache.

It also promotes salivation and dispels facial puffiness, as well as mental disorders, such as mania and depression. Psychospiritually, it supports fluids for dry and withered people, promotes smoothness and coordination, washes away stagnation, tension, anxiety and primal fears.

The insertion is in the skin of the lower lip and has no specific point indications.

Because the chin area in Table 7.1 relates to the Water element in Chinese physiognomy, resting and relaxing can enhance will power or Zhi, the spirit of the Kidneys.

In Figure 7.25, the facial treatment for the chin is outlined. Insert the needle into the area indicated by the dot, then angle it in the direction of the arrow.

2.   The Grin

This area of the face represents the corner of the mouth and the risorius muscle, which retracts the angle of the mouth outward, as in grinning.

In Chinese face reading, it is well known as the courtesan's or concubine's smile. In ancient China, the Emperor only chose young women with upturned mouths for his bed because he knew that these young ladies would be more satisfied and happy with him. The downturned mouth could be trouble and definitely not as fun as their grinning counterparts, while an upturned mouth, with a Cheshire Cat grin and a playful twinkle in the eyes, radiated an aura of mystery.

TABLE 7.1 SUMMARY: THE CHIN	
Muscle	Mentalis; raises and protrudes the lower lip, as in pouting, and wrinkles the skin of the chin
Emotion	Doubt or disdain
Lines/wrinkles	Horizontal chin line
Origin	The anterior part of the lower jaw
Insertion	In the skin of the lower lip on the chin
Needling techniques	Use a 15 mm, 40 gauge needle (#1 Japanese)
Needling (origin)	Needle a special point 0.5 cun lateral to Ren-24 Chengjiang Sauce Receptacle obliquely and then transversely upward toward the lower lip, 0.2–0.3 cun
Needling (insertion)	Needle obliquely and then transversely downward toward the origin of the muscle in the chin, 0.2–0.3 cun
Point location/indications (origin)	0.5 cun lateral to Ren-24 Chengjiang Sauce Receptacle. It expels wind as in Bell's Palsy, windstroke, epilepsy and sudden loss of voice. It eases tension, anxiety and primal fears
Point location/indications (insertion)	A special area in the skin below the lower lip. No specific point indications

For centuries, the oil painting, the Mona Lisa, by Leonardo da Vinci, referred to as *La Gioconda,* because it is believed to be a portrait of Lisa Gherardini, the wife of Francesco del Giocondo, has fascinated art lovers with her mysterious smile and turned-up mouth. To our modern eyes, she may not be beautiful, but, you cannot deny that there is something magical about her. In another era, she would definitely have received an invitation from the Emperor.

Emotion

In an unbalanced state, where the mouth droops downward, the emotions expressed are unhappiness, disappointment, sadness and melancholy. The person wearing this expression is just beginning to be dissatisfied, and is not yet depressed, deeply unhappy or grieving. Something is not right in their lives; perhaps their relationship is unrewarding, their children are leaving home for university, they long for meaning in their lives, more rewarding work, or laughter and sharing among new friends. They are definitely not happy, and most likely lonely and sad.

Lines and Wrinkles

As a consequence of this emotion, small lines, creases or parentheses form vertically at the corners of the mouth. The mouth may turn down slightly

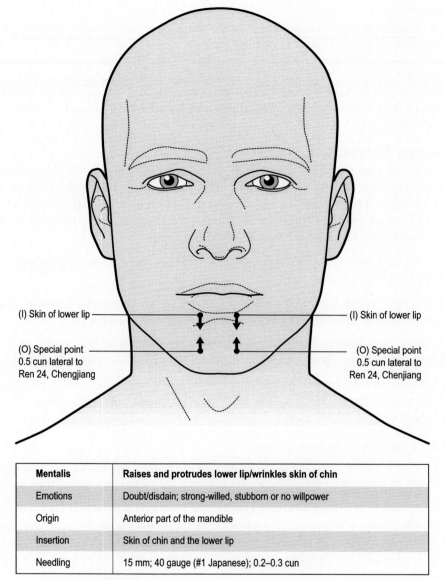

(I) Skin of lower lip — — (I) Skin of lower lip

(O) Special point 0.5 cun lateral to Ren 24, Chengjiang — — (O) Special point 0.5 cun lateral to Ren 24, Chenjiang

Mentalis	Raises and protrudes lower lip/wrinkles skin of chin
Emotions	Doubt/disdain; strong-willed, stubborn or no willpower
Origin	Anterior part of the mandible
Insertion	Skin of chin and the lower lip
Needling	15 mm; 40 gauge (#1 Japanese); 0.2–0.3 cun

Figure 7.25 Needling diagram: The Chin.

before these lines appear. If the sadness goes unchecked, larger marionette or puppet lines could travel down the side of the mouth to meet under the chin in a virtual goatee. Usually this patient hasn't smiled in a long while, and has developed an unconscious habit of repeating this same expression. Needling the face energizes and engages the muscles, which can make the patient more aware of their facial expression and the emotions involved in those expressions.

Origin

The origin of the risorius is located in the fascia over the masseter muscle and is superficial to the platysma or neck muscle.

Insertion

The insertion is in the skin at the corner of the mouth. Therefore, in the movement of the mouth, the skin will wrinkle and form vertical lines at this mobile attachment.

Needling Techniques

This larger area requires a 30 mm, 38 gauge needle for women and 36 gauge needle for men (Japanese #2 or #3 needle). The space between the corners of the mouth and jaw varies, so it is important to evaluate each patient individually. I sometimes use a 36 gauge 30 mm needle with women who have thick skin and larger facial bone structure than the norm.

Once again, always needle the origin first, and then the insertion of the muscle to complete the circuit.

Origin: St-6 Jiache Jawbone; needle obliquely, then transversely toward the insertion of the muscle at the corner of the mouth, 0.3–0.5 cun.

Insertion: St-4 Dicang Earth's Granary; needle this area at the corner of the mouth toward St-6 Jiache Jawbone, obliquely, then transversely 0.3–0.5 cun.

Remember to treat bilaterally and that needle gauge and length are dependent on how large the patient's face is, the thickness of the skin and whether they are male or female. Men tend to have thicker skin and larger faces.

Point Locations and Indications

Origin: St-6 Jiache Jaw Bone, is located one finger's breadth superior and anterior to the angle of the jaw at the prominence of the masseter muscle.

It is one of Sun Si Miao's 13 Ghost Points, and is called Ghost's Bed Guichuang. It treats mania and epilepsy, and is used for Bell's palsy, facial paralysis, windstroke, lockjaw, trigeminal neuralgia, temporomandibular joint dysfunction. It also aids in chewing, opening the mouth, salivation and tension and pain in the jaw.

Insertion: St-4 Dicang Earth's Granary, is located 0.4–0.5 cun lateral to the corners of the mouth below St-3 Juliao Great Bone Hole.

The Golden Mirror, an ancient Chinese text, suggests that St-4 Dicang Earth's Granary is best located below a pulsating vessel. That is why I always have my students palpate each of their St-4 Dicang Earth's Granaries separately, to discern where the most Qi and blood flows and pulsates through the vessels.

They usually discover that each St-4 Dicang Earth's Granary in the left and right sides of the face is in a different location. This is because the face is asymmetrical. I recommend that they needle St-4 Dicang Earth's Granary where they find the strongest pulse. This is usually the most effective and achieves better results.

Earth's Granary receives food and manifests Earthly Qi. It is a local point to eliminate facial wind, paralysis, windstroke, trigeminal neuralgia, facial pain, local mouth and tooth problems, and twitching eyelids.

It is used psychospiritually for people who do not nourish themselves; because of its relationship to food, there are eating imbalances, such as anorexia, bulimia and obesity. In addition, people who mull things over and over, and can't find goodness in their lives, can benefit from this point.

Both St-4 Dicang Earth's Granary and St-6 Jiache Jawbone in Table 7.2 treat the Grin area of the face and can be used for droopy, wry mouth, due to windstroke or Bell's palsy.

In Figure 7.26, the Grin area relates to the corners of the mouth. If a patient is sad, the mouth will turn down slightly.

TABLE 7.2   SUMMARY: THE GRIN

Muscle	Risorius; retracts the angle of the mouth outward, as in a Cheshire Cat grin
Emotion	Unsatisfied, disappointed, unhappy, melancholy
Lines/wrinkles	Vertical lines or parentheses at the corners of the mouth
Origin	In the fascia, overlaying the masseter muscle
Insertion	In the skin, at the corners of the mouth
Needling techniques	Use a 30 mm, 38 or 36 gauge needle (#2 or #3 Japanese)
Needling (origin)	Needle St-6 Jiache Jawbone obliquely, then transversely toward St-4 Dicang Earth's Granary, the muscle insertion, 0.3–0.5 cun
Needling (insertion)	Needle St4 Dicang Earth's Granary obliquely, then transversely toward the muscle origin, St-6 Jiache Jawbone, 0.3–0.5 cun
Point location/indications (origin)	St-6 Jiache Jawbone is located at the prominence of the masseter muscle, when the teeth are clenched. It treats Bell's palsy, windstroke, trigeminal neuralgia, temporomandibular joint dysfunction (TMJ) and jaw tension and pain
Point location/indications (insertion)	St-4 Dicang Earth's Granary is located 0.4–0.5 cun lateral to the corners of the mouth. It is a local point for Bell's palsy, windstroke (wry mouth) and twitching eyelids

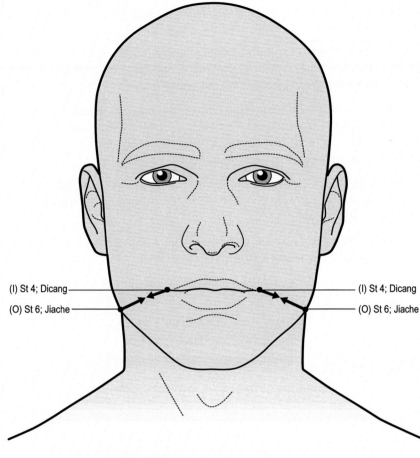

(I) St 4; Dicang

(O) St 6; Jiache

(I) St 4; Dicang

(O) St 6; Jiache

Risorius	Retracts the angle of the mouth outward, as in grinning
Emotions	Dissatisfaction; unhappiness, disappointment
Origin	In the fascia over the masseter muscle
Insertion	Into the skin at the corner of the mouth
Needling	Needling: 30 mm; 38 (#2 Japanese) or 36 gauge (#3 Japanese), 0.3–0.5 cun

Figure 7.26 Needling diagram: The Grin.

3. *The Smile*

This area of the face represents the naso-labial fold, or the smile lines of the face. There are three related muscles involved in making a smile. The levator labii superioris, which has two heads, the infraorbital head, which raises the angle of the mouth, and the zygomatic head which elevates the upper lip laterally, as in a smile. The sister muscle is the levator labii superioris alaeque nasi, which functionally elevates the upper lip and dilates the nostrils.

Fa Ling Lines

In Chinese physiognomy, the naso-labial folds are referred to as Fa Ling lines, and represent our maturity and destiny in the world. The ancient Chinese felt that women, by the age of 40 or 50, and men, in their 30s and 40s, should exhibit some smile lines sweeping downward from the ala nasi, the wings of the nose, to the corners of the mouth. However, modern women in competitive professional careers tend to manifest these lines earlier, like the late Israeli Prime Minister, Golda Meir, and the late Indira Gandhi, who held the same position in India.

The Taoists observed that without these lines a person is still an adolescent, not mature enough to embrace their path or destiny in life. This person couldn't handle power, take responsibility or complete their worldly or spiritual path.

In modern society, we live in a sea of expressionless, Botoxed faces worn by individuals who want to remain perpetual adolescents. I wonder what the ancient Chinese would think about the fear of mortality and aging evidenced by our culture.

Therefore, I educate my patients about the significance of the Fa Ling lines; that they are, at all costs, not to be obliterated or frozen into submission. Gentle Fa Ling lines are beautiful and demonstrate that a person has incorporated the rich experience of their lives and discovered their authentic vocation. There is dignity and exquisite beauty in this expression, which indicates that an individual has smiled and felt happiness in their daily life.

Of course, there are exceptions; a patient may have lost a great deal of weight, and consequently has droopy, saggy smile lines, due to loose skin. This is a constitutional facial situation that can be improved with several courses of treatment.

Emotion

Each of the three muscle heads involved with the smile lines represents different interactive functions, actions and possible emotional expressions. For example, elevating the upper lip, raising the angle of the mouth and dilating the nostrils, can prepare someone for either a sneer or a smile; with this muscular preparation, they can then find an outlet for their contempt or disdain, or in the other extreme, their happiness.

Elevating the upper lip can signal a smile; depressing the mouth, disappointment. The thought and emotion dictates the movement and action of the facial muscle, and the nature of the particular emotional state. This movement occurs instantaneously, but the aftermath of the muscle's activity can linger for a lifetime, unless there is a profound shift psychoemotionally.

Lines and Wrinkles

The lines or wrinkles run vertically, curving around the mouth, and are visible in the naso-labial groove; this area can also be droopy, with untoned, lax flesh, due to hormonal imbalances, lack of appropriate muscular activity (smiling), or loss of the collagen/elastin layer of the skin as part of the natural process of aging.

Origins

1. The origin of the angular head alaeque nasi portion of the muscle is in the upper part of the frontal process of the maxilla.

2. The infra-orbital head originates in the infra-orbital foramen below the orbital ridge of the eye.

3. The zygomatic head is in the malar surface or cheek area of the zygomatic bone.

Remember that the levator labii superioris muscle alaeque nasi has three heads; therefore, there are three distinct origin/insertion pairings. In order to effect a substantial change, it is important to address each pairing.

Insertions

1. The angular alaeque nasi muscle inserts into the skin of the ala nasi at the lateral portion of the nose.

2. The infraorbital head inserts into the skin of the upper lip.

3. The zygomatic portion inserts into the naso-labial groove (smile line) in the skin of the upper lip.

It may be helpful at this point, to review the functions of each one of these components of the levator labii superioris:

- Angular head: elevates upper lip and dilates the nostrils.

- Infra-orbital head: raises the angle of the mouth.

- Zygomatic head: elevates the upper lip laterally.

Needling Techniques

Since there are three distinct areas to target, different needle gauges and sizes will be utilized for each one.

1. For the angular head (alaeque nasi portion), use 15 mm, 40 gauge needles (Japanese #1). This is a very sensitive location; the skin is not thick, and the distance between the origin and insertion is comparatively short.

2. With the infraorbital head, there is a considerable potential for bruising where the infra-orbital nerve emerges from the foramen. Consequently, this is also addressed with 15 mm, 40 gauge needles (Japanese #1).

3. The zygomatic head traverses a larger area and can be needled with a 30 mm, 36 or 38 gauge needle (Japanese #2 or #3). Needle deeper than with the other two heads.

Treatment Protocol

Angular head:

Origin: Bitong M-HN-14; extra point. Needle transversely down toward the ala nasi, 0.2–03 cun.

Insertion: LI-20 Yingxiang Welcome Fragrance; needle transversely upward towards Bitong M-HN-14, 0.2–0.3 cun.

Infra-orbital head:

Origin: St-2 Sibai Four Whites; needle obliquely, then transversely down toward the upper lip, 0.2–0.3 cun.

Insertion: LI-19 Kouheliao Grain Bone Hole; needle obliquely and then transversely up to St-2 Sibai Four Whites, 0.2–0.3 cun.

Zygomatic head:

Origin: SI-18 Quanliao Cheek Bone Hole; needle obliquely and transversely down to the corner of the mouth, 0.3–0.5 cun.

Insertion: A special point; 0.5 cun above St-4 Dicang Earth's Granary in the upper lip. Needle obliquely and transversely up toward the zygomatic bone, 0.3–0.5 cun.

This is a very complete and complex treatment for the naso-labial fold, and it must be performed in its entirety to be effective. The needles are inserted superficially with thin gauges, and therefore, should not feel uncomfortable for the patient. I suggest that you pinch the upper lip gently to distract your patient before needling LI-19 Kouheliao Grain Bone Hole.

Point Locations and Indications

Origin: Angular muscle head, alaeque nasi; Bitong M-HN-14 is an extra point located at the highest part of the naso-labial groove. It treats allergic rhinitis, nasal congestion, nosebleeds, and nasal polyps and boils.

Insertion: LI-20 Yingxiang Welcome Fragrance is located 0.5 cun lateral to the naso-labial groove at the lateral border of the ala nasi. Because LI-20 Yingxiang Welcome Fragrance intersects with the Stomach meridian, it encourages the patient to open the nose and welcome the smell of the Earth element, which is sweetness. It dispels wind heat, facial paralysis, Parkinson's, Bell's palsy, as well as epitaxis, rhinitis and facial swelling.

Psychospiritually, LI-20 Yingxiang Welcome Fragrance clears out toxins from the sinuses and encourages a spiritual fragrance, by restoring an appreciation of beauty and fresh experiences. It has a primal emotional connection to the sense of smell, which is housed in the limbic portion of the brain. Therefore, it can evoke past memories, but it can also encourage new experiences.

Origin: Infra-orbital muscular head: St-2 Sibai Four Whites, is below St-1 Chengqi Tear Container in the depression at the infraobital foramen. It expels

219

wind and consequently treats facial paralysis, twitching eyes, facial pain, and also clears vision and cataracts.

> **CAUTION**
>
> Do not insert or needle deeply into this area, because it can cause injury to the eyeball and the infraorbital nerve, which innervates this foramen. It also bruises easily.

Insertion: A special point 0.5 cun above St-4 Earth's Granary, is used for the insertion of the zygomatic head of this muscle. See the point indications for St-4 Dicang in the section on The Grin earlier in this chapter.

LI-19 Kouheliao Grain Bone Hole, is located below the lateral margin of the nostril, 0.5 cun lateral to Du-26 Shuigou Water Trough. This point eliminates wind, and treats mouth deviation, lockjaw, tremors in the extremities; it also opens the nose, aids rhinitis, epistaxis and loss of smell.

Zygomatic muscle head: SI-18 Quanliao Cheek Bone Hole, is directly below the outer canthus of the eye in the depression on the lower border of the zygomatic bone. It expels wind and clears heat and treats facial paralysis, twitching eyelids, atrophy of the lower eyelids, facial pain and swelling, problems with chewing and yellow sclera in the eye.

Once again, because wind and heat is cleared, the patient may feel more relaxed and less anxious after this area is treated.

In Table 7.3, the smile, or naso-labial fold imbalances are addressed. In ancient China, a person with healthy smile, or Fa Ling lines, was revered for having reached maturity.

Figure 7.27 shows the Needling Diagram for The Smile. Because there are three muscle heads addressed in Figure 7.27, all three areas must be needled to effect a change in the facial landscape.

Facial Exercise

People who do not smile are usually unhappy or resentful, and probably have suppressed anger. In our culture, women have historically not had opportunities to express their anger and disenfranchisement safely without judgment.

I have found that facial exercises can help my patients with issues of smiling. Because these particular exercises are based on isometric muscle movement, they are neutral in nature. I do not discuss the emotional correlations with my patients, at least initially. If they are willing to do the homework, they can usually transform the droopy naso-labial fold, and the attendant emotional states resulting from the imbalance.

One of the functions of this muscle is to elevate the upper lip, as in a sneer; this isometric exercise is initially practiced in two steps:

TABLE 7.3   SUMMARY: THE SMILE

Muscle	The muscle involved in smiling are the levator labii superioris, which has three heads: the infraorbital, which raises the angle of the mouth, the zygomatic, which elevates the upper lip laterally, and the angular head (alaeque nasi), which not only elevates the upper lip, but also dilates the nostrils
Emotion	Contempt, anger, unhappiness
Lines/wrinkles	Vertical lines in the naso-labial groove, curving down from the side of the nose to the corners of the mouth
Origin	Angular head (alaeque nasi): the frontal process of the maxilla
	Infraorbital head: in the infraorbital foramen below the eye
	Zygomatic head: the malar surface of the zygoma
Insertion	Angular head (alaeque nasi): the skin of the ala nasi
	Infraorbital head: the skin of the upper lip
	Zygomatic head: the naso-labial groove in the skin of the upper lip
Needling techniques	Angular head (alaeque nasi): 15 mm, 40 gauge needle (#1 Japanese)
	Infraorbital head: 15 mm, 40 gauge needle (#1 Japanese)
	Zygomatic head: 30 mm, 38 or 36 gauge needle (#2 or #3 Japanese)
Needling (origin)	Angular head (alaeque nasi): needle Bitong M-HN-14 transversely down toward the the ala nasi, 0.2–0.3 cun
	Infraorbital head: Needle St-2 Sibai Grain Bone Hole, transversely down toward the upper lip, 0.2–0.3 cun
	Zygomatic head: Needle SI-18 Qualiao Cheek Bone Hole obliquely, then transversely downward above the mouth corners
Needling (insertion)	Angular head (alaeque nasi): Needle LI-20 Yingxiang Welcome Fragrance transversely upward toward Bitong M-HN-14, 0.2–0.3 cun
	Infraorbital head: Needle LI-19 Kouheliao Grain Bone Hole obliquely, then transversely up to St-2 Sibai Four Whites, 0.2–0.3 cun
	Zygomatic head: Needle a special point 0.5 cun above St-4 Dicang Earth's Granary obliquely, then transversely, up toward the zygoma, 0.3–0.5 cun

Continued

TABLE 7.3 SUMMARY: THE SMILE—cont'd

Point location/ indications (origin)	Angular head (alaeque nasi): Bitong M-HN-14 is located at the highest point of the naso-labial groove at the sulcus of the nose. It treats allergic rhinitis, nasal congestion and nose bleeds
	Infra-orbital head: St-2 Sibai Four Whites is in the depression at the infra-orbital foramen. It treats twitchy eyes, facial paralysis and cataracts
	Zygomatic head: SI-18 Quanliao Cheek Bone Hole is directly below the outer canthus of the eye in the depression on the lower border of the zygoma. It clears heat, treats twitching eyelids, atrophy of the lower eyelids from facial paralysis, and facial pain and swelling
Point location/ indications (insertion)	Angular head (alaeque nasi): LI-20 Yingxiang Welcome Fragrance is located 0.5 cun lateral to the ala nasi. It treats facial paralysis, Parkinson's disease, Bell's palsy, rhinitis and facial swelling. It also encourages an appreciation of beauty
	Infra-orbital head: LI-19 Kouheliao Grain Bone Hole is located 0.5 cun lateral to Du-26 Shuigou Water Trough. It treats rhinitis, deviated mouth, and loss of smell
	Zygomatic head: 0.5. cun above St-4 Dicang Earth's Granary; see the point indications in this chapter under The Grin

'Naso-labial' Sneer/Smile Exercise

1. To begin, both patient and practitioner look into a large mirror together, and sneer. I encourage them to make non-verbal animal sounds, like a cat hissing or the sound of a dog growling, while simultaneously baring the teeth. These primal sounds are often met with embarrassment or a nervous giggle, which usually turns into laughter. I do not force the patient to continue, if they seem reluctant to do so.

The addition of these primitive utterances make this exercise unique and more effective, because it allows people to access the right hemisphere of the brain via the corpus callosum. The right hemisphere is considered to be the half of the brain that is more emotional, creative, non-linear, and non-verbal. In contrast, the left is logical, linear, and rational, and retains the memory of old pain patterns and subsequent emotional resistance.

Using the added vocalizations in this way allows the patient to express and release unpleasant feelings, such as anger or disgust. In fact, the combination of elements is quite potent, and usually elicits a sense of play and much laughter. When the laughter erupts, the exercise has accomplished its task. In my experience, submerged anger is a symptom of suppressed fire element. The laughter not only lifts the naso-labial fold; it also evokes joy,

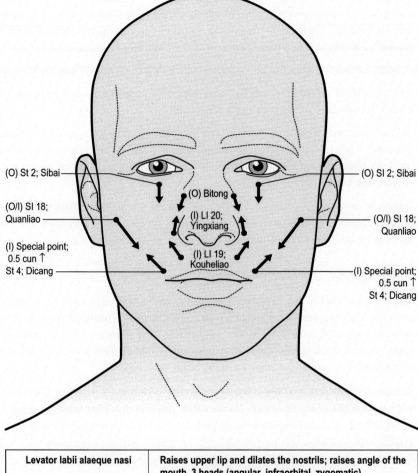

(O) St 2; Sibai

(O/I) SI 18; Quanliao

(I) Special point; 0.5 cun ↑ St 4; Dicang

(O) Bitong

(I) LI 20; Yingxiang

(I) LI 19; Kouheliao

(O) SI 2; Sibai

(O/I) SI 18; Quanliao

(I) Special point; 0.5 cun ↑ St 4; Dicang

Levator labii alaeque nasi	Raises upper lip and dilates the nostrils; raises angle of the mouth. 3 heads (angular, infraorbital, zygomatic)
Emotions	Sadness, anger, disgust
Origin	*Alaeque nasi*: frontal process of maxilla/infraorbital: infraorbital foramen/zygomaticus: malar surface of zygomatic bone
Insertion	Skin of upper lip and the *ala nasi*
Needling	15 mm; 40 gauge (#1 Japanese)/15 mm; 36 or 38 gauge (#2 or #3 Japanese), 0.2–0.3 cun/0.3–0.5 cun

Figure 7.27 Needling diagram: The Smile.

and provides an outlet for the fire of passion. After many years of anti-depressants, being given the permission to sneer for the good cause of lifting the smile lines, in a safe environment, can be quite a gift.

2. The second half of the exercise involves placing the index and middle fingers bilaterally on Bitong, along the side of the nose.

3. Putting steps 1 and 2 together, the patient sneer/smiles, while making the hissing or growling sound, and simultaneously pressing inward and downward on Bitong. They should hold the points for the entire duration of the sound and expression, until they run out of breath.

4. The entire exercise should be repeated 5 to 10 times; twice daily.

I also recommend that they use a tissue or cotton gloves to hold the points, so that the hands do not slip or pull on the skin.

I think that you will find this an effective way to engage your patients in their own process. This is a collaborative effort, and if your patients are not actively involved in their transformational journey, the effectiveness of your treatments will not be as pronounced.

This exercise works only if you as practitioners, are willing to introduce it, and your patients to perform it. This is not an exercise for everyone; use your best judgment to ascertain who may be the best candidates.

4. The Upper and Lower Lips

The orbicularis oris circles around the upper and lower lips and compresses, contracts and protrudes the lips. This sphincter muscle intermingles and converges with several other muscles including the buccinator, levator and depressor anguli oris, the levator and depressor labii inferioris and the zygomaticus muscles.

The buccinator muscle compresses the cheeks when one plays a trumpet; it also aids in the chewing of food. The levator anguli oris elevates the angle of the mouth, while the depressor anguli pulls the mouth downward; the levator labii superioris elevates the upper lip, dilates the nostrils and raises the angle of the mouth, as in a smile. The zygomaticus major muscle draws the angle of the mouth upwards and backwards, as occurs when we laugh, and depressor labii inferioris, in turn, depresses the lower lip to show the lower teeth, as in the expression of irony.

Emotion
The gamut of emotions and actions can be expressed with this sphincter muscle. The lips can pucker, which lends itself to kissing or whistling, or can compress to fit the mouthpiece of a brass instrument. The lips can be pursed in moments of stress, frustration, anxiety or temper. The upper lip elevates in revulsion or to sneer, the corners of the mouth lift to smile or laugh, or lower in moments of disappointment, sadness or despair. The lower lip can pull down to express an ironic or superior air. Thus, this multi-faceted muscle has many expressive options in its emotional repertoire.

Lines and Wrinkles
With the orbicularis oris muscle, lines form around the mouth, the upper and lower lips and likewise at the corners of the mouth. Since this is a circular muscle, lines can form vertically or horizontally to the muscle.

224

In smokers, vertical lip lines eventually become visible because of the way they purse their lips to hold the cigarette in their mouths. Vertical lip lines also result from constitutional causes, such as Lung heat and damp heat in the lower Jiao, which dry out the skin.

In my practice, I do not demand that patients quit smoking in order to have facial acupuncture treatments, but I do educate them about the negative effects of smoking and offer to help them stop if they sincerely want to quit. I also inform them that if they keep smoking, they will need more treatments, and that the results will not be as dynamic.

However, one of my female patients in her 30s was not going to give up smoking. I warned her that I could work on her upper lip lines, but that the effects of the treatments would not last very long because of persistent skin dryness and the puckering and sucking movements she would continue to make when taking a drag on a cigarette.

I have learned that addictive patients tend to resist change and resist releasing unhealthy habits that age them prematurely. However, when confronted with the positive results of 'healthy vanity,' even a confirmed smoker can change her mind!

After two sessions, this patient burst into my clinic, complaining that I was "not doing my job" because the upper lip lines were still prominent, even though they had disappeared for a few days after the previous treatment.

I had her look in the large mirror, and instructed her to take out a cigarette and pretend to smoke it. After a few imaginary puffs, it became obvious to her that the actions of the muscle during the act of smoking were in part responsible for the continued persistence of the undesired lines above her upper lip. While she was ooh-ing and ah-ing over this discovery, I was able to explain to her once again the constitutional imbalances caused by smoking and how they were also contributing to the situation.

I asked her to make a decision about whether she wanted to continue smoking before she returned the next week for another session.

I refer to this as my 'healthy vanity' story because, contrary to what one might have expected, she did stop smoking solely motivated by her looks, and desire to eliminate the undesirable upper lip lines. It really didn't matter to me what changed her mind, because she subsequently learned a great deal about the efficacy of acupuncture, Chinese herbs, diet and healthy aging and became a passionate convert to Chinese medicine!

Horizontal upper lip lines:
I have found that horizontal lines on the upper lip are often associated with a hysterectomy performed in child-bearing years due to fibroids, endometriosis or uterine cancer. This line can also indicate a Caesarian section, sterility both in men and women, a head trauma, or scarring of the uterus by an intrauterine device (IUD).

If there is a history of head trauma, including whiplash, a fall, or hitting the head in any manner, the patient will usually have a blood clot on the tip of the tongue, indicating what the Japanese call *oketsu* or 'stuck' blood.

Since the upper lip relates to the sexual organs, and the philtrum of the upper lip, according to Chinese physiognomy, to longevity, I usually ask to examine the abdominal scar that resulted from the Caesarian section or hysterectomy. I then use Japanese scar therapy distally to release the adhesions, instead of needling the sensitive area on the upper lip. In needling the abdominal scar, the upper lip line becomes very red and full of fresh blood and Qi circulation. There are several benefits that can be achieved in treating the abdominal scar:

1. The upper lip is sensitive, and needling it locally will cause the patient some discomfort.

2. Needling the abdomen affects the upper lip and sexual organs, and treats the cause rather than the symptom.

3. Some scars are horizontal, just above the pubic bone, and others are vertical along the Ren Mai meridian, which disturbs its flow. Needling abdominal scars breaks up adhesions and helps to reestablish the free flow of Qi in the meridians. For example, a horizontal scar above the pubic bone blocks not only the Ren Mai, but also the Kidney, Stomach and Spleen meridians, and will cause constitutional imbalances.

4. An untreated scar in this area will cause secondary problems because the adhesions pull on the organs, muscles and tissues. For example, a horizontal scar can pull on the Bladder, causing frequent urination, a constant feeling of fullness and incontinence. By needling this area, these symptoms will cease in time.

Although teaching Japanese protocols for scar therapy is not within the purview of this facial acupuncture book, it is important to note that by treating an abdominal scar distally, you can evoke constitutional shifts, and that the associated horizontal upper lip line should fade within a course of treatments.

When teaching a seminar some years ago, I noticed a small circle above the right side of a student's upper lip. When I asked her if she had an abdominal scar, she showed me a circular incision on the same side, from a recent tubal ligation. When I treated the scar by Surrounding the Dragon with small intra-dermal needles, the circle on the upper lip turned bright red, mirroring the increased circulation in the abdominal area. Several months later, the scar on her upper lip had vanished.

Nurturance Lines:
Vertical lines surrounding the orbicularis oris muscle on both the upper and lower lips can indicate self-nurturance issues. These lines are not always associated with age, but belong to caretakers who care for others while denying their own needs.

Since the mouth represents the Earth element and receives food and sustenance to support post-natal Qi, issues like anorexia, bulimia, constant worry or an inability to find sweetness or goodness in anything can also arise. These lip lines are usually more pronounced in women. However, both men and women who care for elderly parents can develop these vertical lines around their mouths.

We live in a society in which there is little down time to relax, sleep, eat, be alone, to have quiet and rest. These nurturance lines are not always related to age, but are more likely to reflect the universal condition of imbalance and depletion prevalent in our world today.

Corner of Mouth Lines:
The orbicularis oris sphincter muscle, like the orbicularis oculi, has many potential imbalances that can manifest as lines, wrinkles, pouches, and sagging at the corners of the mouth. These facial features are an important factor in the expression of a variety of emotions – including dissatisfaction, sadness, disgust and grief – that can lead to constitutional weaknesses and TCM patterns.

Origin
The origin of the orbicularis oris muscle is found in front of the maxilla and mandible.

Insertion
The insertion of this muscle is situated in the muscle fibers near and above the corners of the mouth.

Needling Techniques
The area around the mouth is extremely sensitive and 30 mm, 40 gauge or lower needles (#1 Japanese) are recommended. If the patient has a large area around the mouth, use a thicker gauge needle.

In this case, there are two bilateral points of origin located in the bones of the maxilla and mandible. The insertion is in the skin near and above the corners of the mouth around and near St-4 Dicang Earth's Granary. By first needling the origin of the muscles, and threading toward St-4 Dicang Earth's Granary, the insertion of the muscle is implied without inserting extra needles, which is greatly appreciated by the patient in this delicate mouth area.

The Origins and Insertions:
1. A special point 0.5 cun lateral to Jiachenjiang M-HN-18. Needle both origin points in the mandible transversely 0.2–0.3 cun toward St-4 Dicang Earth's Granary at the corner of the mouth, which stimulates the insertion of the muscle.

2. Needle LI-19 Kouheliao Grain Bone Hole transversely 0.2–0.3 cun from the mandible toward St-4 Dicang Earth's Granary, which stimulates the

227

muscle insertion above the upper lip near the corner of the mouth. Needle bilaterally.

Because the orbicularis oris is a circular sphincter muscle, the origin and insertion points require needling with the intention of a continuous loop that informs many muscle fibers around the mouth. I would begin by first needling the lower jaw and then the maxilla in the upper lip. Remember to gently pinch in the LI-19 Kouheliao Grain Bone Hole area to distract your patient from any needling discomfort.

Point Locations and Indications: Origins and Insertions

The special point is located 0.5 cun lateral to Jiachengjiang M-HN-18, which is located 1 cun lateral to Ren 24 Chengjiang Sauce Receptacle. Since this point is so close to Jiachengjiang M-HN-18, it has similar indications, such as facial paralysis, trigeminal neuralgia, face and tooth pain, and gum swelling.

In Table 7.4, vertical upper lip lines relate to Kidney Yin deficiency, and the length and definition of the philtrum is associated with longevity.

TABLE 7.4 SUMMARY: UPPER AND LOWER LIPS

Muscle	Orbicularis oris; circles around the upper and lower lips, compresses, contracts and protrudes the lips
Emotion	Anxiety, frustration (pursed lips), revulsion, sneering (elevated upper lip), smiling (corners of the mouth elevate), despair, disappointment (corners of the mouth lower), irony (lower lip pulls down)
Lines/wrinkles	Vertical lines above and below the lips; horizontal lines above the lips, as well as vertical lines at the corners of the mouth
Origin	In the frontal area of the maxilla and mandible
Insertion	Muscle fibers near and above the corners of the mouth
Needling techniques	Use a 30 mm, 40 gauge needle (#1 Japanese)
Needling (origin)	Needle a special point 0.5 cun lateral to Jiachengjiang M-HN-18 transversely 0.2–0.3 cun upward toward St-4 Dicang Earth's Granary
Needling (origin)	Needle LI-19 Kouheliao Grain Bone Hole transversely 0.2–0.3 cun downward toward St-4 Dicang Earth's Granary
Point location/indications (origin/insertion)	LI-19 Kouheliao Grain Bone Hole has already been introduced in The Grin portion of this chapter. The special point is 0.5 cun lateral to Jiachengjiang M-HN-18, 1 cun lateral to Ren-24 Chengjiang Sauce Receptacle. It treats facial paralysis, trigeminal neuralgia, face and tooth pain

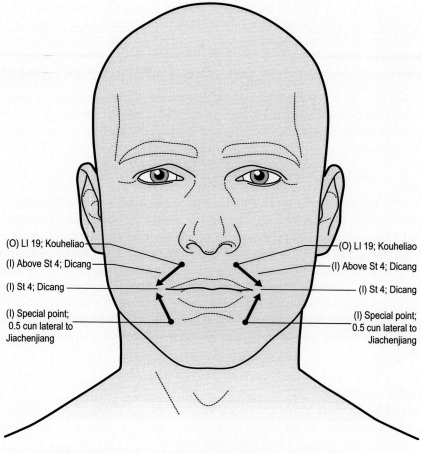

(O) LI 19; Kouheliao
(I) Above St 4; Dicang
(I) St 4; Dicang
(I) Special point;
  0.5 cun lateral to
  Jiachenjiang

(O) LI 19; Kouheliao
(I) Above St 4; Dicang
(I) St 4; Dicang
(I) Special point;
  0.5 cun lateral to
  Jiachenjiang

Orbicularis oris	A sphincter muscle that contracts, compresses and protrudes the lips
Emotions	Associated with habits, hormones and the sexual organs; impotence, menopause, Kidney Yin deficiency, nourishment issues
Origin	In the frontal areas of both maxilla and mandible
Insertion	Muscle fibers near and above the corners of the mouth
Needling	15 mm; 40 gauge (#1 Japanese), 0.2–0.3 cun

Figure 7.28   Needling diagram: Upper and Lower Lips.

In Figure 7.28, this useful technique uses only one needle for each muscle origin, and the insertion site, St-4 Dicang Earth's Granary, is implied by the direction and angle of the needle.

5.   The Cheeks

The buccinator muscle compresses the cheeks and expels air between the lips as in blowing a trumpet. The buccinator is also an important muscle in

229

mastication. It holds food in the mouth while chewing or, if out of balance or untoned, allows food to fall out of the mouth. This syndrome is often seen in elderly people who have dentures, or people who have had considerable dental work.

This muscle is deeper than the other facial muscles. It is overlaid by: the risorius muscle, which retracts the angle of the mouth as in grinning; the orbicularis oris muscle, which encircles the mouth; the masseter, which elevates the jaw and clenches the teeth; and the insertion of the platysma neck muscle, among others.

Emotion

Generally, the buccinator is not considered an expressive muscle, but one that is used for chewing. Because so many other muscles overlay and intermingle with the buccinator muscle, it is involved in several facial expressions. For example, the act of compressing the cheeks can be the precursor to whistling, blowing a kiss to a loved one, sucking a lemon or (the action of) an infant suckling at its mother's breast. Emotionally, sucking a lemon can convey a sour, superior or disdainful attitude, while the blowing of a kiss signals affection, playfulness or love. Of course, these emotional readings depend upon cultural context. Sucking and kissing motions and noises can have different meanings.

Lines and Wrinkles

The wrinkle can manifest as a vertical line starting at St-5 Daying Great Reception, and extending up the cheek area. This wrinkle is often seen in smokers because of constitutional Lung heat and dryness.

However, the most common complaint is hollow, sunken cheeks that make the patient look gaunt and unwell. Sunken cheeks may be caused by: waning hormones, which cause the collagen/elastin layer of the skin to lose thickness and tonicity; dental work; pulled teeth; dentures; eating disorders such as anorexia, commonly seen in undernourished fashion models; chronically ill people, with acquired immunodeficiency syndrome (AIDS) or cancer; and Jing-deficient mothers after a difficult childbirth.

When the buccinator muscle is needled, it plumps up the cheek area. Treating the buccinator develops the cheek, and, in a few sessions, makes the patient look fresher and younger.

Treating this muscle also helps older people keeps food in their mouths while they are eating. It also presses food against the cheeks to keep food from accumulating in the mouth.

A dimple can form in the buccinator muscle when a person is smiling. Over time, with a loss of collagen elastin, smoking, aging and skin dryness, the dimple may become a deep indentation, line or wrinkle. What was previously viewed as charming can look like a hole in the skin if it is not treated with facial acupuncture.

Origin
The origin of the buccinator muscle is at the junction of the maxilla and mandible at the level of the molar teeth.

Insertion
The insertion is in the muscle fibers that blend and intermingle with the orbicularis oris muscle at the corner of the mouth. This sphincter muscle has many possibilities for expressive muscle movement, and makes this insertion site extremely mobile, and thus rich with potential for developing lines and wrinkles.

Needling Techniques
The buccinator is one of the deepest muscles in the face and needs a deeper insertion, 0.5 cun, and a larger needle to traverse the area between the jaw and the corner of the mouth. I recommend a 38 to 36 gauge needle, 30 mm (#2 or #3 Japanese). The thicker needle is used for thicker skin and larger faces.

Origin: St-7 Xiaguan Below the Joint is needled perpendicularly first to a depth of at least 0.3–0.5 cun; then it is needled transversely toward the muscle's insertion, at the corner of the mouth. You do not want any more needle depth unless the patient has unusually thick skin, or strong bone structure, as in an Earth element type.

Insertion: The insertion is located in the muscle fibers 1 cun lateral to St-4 Dicang Earth's Granary. Needle 0.3–0.5 cun perpendicularly, and angle the needle transversely toward St-7 Xiaguan Below the Joint. Make sure that you use a longer 30 mm needle, and needle bilaterally.

Point Locations and Indications
Origin: St-7 Xiaguan, Below the Joint, is located with the mouth closed on the inferior border of the zygomatic arch, in the depression anterior to the mandible's condyloid process. St-7 Xiaguan Below the Joint is indicated for bruxism, temporomandibular joint dysfunction, lockjaw, trigeminal neuralgia, facial paralysis, pain and swelling in the upper teeth, deafness and hemiplegia.

Insertion: A special point 1 cun lateral to St-4 Dicang Earth's Granary has similar indications, and can be reviewed under the Grin portion of this chapter.

Hollow, sunken cheeks, referred to in Table 7.5, are commonly seen in people with eating disorders, such as anorexia and bulimia.

The buccinator muscle in Figure 7.29 lies deep within the cheek area. If balanced, it holds food in the mouth while chewing; when unbalanced, food falls out of the mouth.

TABLE 7.5 SUMMARY: THE CHEEKS

Muscle	Buccinator; compresses the cheeks, expels air between the lips, and aids in chewing food
Emotion	Superior, sour attitude (sucking in the cheeks like on a lemon), affection/playfulness (blowing a kiss to a loved one)
Lines/wrinkles	Vertical wrinkle from St-5 Daying Great Receptacle up the cheeks, sunken cheeks
Origin	At the level of the maxilla and mandible near the molar teeth
Insertion	Muscle fibers that intermingle with the orbicularis oris at the corner of the mouth
Needling techniques	Use a 30 mm, 38 or 36 gauge needle (#2 or #3 Japanese)
Needling (origin)	Needle St-7 Xiaguan Below the Joint perpendicularly, 0.3–0.5 cun, then transversely toward the muscle's insertion, lateral to the corner of the mouth
Needling (insertion)	Needle a special point 1 cun lateral to St-4 Dicang Earth's Granary, 0.3–0.5 cun perpendicularly, and then transversely toward St-7 Xiaguan Below the Joint
Point location/indications (origin)	St-7 Xiaguan, Below the Joint, is located, with the mouth closed, in the depression anterior to the condyloid process of the jaw. It treats bruxism, TMJ, lockjaw, trigeminal neuralgia, facial paralysis and deafness
Point location/indications (insertion)	The special point 1 cun later to St-4 Dicang Earth's Granary has similar indications to St-4 Dicang (see The Grin section in this chapter)

6. The Laugh

The zygomaticus major muscle draws the corners of the mouth outward and upwards, as in a laugh. This is not just a smile, but a spontaneous belly laugh that fosters joy and delight. Right now, if you were to draw the corners of your mouth outward toward your ears, showing your teeth, while simultaneously exclaiming "Aha" several times, you would probably laugh out loud!

Even though you might feel silly doing this laughing exercise, the Shen would still dance and shine from your eyes.

Emotion
The act of moving the zygomaticus major muscle while making the accompanying sound engages the emotion of joy and encourages the expression of laughter.

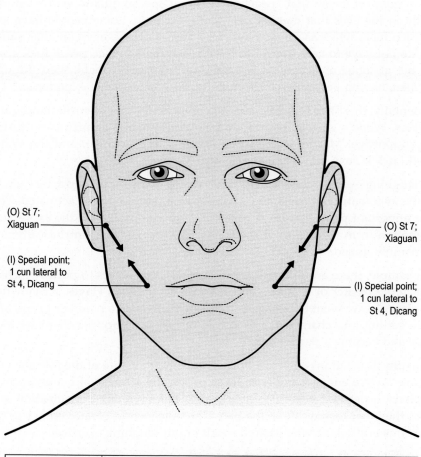

(O) St 7;
Xiaguan

(I) Special point;
1 cun lateral to
St 4, Dicang

(O) St 7;
Xiaguan

(I) Special point;
1 cun lateral to
St 4, Dicang

Buccinator	Compresses the cheeks, expels air between the lips, as in blowing a trumpet, and aids in mastication (chewing)
Emotions	Disdain, affection, love or self-loathing. Chronic illness, dental work, aging, eating disorders
Origin	Junction of the maxilla and mandible at the level of the molar teeth
Insertion	Muscle fibers at the angle of the mouth that blend with the orbicularis oris
Needling	30 mm; 38 or 36 gauge (Japanese #2 or #3), 0.3–0.5 cun

Figure 7.29 Needling diagram: The Cheeks.

If a patient has difficulty laughing, there usually is an imbalance in the zygomaticus muscle, as well as in the Fire element, because they may exhibit very little sparkle or Shen in the eyes. According to Lillian Bridges in *Face Reading in Chinese Medicine*, this glitter relates to "Sparkling Peach Luck" which is "pure fire energy at its brightest. People who have this kind of peach luck are seen as fun, comical, charming and delightful … They laugh and smile easily, their eyes are bright, and their smiles are huge."

233

Lillian goes on to say that "peach luck is that special quality expressed primarily in the eyes that magnetizes others to you … Some people have lots of peach luck, whereas others have very little. Luckily, everyone has some. You do not have to be beautiful to have peach luck. In fact, peach luck gives you the glamour of beauty. It is a show of your spirit manifested through the Shen, having been filtered through the Five Elements of experience."[7]

Elementally, this Shen has different appearances; the Fire element dances and sparkles, Wood's gaze is intense, probing and direct, the Earth is nurturing and supportive, Metal's look can be dreamy and sensitive, and the Water Peach Luck is sexy, seductive and soulful.[8]

The laughing exercise connects the outer world to the inner world; by exercising the zygomaticus muscle, the emotions or inner life can be activated. This is an important point that bears repeating: we cannot divorce the expression of emotion from the action of the facial muscles. They are intrinsically and inseparably linked.

For example, there are different techniques used by actors to portray a character in the theater or in film. The American actor Helen Hayes, a renowned thespian, always went backstage before a performance to hold her props, and while getting into character and putting on her makeup, the character took shape and became a part of her.

These physical actions connected her to the emotional life of the role she was playing. Active engagement with these props, the artifacts of her character's imaginary existence, served to spark Ms. Hayes' creative imagination and evoke the inner feeling life of the part. The outer world connected her to the inner; this is similar to the desired result of our laughing exercise.

Conversely, the Stanislavsky Method encourages the actor to first produce the feelings of the character, and then the inner world informs the outer reality. It doesn't really matter whether the emotion results from a particular neurochemical response, or whether it is triggered by an exercise involving intention and muscle movements.

Therefore, an exercise of this kind, especially when it targets the expressive muscles of the face, is very effective for toning the facial muscles and for lifting the spirits.

Lines and Wrinkles

Zygomaticus lines, wrinkles, crevices and pouches form vertically to the muscle when a person is unhappy and does not laugh. The muscle then loses its tonicity and droops around the SI-18 Quanliao Cheek Bone Hole area directly under the cheek bones.

If the skin is dry, the hormones are unbalanced, or the person is extremely suntanned or smokes, vertical lines will form from SI-18 Quanliao Cheek Bone Hole down to St-6 Jiache Jawbone.

Often, the corners of the mouth have been turned down for a long time and the cheekbones do not look lifted and sculpted. If this is the case, the cheeks sag and eventually form jowls. Additionally, with the mouth turned down in a sad expression, lines form vertically at the corners. There is little light emanating from their eyes – no joy or a Shen-less look, as in a person who has suffered loss.

Origin

The origin of the muscle is in the anterior portion of the zygomatic bone. This is the area that, when needled, gives a look of higher cheek bones. But, without attending to the muscle structure, this area will not look lifted. Also, laughter on a regular basis helps keeps this muscle toned.

Insertion

The insertion is found in the skin at the corner of the mouth, where it mingles with the orbicularis oris muscle.

Needling Techniques

Use a 30 mm, 38 or 36 gauge needle (#2 or #3 Japanese) to traverse this larger area on the face. Remember to needle the origin and then the insertion of each muscle, bilaterally, on the face.

Origin: The origin of the muscle is needled first at SI-18 Quanliao Cheek Bone Hole perpendicularly, 0.3–0.5 cun, and then transversely toward the mouth.

Insertion: The insertion of the muscle is in the skin at the corner of the mouth St-4 Dicang Earth's Granary. Insert the needle perpendicularly, then angle it transversely toward the cheek bones, its point of origin. Make sure that you complete the circuit by needling the origin and insertion of the muscle on the same side, then bilaterally.

Needling the origin and insertion sculpts the cheeks and lifts the zygomaticus muscle, as well as the corners of the mouth.

Point Location and Indications

SI-18 Quanliao Cheek Bone Hole is located below the outer canthus of the eye at the lower border of the zygomatic arch. The indications for this point have been covered in the Smile portion of this chapter

SI-18 Quanliao Cheek Bone Hole is related to the Fire element, and when needled, it releases heat in the cheek area. If this point bleeds after needling, it may be releasing old heat and blood. Do not assume that it will bruise because it is bleeding.

St-4 Dicang is called Earth's Granary because it is situated at the corner of the mouth, which receives food for nourishment into the body, and represents earthly Qi.

TABLE 7.6 SUMMARY: THE LAUGH	
Muscle	Zygomaticus; draws the corners of the mouth outward toward the ears, and upward, as in a laugh
Emotion	Joy, laughter, or a sad, Shen-less look
Lines/wrinkles	Vertical lines and pouches from St-6 Jiache Jawbone up to SI-18 Qianliao Cheek Bone Hole; sagging cheekbones, which lead to jowls
Origin	Anterior part of the zygomatic bone
Insertion	Skin at the corner of the mouth
Needling techniques	Use a 30 mm, 38 or 36 gauge needle (#2 or #3 Japanese)
Needling (origin)	Needle SI-18 Qianliao Cheek Bone Hole perpendicularly 0.3–0.5 cun, then transversely down toward the mouth
Needling (insertion)	Needle St-4 Dicang Earth's Granary perpendicularly 0.3–0.5 cun, then transversely up toward the cheekbone area
Point location/indications (origin)	SI-18 Qianliao is located directly below the outer canthus of the eye in the depression at the lower border of the zygomatic bone. The indications have been covered in The Smile portion of this chapter
Point location/indications (insertion)	St-4 Dicang Earth's Granary is located 0.4 cun lateral to the corner of the mouth. The indications can be found in The Grin section of this chapter

The Fire element is the Mother of Earth in the Five Element generation cycle, and it is important for healthy digestion, not only of food, but also the assimilation of ideas and emotional states.

In Table 7.6, the zygomaticus muscle functionally facilitates laughter, which brightens the Shen, eases tension, and supports 'healthy aging.'

Treating the Laugh in Figure 7.30 lifts and sculpts the cheek bones. It is not necessary to needle SI-18 Quanliao Cheek Bone Hole upward to achieve this desired effect, when using the origin/insertion of the muscle.

7. Crow's Feet

The muscle used to treat crow's feet is the temporoparietalis, which tightens the scalp and draws back the skin of the temples. It is what we call an artifact muscle – like the appendix, it is not considered necessary for our modern day anatomy. When this muscle weakens or becomes inflexible, it creates wrinkles at the corners of the eyes. The temporoparietalis is a small muscle that fans out over the temples and lies under the larger temporalis muscle.

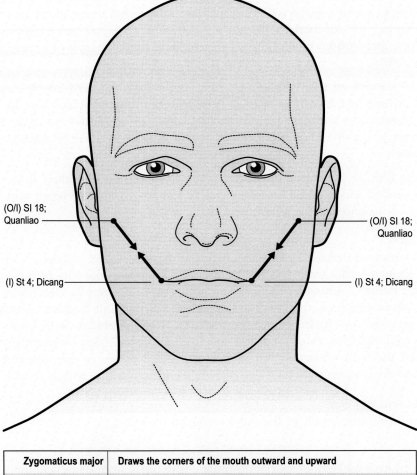

(O/I) SI 18; Quanliao

(O/I) SI 18; Quanliao

(I) St 4; Dicang

(I) St 4; Dicang

Zygomaticus major	Draws the corners of the mouth outward and upward
Emotions	Joy, laughter; joyless, Shen-less
Origin	In the anterior portion of the zygomatic bone
Insertion	In the skin at the angle of the mouth, mingling with the orbicularis oris
Needling	30 mm; 38 (#2 Japanese) or 36 (#3 Japanese), 0.3–0.5 cun

Figure 7.30 Needling diagram: The Laugh.

I always ask acupuncturists who attend my seminars which of them can wiggle their ears. This is a talent that has been lost in most people, and strangely enough, it seems to prevent the development of crow's feet.

In pre-historic times, we human beings needed to be more vigilant about unexpected noises and sounds in order to ensure our survival. It is possible that our ancestors' ears might have cocked like a spaniel's do when it hears a bird, so it can flush the bird out of the marshes.

As more highly developed *Homo sapiens*, we have lost some of our primal abilities to survive in the wild. But we have adapted to living in urban environments. Our survival challenges are different. Now we must cope with negative perceptions of aging, peer pressure and rigid concepts of beauty and desirability.

I have discovered that people who can wiggle their ears have fewer crow's feet, or lines at the corners of their eyes. It doesn't matter what their age is! Of course, there are other factors, such as exposure to ultraviolet light, skin dryness, or habitual squinting – factors that are exacerbated by sunny, dry climates.

Gentle lines at the corners of the eyes are desirable because they show we have smiled and laughed, but deep crow's feet are usually the result of more severe imbalances in the temporoparietalis muscle.

Emotion

This muscle is defined more by its function than a specific emotion, because it is located in the scalp and not on the face. However, the side of the head relates to the Gall Bladder meridian and the temporalis muscle. Because of its location in this area, the emotional landscape of the Gall Bladder, which is characterized by frustration, anger, resentment and problems with decision-making, might be considered relevant to this muscle. I have certainly witnessed the frustration and impatience of my colleagues as they attempt to engage the temporoparietalis muscle, while endeavoring to wiggle their ears!

Lines and Wrinkles

Lines form horizontally at the outer corner of the eyes.

Origin

The origin of the temporoparietalis muscle is in the temporal fascia above and anterior to the ear.

Insertion

The insertion is in the temporal fascia at the side of the head.

Needling Techniques

Needle the scalp, using a 30 mm or 40 mm, 36–32 gauge needle in order to engage this muscle, 0.3–0.5 cun.

Origin and insertion: GB-7 Qubin Temporal Hairline Curve; needle transversely back toward the scalp and up toward GB-8 Shuaigou Valley Lead, 0.3–0.5 cun.

Because we are engaging both the skin of the pre-auricular hairline and the galea aponeurotica, it is possible to address both the origin and insertion of the muscle with a single needle. It is not necessary to use two needles; needling the scalp is very powerful and effective.

Point Location and Indications

GB-7 Qubin Temporal Hairline Curve is just above the posterior border of the pre-auricular hairline, about one finger's breadth anterior to TH-20 Jiaosun Angle Vertex, just above the vertex of the ear. GB-7 Qubin Temporal Hairline Curve benefits the jaw, eliminates wind, and treats facial paralysis, Bell's palsy, trismus, temporal pain and headache, temporomandibular joint dysfunction, and lockjaw.

GB-8 Shuaigou Valley Lead is above the apex of the ear, 1 cun above TH-20 Jiaosun Angle Vertex. It is a good local point for migraine headaches; it clears wind, Liver Yang Rising, Liver fire, and treats tinnitus, deafness, dizziness, vertigo, vomiting, convulsions, facial paralysis and eye disorders.

Psychospiritually, it aids in grounding the patient in order to assimilate information, to calm anxiety, and alleviate acute and chronic childhood fear. It also treats addictions, alcoholism and obsessive–compulsive disorder.

Crow's feet, or lines at the corners of the eye, are not only caused by sun exposure, dry, or aged skin, but also by an imbalance in the temporoparietalis muscle. See Table 7.7.

TABLE 7.7   SUMMARY: CROW'S FEET

Muscle	Temporoparietalis; tightens the scalp, and draws back the skin of the temples
Emotion	Relates to the Gall Bladder channel and can express anger and frustration
Lines/wrinkles	Horizontal lines at the outer canthus of the eye
Origin	In the fascia of the temples in front of and above the ear
Insertion	In the fascia of the temples at the side of the head
Needling techniques	Use a 30 or 40 mm, 36–32 gauge needle (#3–#5 Japanese)
Needling (origin and insertion)	Needle GB-7 Qubin Temporal Hairline Curve transversely back and up toward GB-8 Shuaigou Valley Lead, 0.3–0.5 cun
Point location/indications (origin)	GB-7 Qubin Temporal Hairline Curve is located just above the posterior border of the pre-auricular hairline, just anterior to TH-20 Jiaosun Angle Vertex. It benefits the jaw, treats TMJ, temporal pain and headache, and facial paralysis
Point location/indications (insertion)	GB-8 Shuaigou Valley Lead is 1 cun above the apex of the ear; it treats migraine headaches, tinnitus, deafness, convulsions, facial paralysis and eye imbalances

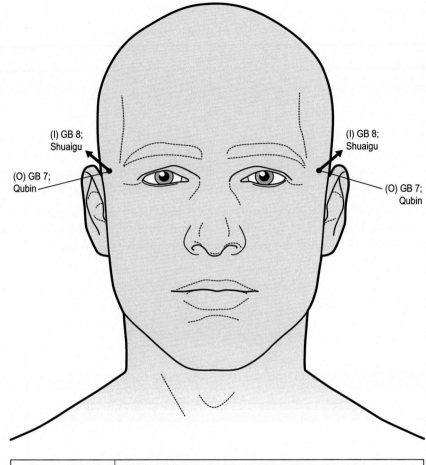

Temporoparietalis	Tightens the scalp and draws back the skin of the temples
Emotions	Associated with the Gall Bladder; frustration, anger, resentment
Origin	In the temporal fascia above and anterior to the ear
Insertion	In the temporal fascia at the side of the head
Needling	30 or 40 mm; 38 gauge (#2 Japanese) or 36 (#3 Japanese), 0.3–0.5 cun

Figure 7.31 Needling diagram: Crow's Feet.

In Figure 7.31, needling GB-7 Qubin Temporal Hairline Curve transversely up toward to GB-8 Shuaigou Valley Lead in the scalp not only treats crow's feet, and also wind and facial paralysis.

8. *Eye Bags*

In my seminars, I am fond of saying that all eye bags are not created equal. Some of them are Gucci, some Pucci, while others are Samsonite. Bags under the eyes are like suitcases, because we carry them with us wherever we travel in life. They have a particular elemental class, quality and connection to our genetics, lifestyle, habits and emotions. The palpebral portion of the orbicularis oculi muscle closes the lower eyelid, as in blinking.

Emotion

Lines or bags under the eyes can indicate grief or sorrow. Puffiness under the eye may indicate unexpressed tears. An involuntary twitch or blink may manifest as wind, which can indicate an aversion to wind and an unwillingness to change. This wind could also signal imminent changes in a patient's life. A twitch can also be a sign of Bell's palsy, windstroke or facial paralysis.

Eye Bags, Lines and Wrinkles

In Chinese physiognomy, several horizontal lines directly under the eyes are called lost love lines. In gently questioning the patient who possesses these lines, I usually discover that they have just broken up with the love of their life, or recently experienced the loss of a loved one. I have seen these lines disappear when a patient comes to terms with the loss.

Pouches, puffiness, dark circles and lines under the eyes are generally part of the landscape of aging, as well as symptoms of imbalance, in this sphincter muscle, which includes both an orbital and a lacrimal component. This large circular muscle also merges and intersects with several other facial muscles.

Eye bags usually have constitutional origins, relating to the Five Elements and the Zang-fu organ systems. By observing the terrain of the lower eyelids in a patient's face, the imbalances in these organs can be diagnosed.

For example, puffy bags without darkness or discoloration under the eyes can relate to systemic damp, the Earth element and the Spleen's transformation and transportation of Qi, blood and fluids.

Non-puffy, dark circles under the eyes can indicate several imbalances; however, if there is no genetic Jing deficiency, they usually relate to the Wood element. Because the Liver stores blood at night when we sleep, these dark circles often appear under the eyes of a patient who burns the candle at both ends, stays up late at night, and doesn't get enough sleep.

The Japanese relate this syndrome to systemic blood stagnation, referred to as *oketsu* or stuck blood. The Liver is not spreading and storing the blood properly, which congests the Qi and blood. A panda bear look, with dark circles around the entire eye, can indicate that hepatitis has affected both the Liver and Spleen or an inherited Jing deficiency. I always ask a patient if they were born with the dark circles and whether anyone in their family also had dark circles. Usually both Kidney pulses are deficient, and there are signs and symptoms of adrenal exhaustion. This differentiates Wood element dark circles from those relating to the Water element.

In my experience, dark circles that are also puffy can indicate Kidney deficiency. It takes time for the Kidneys in a basically healthy person to become deficient. As we age, the Kidney function declines, if we have not fortified ourselves with longevity tonics, diet, exercise, acupuncture, massage, herbs, rest and a positive outlook on life.

My observations are not judgments, but part of the Four Exams in Chinese Medicine. I substantiate my findings with diagnostics using tongue, pulse, hara and palpation techniques. Do not assume that all eye bags are the same; I encourage you to be curious, and discern for yourselves the root causes of these facial syndromes.

Origin
The origin is in the palpebral portion of the muscle, from the palpebral ligament.

Insertion
The insertion of the muscle is located in the palpebral fibers that interlace at the lateral angle of the eye.

Needling Techniques
In needling Qiuhou M-HN-8, first locate the anatomical landmark, an indentation in the lower orbital ridge of the eye, which is the exact area to be needled. I generally palpate and locate Qiuhou M-HN-8 before I needle within the orbital ridge. Use a 30 mm, 40 gauge needle (#1 Japanese).

I do not needle this point while the patient closes their eyes, and rolls them back into their head, as is indicated in most acupuncture manuals. While I understand the principle involved, I find this unnecessary. Instead, I have the patient keep their eyes closed while I insert the needle gently and superficially, straight down toward the treatment table. I carefully extract and discard the tube, and slowly continue to needle straight down. Since I cannot be sure prior to needling this point how much room there is between the eye orbit and the eye itself, I explore the space gently, until I feel that I have reached the spatial limit.

In my experience, the right and left sides of the face are asymmetrical, and consequently the space within the eye orbit is not the same. Therefore, I do not assume that Qiuhou M-HN-8 will be needled to the same depth for both eyes.

Origin and insertion: The origin and insertion are the same. Use a larger 30 mm 40 gauge #1 Japanese. I use a longer needle because I don't know how deeply I can insert a needle into the two Qiuhou M-HN-8 points.

CAUTION

If you have not needled this point before, please seek out supervision from an experienced practitioner. When you remove the needle, hold the point with a cotton ball for thirty seconds to prevent bruising.

TABLE 7.8   SUMMARY: EYE BAGS

Muscle	The palpebral portion of the orbicularis oculi muscle closes the lower eyelids, as in blinking
Emotion	Grief, sorrow
Lines/wrinkles	Horizontal lines directly under the eyes, puffy bags, dark circles under the eyes
Origin	In the palpebral part of the muscle
Insertion	The palpebral fibers at the lateral angle under the eye
Needling techniques	Use a 30 mm, 40 gauge needle (#1 Japanese)
Needling (origin and insertion)	Carefully, slowly, needle Qiuhou M-HN-8 Behind the Ball transversely down toward the massage table
Point location/ indications	Qiuhou is located lateral to St-1 Chengqi Tear Container, and is found at the lower border of the eye orbit at the later and medial ¾ of the infrorbital margin. It disperses puffiness, inflammation and stagnation under the eye, treats glaucoma and optic nerve atrophy

Point Locations and Indications

The extra point Qiuhou M-HN-8 is located lateral to St-1 Chengqi Tear Container at the lower border of the eye orbit at the lateral ¼ and medial ¾ of the infraorbital margin.

Qiuhou M-HN-8 benefits the eye and treats all eye diseases, such as glaucoma, optic nerve atrophy and shortsightedness. It also disperses puffiness, inflammation and stagnation under the eye.

The area within the eye orbit shown in Table 7.8 treats eye bags, as well as ocular computer stress syndrome (OCSS) with eye inflammation, headaches, stress and irritability.

The right and left sides of the face in Figure 7.32 are not symmetrical, nor are the spaces between the eye and the eye orbit the same. Needle the extra point Qiuhou, for eye bags, slowly and carefully.

9.   Droopy Eyelids/Sagging Eyebrows

Most patients have an aversion to saggy eyelids, and women in particular are horrified to see that they are inheriting their mother's droopy eyelids! The muscle involved is the orbital portion of the orbicularis oculi muscle. The orbital branch arches around the upper eyelids within the orbital muscle fibers, and forcibly closes the eyelids as in winking an eye.

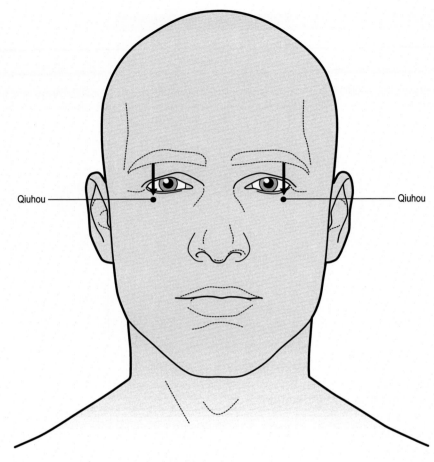

Qiuhou — — Qiuhou

Orbicularis oculi	The palpebral portion which closes the lower eyelids, as in blinking
Emotions	Grief, stress; wind in the eyes; aversion to change. This is also linked to internal imbalances
Origin/insertion	(O) the palpebral part of the muscle, from the palpebral ligament; (I) the palpebral fibers that interlace at the lateral angle of the eye
Needling	30 mm; 40 gauge (#1 Japanese)

Figure 7.32   Needling diagram: Eye Bags.

Emotion

Emotionally, the eyebrows can lower in sadness, disappointment, sleepiness, disagreement, disapproval, disgust, dread or worry. However, droopy eyelids can also result from constitutional disharmony; usually the Spleen Qi is deficient, and the muscle is prolapsing. Droopy eyelids can also result from chronic worry, which damages the Spleen. One syndrome feeds the other – as we discussed earlier – the Shen leads the Qi.

Lines and Wrinkles

I have discovered that when the entire scalp or galea aponeurotica is tense from the frontalis muscle to the occipitalis muscle, the eyebrows will sag because the scalp is tight and there is no balance in the tonicity of the muscle.

This imbalance can also cause chronic sinus problems, due to systemic puffiness of the upper eyelids, the result of constitutional Spleen/Earth or Lung/Metal imbalances.

Needling Techniques

Origin: An extra point, Upper Shangming Upper Brightness is needled transversely upward 0.2 cun under the eyebrow toward the extra point YuYao M-HN-6.

Insertion: GB-14 Yangbai Yang White is needled transversely downward 0.2 cun toward YuYao M-HN-6.

To needle Upper Shangming Upper Brightness effectively, have your patient close their eyes, and locate Upper Shangming under YuYao M-HN-6 on the superciliary arch of the eyebrows. If the eyebrows are sagging over Upper Shangming, hold the brow up with your non-dominant hand so you can needle this point. Make sure that you first locate the foramen under the superciliary arch. Release the needle from the tube, hold up the eyebrow, and needle this point upwards transversely with your dominant hand while still holding the eyebrow up. It is important to needle transversely, not obliquely, because this area is very shallow and delicate.

One of the keys to successfully needling this point is to hold the needle with your thumb and index finger on each side of the needle. Do not hold it vertically, above and below the needle. Holding the needle on the sides facilitates an easier, more transverse insertion, because your fingers will not be in the way of the needle.

The eyebrow areas will be different, and both must be needled. The needling technique is delicate, which can make it difficult. I always demonstrate this technique in my seminars before students practice it, because this area can bruise easily and the technique is unusual.

Point Locations and Indications

Origin: Upper Shangming Upper Brightness is an extra point located in the indentation directly under the eyebrow below YuYao M-HN-6. It is used to lift droopy, hooded eyelids, so that the patient can see not only physically, but also psychospiritually. It can also disperse puffiness and damp in this area, but these conditions must be addressed constitutionally as well.

Insertion: GB-14 Yangbai Yang White is located one cun directly above the middle of the eyebrow, and above the pupil of the eye when one is looking straight ahead. It eliminates wind, and therefore treats facial paralysis, Liver

TABLE 7.9   SUMMARY: DROOPY EYELIDS

Muscle	The orbital portion of the orbicularis oculi muscle, which closes the upper eyelids as in winking
Emotion	Worry, sadness, disapproval, disappointment
Lines/wrinkles	Sagging, puffy upper eyelids
Origin	The orbital portion of the medial orbital eye margin
Insertion	The orbital fibers that arch around the upper eyelids
Needling techniques	Use a 15 mm, 40 gauge needle (#1 Japanese)
Needling (origin)	Needle Upper Shangming transversely up into the indentation directly under the eyebrow below YuYao M-HN-6, 0.2 cun
Needling (insertion)	Needle GB-14 Yangbai Yang White transversely down toward YuYao M-HN-6, 0.2 cun
Point location/indications (origin)	The extra point Upper Shangming is in the indentation directly under the eyebrow below YuYao M-HN-6. It lifts droopy eyelids, disperses puffiness and allows the patient to see
Point location/indications (insertion)	GB-14 Yangbai Yang White is 1 cun directly above the middle of the eyebrow; it treats facial paralysis, unilateral headaches, droopy and twitching eyelids, and clears vision

Yang Rising, unilateral headaches, droopy eyelids, clears the vision, treats twitching eyelids and Bell's palsy.

Psychospiritually, it encourages decision-making, clarity and calmness, and clears the Wood element.

Hooded, sagging eyelids may be genetic and related to constitutional imbalances in Taiyin, Spleen and Lung meridians. See Table 7.9.

For sagging eyebrows in Figure 7.33, check the three anatomical landmarks or indentations above and below the eyebrow. Upper Shangming Upper Brightness is below the eyebrow, YuYao is in the middle, and GB-14 Yangbai Yang White is above the eyebrow.

10.   The Frown

The frown lines between the eyebrows are customarily the first facial wrinkles to be Botoxed by cosmetic surgeons. The corrugator supercilii muscle, which draws the eyebrows down to produce this frown, is one of the most injected sites on the face.

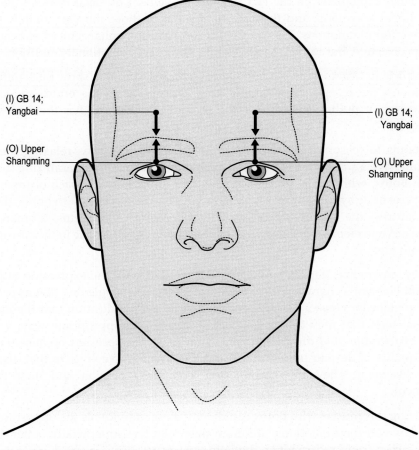

(I) GB 14;
Yangbai

(O) Upper
Shangming

(I) GB 14;
Yangbai

(O) Upper
Shangming

Orbicularis oculi	The orbital portion, which arches around the upper eyelid within the orbital muscle fibers, and closes the eyelids, as in winking
Emotions	Sadness, disappointment, disapproval, dread, worry
Origin	The orbital portion which emanates from the medial orbital eye margin
Insertion	The orbital fibers which arch around the upper eyelid
Needling	15 mm; 40 gauge (#1 Japanese), 0.2 cun

Figure 7.33 Needling diagram: Droopy Eyelids.

A Maryland dermatologist, Eric Finzi M.D., had noticed that a number of clinically depressed patients had noticeable glabellar wrinkles. Finzi speculated that Botox might be helpful in immobilizing that facial muscle and preventing the depressed patients from frowning. In a study of 10 women, Finzi found that nine of them no longer exhibited symptoms of depression 2 months following Botox injections.[9] None of the study participants had previously responded to standard treatments for depression, i.e. psychotherapy and/or drug treatments.

247

Dr. Finzi capitalized on the fact that the movement of facial muscles elicits emotional responses, and that immobilization of those muscles inhibits the expression of emotions. This study did not have the enhancement of beauty as its objective, but rather the alleviation of a psychoemotional condition.

An article in *Newsweek* cites a number of similar studies that show that smiling promotes the release of mood-elevating endorphins in the brain, and that frowning, or pulling the corners of the mouth downward, has the opposite effect.[10]

It stands to reason that needling the frown lines, and thus relaxing them, would have a similar effect on facial expression and mood as paralyzing them with Botox, without the toxic chemicals. The allopathic approach of treating the presenting symptom, which, in this case is the frown line, with Botox, does not address the underlying cause. The underlying cause stems, ultimately, from a Wood element disharmony, and the resulting imbalance in the corrugator muscle.

In my experience, depression masks a discomfort with the expression of the Wood element's characteristic emotion of anger. The single line that appears in the glabellar crease, the 'suspended sword,' is an indication that the individual feels that they cannot connect, in a safe and appropriate way, with their frustration and disappointment. They become depressed because there is a quality of despair in their lives, and they cannot give voice to that disenfranchisement. They are disconnected from their passion and their Fire element.

Freezing this muscle with Botox could deny these individuals the opportunity to transcend their emotions; although they may feel superficially better, the depression could return when the Botox wears off.

I have experienced this to be true in my practice; however, facial acupuncture does not provide an instantaneous result like Botox, but is an organic process that works at a constitutional level, within the flow of a treatment series. Because the face is so expressive, the evocation of emotion and spirit can effect a change not only in the patient's look, but also their *out*look. These treatments are a transformative step toward quality of life and aliveness.

Emotions

The frown can telegraph suffering, anger, frustration, impatience, or deep concentration. In Chinese physiognomy, this area is called the Seat of the Stamp, which relates to the paternal line, and the impact of the father upon his child. And, as previously noted in this chapter, is referred to as a 'suspended sword.'

Lines and Wrinkles

The corrugator supercilii muscle causes vertical lines between the eyebrows, and similar vertical lines upward and across the forehead. The 'suspended sword,' a long deep line between the eyebrows, relates to internalized anger; the person who develops this sort of line on their face usually has difficulty in speaking out and claiming their own voice or personal power. They turn their blame and anger in on themselves.

Two lines between the eyebrows denote damp heat in the Gall Bladder. Since the Gall Bladder is a Yang organ, the characteristic emotions of anger, annoyance and impatience are directed outward toward an external stimulus.

In my practice, I have witnessed the single line of the 'suspended sword' transformed into the twin lines of the Gall Bladder. Even though this denotes progress, the patient who previously suffered in silence now expresses their annoyance outwardly, but has no idea why they are so perturbed. It is a generalized anger, because the feelings have been submerged for so long. Unfortunately, you, as the practitioner, may be the immediate target for these emotions.

In this case, it is important to clarify that you are not responsible for their emotions, and to set boundaries around emotional outbursts. I recommend homework for these patients, such as qigong, martial arts, African or Brazilian dance, with live drumming, vigorous walking, acting classes, voice lessons, and other creative therapies. I also recommend that they consult a therapist, and other healthcare practitioners who may be able to help facilitate their release of old, unconscious frustrations.

When a patient's emotional expression shifts from internalized to externalized anger, it can be disconcerting, both for patient and practitioner. It could be likened to a different outcome to that famous scene from the classic Grimm's fairy tale of Sleeping Beauty: if, after being awakened by the handsome Prince Charming with a loving kiss, instead of melting into his arms, the heroine returns his tenderness with a hard uppercut to his jaw, shouting, "How dare you keep me waiting so long!" he would have no way of seeing that one coming.

However, *you* are now forewarned, and have some knowledge of the potential consequences of awakening frozen Jing in this crucial area between the brows.

I continue to treat patients who are undergoing this particular transition constitutionally, using psychospiritual and Shen points, topical and internal herbal therapies, and of course, facial acupuncture.

This work is transformative, and consciousness shifts may happen rather unexpectedly when you're working with the most emotive part of the body, the face!

Origin
The origin of this muscle is in the medial portion of the supraorbital ridge of the eyebrow.

Insertion

The insertion is in the skin of the medial half of the eyebrow.

Needling Techniques

Use a 15 mm 40 gauge or smaller (#1 Japanese) to needle into the eyebrow area. Since this is a very sensitive area, with little flesh over the bone, it is usually not necessary to use a thicker, longer gauge needle. However, if the patient has a large, wide brow area, and is fleshy, you will need to use a longer, thicker needle.

Origin: Needle the extra point, YuYao M-HN-6 transversely toward the medial aspect of the eyebrow; the depth of insertion is 0.2–0.3 cun, since, as previously noted, this is not usually a particularly fleshy area of the face.

Insertion: Needle Bl-2 Zanzhu Collecting Bamboo ring transversely toward YuYao M-HN-6; once again, the needle depth is 0.2–0.3 cun.

Point Locations and Indications

YuYao M-HN-6 is an extra point located in the center of eyebrow, in the depression directly above the pupil of the eye when the individual is looking straight ahead.

YuYao benefits the eyes, calms redness, swelling, eye pain, twitching eyelids, frontal headaches and supraorbital pain.

Bl-2 Zanzhu Collecting Bamboo, is located in the medial extremity of the eyebrow. It expels wind, brightens the eyes, soothes the Liver, treats redness and twitching, clears the head, treats manic–depressive behavior and loss of consciousness.

According to the ancient Chinese, when bamboo is harvested and bound, the resulting arrangement resembles a large eyebrow.

Some patients frown (Table 7.10) because it gives them an intense quality and concentration skills that they need in their lives. Please honor their choice to keep the vertical wrinkles between their eyebrows.

In treating The Frown in Figure 7.34, remember that there is very little flesh on the eyebrows; needle transversely into the points to save your patient from discomfort.

11.   The Forehead

According to Western medicine, the frontalis muscle raises the forehead in fright, shock and surprise, and wrinkles the skin on the forehead horizontally.

Emotions

In Chinese medicine, raising the eyebrows and wrinkling the forehead is a sign of disturbed Shen characterized by fire and heat rising to this part of the face.

TABLE 7.10 SUMMARY: THE FROWN

Muscle	Corrugator supercilii; draws the eyebrows down medially to produce a frown
Emotion	Frustration, impatience, anger, suffering
Lines/wrinkles	Vertical lines between the eyebrows
Origin	The medial part of the eyebrow
Insertion	In the skin of the medial half of the eyebrow
Needling techniques	Use a 15 mm, 40 gauge needle (#1 Japanese)
Needling (origin)	Needle the extra point YuYao M-HN-6 transversely toward the medial part of the eyebrow, 0.2–0.3 cun
Needling (insertion)	Needle Bl-2 Zanzhu Collecting Bamboo transversely toward YuYao M-HN-6, 0.2–0.3 cun
Point location/indications (origin)	YuYao M-HN-6 is located in the center of the eyebrow. It calms eye swelling, redness and pain, as well as twitching eyelids, and treats frontal headaches
Point location/indications (insertion)	Bl-2 Zanzhu Collecting Bamboo is located in the medial extremity of the eyebrow. It treats eye redness and twitching, soothes Liver Qi and manic-depression

Lines and Wrinkles

Many years after prolonged stress or a traumatic event, people still habitually wear their fright and surprise on their foreheads, etched there in the form of horizontal lines, wrinkles and muscle tension. These muscles are referred to as myotatic units because they both insert into the scalp and synergistically affect muscle movement. Therefore, the bellies of the frontalis and occipitalis muscles function in tandem with each other, and any contracture or habitual wrinkling of the forehead can cause tension, headaches and pain in the occipital and cervical areas of the head and neck.

Since all the Yang meridians rise up to the face and head, especially the Bladder, Gall Bladder and Stomach meridians, which traverse the forehead area, it is important to anchor and ground the Yang constitutionally before needling. This prevents unwanted headaches, hot flashes, hypertension, anxiety, shallow breathing and disturbed Shen.

For this reason, do not thread all the lines in the forehead in a single treatment.

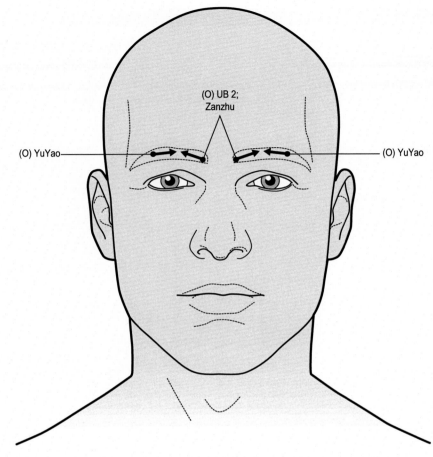

(O) UB 2; Zanzhu

(O) YuYao

(O) YuYao

Corrugator supercilii	Draws eyebrows downward and medially
Emotions	Suffering, anger, concentration, frustration, impatience, depression
Origin	Medial part of the supraorbital ridge
Insertion	Skin of medial half of the eyebrow
Needling	15 mm; 40 gauge or smaller (#1 Japanese), 0.2–0.3 cun

Figure 7.34 Needling diagram: The Frown.

Origin
The origin of the frontalis muscle is in the epicranial aponeurosis, at the level of the coronal suture.

Insertion
The insertion is on the forehead above the eyebrows. In treating forehead lines, it is important to discern the level of tension in the entire scalp, the galea aponeurotica. The galea aponeurotica covers the frontalis forehead muscle and occipitalis muscle at the back of the head.

Remember that the Shen leads the Qi, and that thought and emotions are the precursors to muscle movement, which, in turn, causes the lifting of the forehead in fright and surprise. This is why I use Shen and psychospiritual points constitutionally in the treatment of my patients.

Unresolved trauma can lodge in the forehead from an event that happened many years prior to their initial Constitutional Facial Acupuncture treatment. Being aware of this stored muscle memory is very important for the efficacy of the facial acupuncture treatments.

We are fortunate that Chinese medicine treats the entire person on all levels, and that we, as acupuncturists are facilitators of this evolutionary process, not only for our patients but also for ourselves.

Needling Techniques

This area above the eyebrow only requires a 15 mm 40 gauge needle, or smaller (#1 Japanese). If you are treating an Earth element type, with the characteristic thick skin, then you will need a 30 mm, 38 or 36 gauge needle (#2 or #3 Japanese). Use your judgment; you do not need to inflict unnecessary pain upon your patient with this protocol to effect a change in the facial terrain.

Origin: GB-14 Yangbai Yang White is needled transversely at a depth of 0.2–0.3 cun, toward the lateral end of the eyebrow.

Insertion: TH-23 Sizhukong Silk Bamboo Hollow is also needled transversely toward GB-14 Yangbai, 0.2–0.3 cun. Needle both the origin and insertion for one eyebrow, before moving on to the other eyebrow, to complete the circuit. Do not wait too long, talk to your patient before you complete this process. Taking too long to complete the treatment can disturb the Shen if 1) the patient's Yang is not sufficiently grounded with constitutional treatment points; or 2) the right and left hemispheres of the brain are not balanced by the needling of both sides of the face in a timely fashion.

Point Locations and Indications

GB-14 Yangbai Yang White is located directly above the midpoint of the eyebrow. The point indications for have been previously discussed in this chapter under the section on Droopy Eye and Sagging Eyebrow.

TH-23 Sizhukong Silk Bamboo Hollow, is in the depression at the lateral end of the eyebrow. It treats facial paralysis, headache around the eyes, blurred vision, pain, redness, and twitching of the eyelids.

Psychospiritually, Silk Bamboo Hollow directs Shen inward, and is good for people defined solely by their outer relationships. It warms the Spirit and helps to make individuals less superficial, more authentic and heart-centered in their behavior toward others.

Silk is precious, like Spirit, and a Hollow provides access to an interior space where people can become more self-reflective. If there is insanity, this essence

TABLE 7.11 SUMMARY: THE FOREHEAD

Muscle	Frontalis; raises the eyebrows and wrinkles the skin of the forehead
Emotion	Fright, surprise, anxiety
Lines/wrinkles	Horizontal lines across the forehead
Origin	The epicranial aponeurosis, at the coronal suture
Insertion	In the skin of the frontal area above the eyebrows
Needling techniques	Use a 15 mm, 40 gauge needle (#1 Japanese)
Needling (origin)	Needle GB-14 Yangbai Yang White transversely 0.2–0.3 cun toward the lateral end of the eyebrow
Needling (insertion)	Needle TH-23 Sizhukong Silk Bamboo Hollow transversely 0.2–0.3 cun toward GB-14 Yangbai Yang White
Point location/indications (origin)	GB-14 Yangbai Yang White is located above the midpoint of the eyebrow; see point indications in the Droopy Eyelids/Sagging Eyebrow portion of this chapter
Point location/indications (insertion)	TH-23 Sizhukong Silk Bamboo Hollow is in the depression at the lateral end of the eyebrow. It treats blurry eyes, pain, redness, twitching eyelids, facial paralysis and headache. Psychospiritually, the hollow directs the Shen inward, consolidating essence back to the Kidneys

needs to be warmed, because these patients manifest both internal cold and external heat.

Be careful treating lines and tension on the foreheads of patients with hypertension, because the Yang could rise and disturb the Shen (Table 7.11).

When needling the forehead in Figure 7.35, use St-44 Neiting Inner Court to constitutionally anchor and prevent wind and heat from rising to the face.

12. The Neck

The platysma is a long quadrangular muscle which contracts and pulls the corners of the mouth down, raises the skin of the chest, and wrinkles the neck horizontally. It is located in the fascia of the upper pectoralis and deltoideus muscles, and extends up the length of the neck, under the chin, to the angle of the mouth.

It is so thin that a pathologist will peel it away immediately during the dissection of a cadaver. Despite its apparent fragility, the platysma is a significant structural aspect of the facial musculature, which means that it can be toned and lifted with Constitutional Facial Acupuncture treatments.

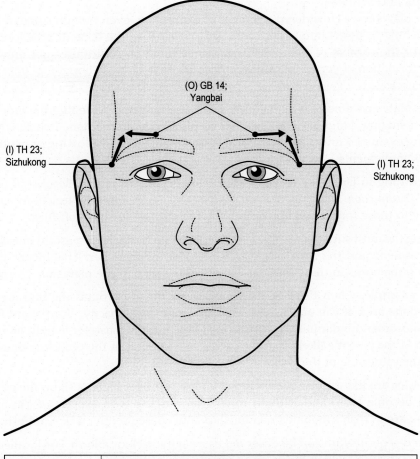

Frontalis	Raises the eyebrows in fright or surprise and wrinkles the forehead
Emotions	Fright, shock, surprise; disturbed Shen
Origin	In the epicranial aponeurosis, at the level of the coronal suture
Insertion	In the skin of the frontal region above the eyebrows
Needling	15 mm; 40 or 38 gauge (#1 or #2 Japanese), 0.2–0.3 cun

Figure 7.35 Needling diagram: The Forehead.

Emotion

Its emotional repertoire includes anxiety, sadness, grief, dissatisfaction, suffering and irony, and even horror. Lying in the subcutaneous fascia of the lower face and neck, these fibers intermingle with the orbicularis oris muscle, which encircles the mouth. They also attach to the corners of the mouth, and blend with other facial muscles, such as the depressors, both labii and inferioris, which depress the mouth and lower lip to exhibit irony and deep grief.

Lines and Wrinkles

The platysma is considered a muscle of expression, even though some of the attachments insert into superficial fascia rather than the bone. It functions to lower the corners of the mouth, and, consequently, contributes not only to the formation of vertical wrinkles in that location, but also horizontal lines on the neck.

The platysma muscle is active only when opening and widening the mouth, as in singing, laughing and also, not so pleasantly, in the dental chair when being examined or drilled. It is not actively involved in swallowing or in other neck movements.

According to Dr. Janet Travell in her book on trigger points, *Myofascial Pain and Dysfunction: The Trigger Point Manual, Vol. 1*, this muscle functions similarly to those found in a horse's neck, which it uses to shake off flies.[11]

Being the most superficial muscle, it overlays the sternocleidomastoid muscles, the scalene and the mastication muscles, like the masseter. This means that any imbalances in these muscles can affect the tone of the platysma.

For example, when there is a tight masseter muscle around the St-6 Jiache Jawbone area, it can affect the platysma's tone and tenacity. If a patient has temporomandibular joint dysfunction (TMJ), and the masseter is tight on one side of the jaw, it's likely that they will have sagging in the platysma muscle on the same side of the neck.

Muscles are like rubber bands. If one end of a rubber band is tight, the other will become loose and without tone. The muscle's twin aspects of Yin and Yang are in disharmonious relationship and, consequently, lack equilibrium.

This disequilibrium can be observed as a saggy neck or a loose cord, called a 'turkey wattle', which forms on the same side of the neck as the constrained masseter muscle. Also, be aware that any trauma or accident, like whiplash, which affects the muscles and fascia at the back of the neck, can contribute to imbalances in the platysma.

Make sure that there are no subluxations in the cervical vertebrae, which can also create sagging of the platysma. I refer my patients out to an osteopath or a chiropractor if I detect misalignments in the neck area.

Palpate and balance the entire neck – front, back and sides – and treat the muscles involved in the imbalances for the best results.

The origin and insertion protocols that I have created for this large neck muscle are very effective, and feature some unusual needling techniques. They will need to be practiced to achieve mastery. Please perform all the recommended steps within this protocol.

Since the platysma covers such a large area on the chest and neck, there are five origin and insertion sites. For the sake of clarity, I will pair each of these sites separately on the chest, chin, neck, corners of the mouth and jaw.

Origin

The origin of this muscle is in the fascia of the upper pectoralis and deltoideus muscles.

Insertion

The insertion is in the fibers that interlace at the angle of the mouth, jaw and mandible.

Needling Techniques

1.   The Chest: St-13 Qihu Qi Door; needle bilaterally and obliquely, then transversely 0.3–0.5 cun outward toward the shoulder. Do not needle this area perpendicularly, because deep needling can cause a pneumothorax. I have never seen or experienced such an occurrence in the needling of this particular point, but it is always advisable to err on the side of caution.

Use a 30 mm, 36 or 38 gauge needle (#2 or #3 Japanese) to traverse this area under the clavicle, and one needle to access both the origin and insertion. The needles involved should grab when pulled backward after needling; this grabbing sensation is similar to De qi. The muscle involved is the subclavius, which positively affects the brachial plexus and prevents thoracic outlet syndrome.

Releasing this area will alleviate symptoms, such as a frozen shoulder, or any numbness or tingling down the arm. You are literally opening up the Qi in this area, hence the name Qi Door.

2.   The Chin: Needle the extra point Jiachengjiang M-HN-4 bilaterally and transversely outwards about 0.2–0.3 cun. Use a 15 mm 40 gauge or smaller needle (#1 Japanese). This technique traverses the depressor labii inferioris muscle, which pulls down the lower lip to express irony.

3.   The Jaw: The origin of this area is St-5 Daying Great Reception and the insertion is St-4 Dicang Earth's Granary at the corners of the mouth. Remember that the muscle fibers at the corners of the mouth insert into the skin and blend with the muscles at the angle of the mouth.

Origin: Needle St-5 Daying Great Reception obliquely 0.3–0.5 cun and then transversely upward toward the corners of the mouth. Use a 30 mm 38 or 36 gauge needle (#2 or #3 Japanese) to cover this larger area.

Insertion: Needle St-4 Dicang Earth's Granary obliquely 0.3–0.5 cun, then transversely downward toward St-5 Daying Great Reception.

Always needle the origin followed by the insertion of the muscle on the same side of the face, and then repeat the procedure on the other side to complete the energetic circuit of the paired muscles. Use a 30 mm 38 or 36 gauge (#2 or #3 Japanese) when you needle this area.

4.   Origin/insertion, Areas 4 and 5: 'Wrapping Around the Bone' Technique. These two areas will require you to master an unusual needling technique that I call 'Wrapping Around the Bone.' This technique uses one needle to access

both the jaw and its muscle attachments and tendons. Needle both the origin of the muscle located on the mandible, and the insertion in the fascia under the jaw.

Reminder: Before needling, be sure to give your patient homeopathic arnica 6C to prevent acute bruising. I recommend that you practice this technique on yourself before attempting to needle your patients.

A saggy, drooping neck with horizontal lines across it, coupled with vertical lines at the corners of the mouth, is difficult to treat effectively. This is why I work with muscle structure, and created this particular technique to address that issue.

If you have a patient whose neck is noticeably sagging, and they also have many horizontal lines across their neck, it is wise to treat the platysma muscle first, prior to threading the lines. This is an exception to the Wrinkle Rule found in Chapter 6.

If you do not first address the muscle, the continued sagging will further exacerbate the wrinkles in the skin of the neck.

I have seen patients whose skin was so flaccid that it covered their ears so that they could not hear me after they lay down on the massage table. This degree of sagging is a strong indication that treating the platysma muscle should be your first priority; only after the sagging has been alleviated is it appropriate to move on to threading the lines on the neck.

In these extreme cases, toning the neck muscle can require more than one series of treatments. In order to achieve significant results, neck treatment must be accompanied by constitutional treatments, lifestyle changes, dietary adjustments, and both topical and internal Chinese herbs.

The good news is that these acu-muscle treatment points are very effective; in utilizing muscle structure, we address the fundamental imbalances that contribute to these particular signs of aging.

Patients sag for many reasons, such as weight loss, Spleen Qi deficiency, hereditary collagen/elastin deficiency, weak ligaments and tendons, not enough dietary protein, waning hormones, trauma, accidents, and extreme grief, among other reasons.

The Medial Jaw Bone; 'Wrapping Around the Bone' Technique A: A special point, St-4 ¾ Dicang+ Earth's Granary, is directly below Dicang Earth's Granary on the edge of the mandible and on the top of the jaw bone.

Both the origin and insertion of the muscle are addressed with one needle. The origin is inserted into the area slightly above the jawbone, and the insertion into the skin slightly under the jaw.

Instructions: Insert the needle perpendicularly, 0.3–0.5 cun, into the special point, St-4¾ Dicang+; angle it transversely down over the chin toward the massage table. You will feel the needle under your fingers. Make sure that you have a sufficient length of needle to perform the 'Wrapping Around the Bone' Technique. Wrap the needle under the jaw, angling it toward SI-17 Tianrong Celestial Countenance.

This unique needling technique of 'Wrapping Around the Bone', accesses not only the acupuncture point, but also the area and muscle attachments under the chin. Use at least a 30 mm, 38 or 36 gauge needle (#2 or #3 Japanese). If you choose to attempt this with a smaller gauge needle, the needle may bend, and it could become entwined in the muscle – the muscles around the jaw are particularly strong. In this case, you can insert another needle to release the stuck needle.

If you are treating a sensitive patient, do not think that a smaller needle size in this area will suffice, because it will not. Look to your needling techniques, and practice them on yourself first until you are confident of them.

Make sure that the patient is breathing in their Dantien, and not in a shallow fashion, or they will likely hyperventilate. If you have them sigh when they exhale, they will be less sensitive to the needles.

If you have a patient with a large jaw and thick skin, use a thicker, higher gauge needle.

Lateral Jaw Bone; 'Wrapping Around the Bone," Technique B: **A special point above SI-17** Tianrong Celestial Countenance is located above and on the edge of the angle of the jaw. Once again, both the origin and insertion are addressed with a single needle.

Instructions: Needle perpendicularly 0.3–0.5 cun, then transversely down over the chin toward the massage table. Once again, use your non-dominant hand to feel the passage of the needle under the skin so that you can then wrap the needle around and under the bone. Angle it inward toward the chin or the center of the face.

Point Location and Indications
The Chest: St-13 Qihu Qi Door is located in the depression at the midpoint of the inferior border of the clavicle, 4 cun lateral to the Ren meridian. It also may be found 2 cun lateral to Ki-27 Shufu Storage Warehouse.

It clears heat, treats rebellious Qi and opens the chest, and it is a local point for the treatment of asthma, bronchitis, respiratory issues and wheezing. It also calms hiccoughs, and treats vomiting blood, an inability to turn the head, and eases chest congestion.

The name, Qi Door, implies that this point can serve as a portal through which emotions may be released and beneficial energies may enter the body. People who are always hesitating have this door partially open or closed and consequently, nothing may enter or exit. Psychospiritually, this point permits the passage of energy. However, the door swings both ways, and can either nurture a person who needs to receive mothering, or can close if a person rejects that longed-for help and/or compassion.

> **CAUTION**
>
> Deep or perpendicular insertion in this area can affect the subclavian vessels and may also puncture the lung. Consequently, I have recommended only an oblique, superficial insertion and then transverse needling of this point.

The Chin: The extra point, Jiachengjiang M-HN-18 is located 1 cun lateral to Ren-24 Chengjiang Sauce Receptacle, and the indications have been outlined in the section on the Upper and Lower Lip section earlier in this chapter.

The Mouth and Jaw: St-5 Daying Great Reception is located in the depression at the anterior border of the masseter muscle. I recommend that you have your patients clench their jaws in order to locate this point.

> **CAUTION**
>
> Avoid excessive stimulation of this point because it can damage the facial artery and vein. This point eliminates facial wind and redness, and swelling in the face and cheeks. It also treats temporomandibular joint dysfunction (TMJ), facial paralysis, windstroke with aphasia, twitching lip, lockjaw, and other wind-related syndromes.

Information on St-4 Dicang Earth's Granary, can be found earlier in this chapter, in the section on The Grin, Corners of the Mouth.

The medial jaw bone: St-4 ¾ Dicang+ Earth's Granary is also covered in the section on The Grin, found earlier in this chapter. Since this special point is in alignment with Dicang, the indications are similar. The area around the mouth concentrates on nourishment and post-natal Qi issues.

The lateral jaw bone: the location for this special point SI-17 Tianrong Celestial Countenance is slightly above and posterior to the angle of the mandible, in the depression on the anterior portion of the sternocleidomastoideus (SCM) muscle.

It resolves damp heat and phlegm, regulates rebellious Qi, as in a goiter, an inability to speak, tinnitus, deafness, acute asthma attacks and bruxism. The *Spiritual Axis* originally documented SI-17 Tianrong Celestial Countenance as a Gall Bladder point; in the 10th century, the *Systemic Classic of Acupuncture and Moxibustion* said that it belonged to the Small Intestine channel. It is considered a Windows of the Sky point, which affects the orifices of the head and face. They are the great windows through which Divine Heavenly Qi moves.

When this Qi is chaotic, convulsions, dizziness, schizophrenia, and loss of speech and hearing can ensue. Psychospiritually, everything is a heavenly creation. This point refines the dross of earthly existence and transforms it into inner purity and essence. If this window is clear and clean, we can see the divine spark in all creatures. When it is blocked, it is difficult to find goodness in anything, especially ourselves.

Be aware that treating a saggy neck (Table 7.12) may take two treatment series, if the patient is not constitutionally healthy.

At the end of this chapter (Table 7.13), each of the 12 areas, the muscle involvement, plus origin and insertion sites are summarized to clarify the Constitutional Facial Acupuncture needling protocol.

The 'Wrapping Around the Bone' technique in Figure 7.36 uses one needle to lift and tone the neck's 'turkey wattles' and jowls, by addressing the muscle, ligaments and tendons above and below the jaw area.

TABLE 7.12 SUMMARY: THE NECK

Muscle	Platysma; contracts and pulls down the curves of the mouth and lifts the skin of the chin
Emotion	Grief, irony, suffering, sadness
Lines/wrinkles	Horizontal lines on the neck
Origin	In the fascia of the chest
Insertion	Fibers below the chin, at the mouth corners and jaw
Needling Techniques	
1. Chest	
Origin/insertion	Needle St-13 Qihu Qi Door obliquely then transversely 0.3–0.5 cun outward toward the shoulder; use a 30 mm, 38 or 36 gauge needle (#2 or #3 Japanese)
2. Chin	
Origin/insertion	Needle Jiachengjiang M-HN-4 transversely outwards 0.2–0.3 cun; use a 15 mm, 40 gauge needle (#1 Japanese)
3. Jaw	
Origin	Needle St-5 Daying Great Reception obliquely 0.3–0.5 cun, then transversely upward toward the corners of the mouth; use a 30 mm, 38 or 36 gauge needle (#2 or #3 Japanese)
Insertion	Needle St-4 Dicang Earth's Granary 0.3–0.5 cun obliquely then transversely downwards toward St-5 Daying Great Reception
4. Medial jaw	'Wrapping Around the Bone,' technique A

Continued   261

TABLE 7.12 SUMMARY: THE NECK—cont'd

Origin/insertion	Needle a special point, St-4¾ Dicang+ Earth's Granary; use a 30 mm, 38 or 36 gauge needle (#2 or #3 Japanese)
5. Lateral jaw	'Wrapping Around the Bone,' technique B
Origin/insertion	Needle a special point above SI-17 Tianrong Celestial Countenance perpendicularly 0.3–0.5 cun, angle transversely and downward toward the table, then inward toward the chin; use a 30 mm, 38 or 36 gauge needle (#2 or #3 Japanese)

Point Location/Indications

1. Chest	St-13 Qihu Qi Door; in the depression 4 cun lateral to Ren Mai under the clavicle; it clears heat, calms hiccoughs, and treats respiratory issues
2. Chin	Jiachengjiang M-HN-18; 1 cun lateral to Ren-24 Chengjiang Sauce Receptacle. For indications see the Upper and Lower Lip section in this chapter
3. Jaw and mouth	St-5 Daying Great Reception; in the depression at the anterior border of the masseter muscle. It treats TMJ, facial paralysis, twitching lips and lockjaw. St-4 Dicang Earth's Granary is lateral to the corner of the mouth; see The Grin section in this chapter
4. Medial jaw	'Wrapping Around the Bone,' technique A; a special point St 4¾ Dicang+ Earth's Granary, directly below St-4 Dicang, just above the jaw. The indications are similar to Dicang in The Grin portion of this chapter
5. Lateral jaw	'Wrapping Around the Bone,' technique B; above SI-17 Tianrong Celestial Countenance, just above the anterior and posterior angle of the jaw. It treats tinnitus, deafness, bruxism and goiters

Conclusion

In treating your patient with this origin/insertion protocol, please do not needle all the facial areas at once. Have your patient choose an area of the face that they wish to target, such as the forehead, neck, droopy eyes or mouth. When you observe noticeable improvement in the area you have been treating, then move on to the next one. Review Chapter 6, which discusses the 'Wrinkle Rule' and other pertinent information. You either treat the muscle imbalance or thread a needle through a line or wrinkle, which remains in the skin after you assess the face.

Do not treat the muscle and thread the line or wrinkle at the same time, because it will be too much for your patient. Remember that you have an entire treatment series, of 12–15 (up to 20) sessions, and overloading the face

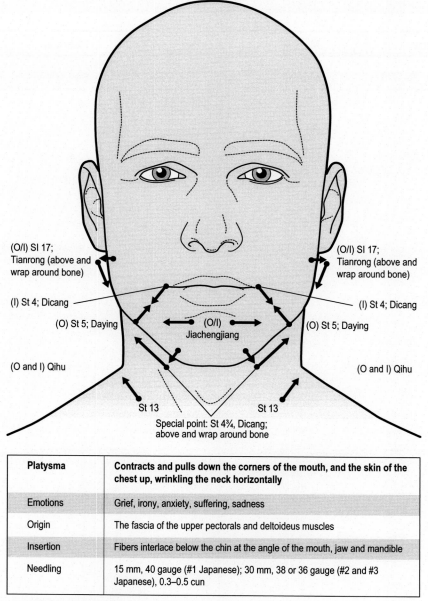

Platysma	Contracts and pulls down the corners of the mouth, and the skin of the chest up, wrinkling the neck horizontally
Emotions	Grief, irony, anxiety, suffering, sadness
Origin	The fascia of the upper pectorals and deltoideus muscles
Insertion	Fibers interlace below the chin at the angle of the mouth, jaw and mandible
Needling	15 mm, 40 gauge (#1 Japanese); 30 mm, 38 or 36 gauge (#2 and #3 Japanese), 0.3–0.5 cun

Figure 7.36 Needling diagram: The Neck.

with needles is unnecessary, especially when working with muscle structure. For example, if a patient has lines in the naso-labial fold, and, when you assess the face, these lines are still visible, thread a needle superficially from the corners of the mouth up to the nose, LI-20 Yingxiang Welcome Fragrance area. If the line disappears during your assessment, use the origin/insertion technique.

TABLE 7.13   SUMMARY: THE FACIAL LANDSCAPE – 12 AREAS

Area	Muscle	Origin	Insertion
1. The Chin	Mentalis	Special point; 0.5 cun lateral to Ren 24, Chengjiang	Skin of lower lip
2. The Grin	Risorius	St-6 Jiache	St-4 Dicang
3. The Smile; naso-labial fold	Levator labii superioris alaeque nasi	Bitong St-2 Sibai SI-18 Quanliao	LI-20 Yingxiang LI-19 Kouheliao special point 0.5 cun above St-4 Dicang
4. Upper and lower lips	Orbicularis oris	LI-19 Kouheliao special point 0.5 cun lateral to Jiachengjiang	Above St-4 Dicang St-4 Dicang
5. Sunken cheeks	Buccinator	St 7 Xiaguan	Special point; 1 cun lateral to St-4 Dicang
6. The Laugh	Zygomaticus major	SI-18 Quanliao	St-4 Dicang
7. Crow's feet	Temporoparietalis	GB-7 Qubin	GB-8 Shuaigu
8. Under eye bags	Orbicularis oculi; palpebral portion	Qiuhou	Same
9. Droopy eyelids/ sagging eyebrows	Orbicularis oculi; orbital portion	Upper Shangming	GB 14 Yangbai
10. The Frown	Corrugator supercilii	YuYao	Bl 2 Zanzhu
11. The Forehead	Frontalis	GB 14 Yangbai	TH 23 Sizhukong
12. The Neck	Platysma	St-13 Qihu	Same
		Jiachengjiang	Same
		St-5 Daying	St-4 Dicang
		St-4 ¾	Same
		SI-17 Tianrong	Same

This facial approach is very effective because it employs acupuncture points in tandem with muscle structure. You can treat the muscle and thread an area of the face if they are not the same area. For example, if a patient has a saggy neck, utilize the platysma acu-muscle treatment; and, if they also have a Liver line between the eyebrows, one that is in the skin, thread the line. This is an elegant treatment, not too much, and also effective. It gives their body a chance to heal and change, without being subjected to the stress of excessive needle insertions.

In Chapter 9, I introduce the topical Chinese modular herbal remedies, which enhance and promote the efficacy of the Constitutional Facial Acupuncture treatment protocols.

REFERENCES

1. Cain S. Quiet: The Power of Introverts in a World that just Can't Stop Talking. New York, NY: Crown Publishers; 2012.

2. Gladwell M. Blink: The Power of Thinking without Thinking. New York, NY: Little, Brown & Co.; 2005. p. 199–200.

3. Text in English translation found at http://www.gutenberg.org/files/14988/14988-h/14988-h.htm, p. 185.

4. Bridges L. Face Reading in Chinese Medicine. 2nd ed. London, UK: Elsevier; 2012. p. 148.

5. Ekman P. Darwin, deception and facial expression. In: Ekman P, Davidson R, De Waals F, editors. Annals of the New York Academy of Sciences, vol. 1000. New York: New York Academy of Sciences; 2003a. p. 205–21. doi:10.1196/annals.1280.010; reference located in Darwin the detective: Observable facial muscle contractions reveal emotional high-stakes lies, Evolution and Human Behavior, doi:10.1016/j.evolhumbehav.2011.12.003, Elsevier, UK.

6. "Botox injections put a crease in emotional evaluations," reported at http://www.sciencenews.org/view/generic/id/60844, Friday, July 2, 2010, Bruce Bower, contributor.

7. Bridges L, op. cit., p. 235.

8. See Table 9.1, "Signs of Peach Luck", Ibid., p. 239.

9. Finzi E, Wasserman E. Treatment of Depression with Botulinum Toxin A: A Case Series, reported in Dermatologic Surgery. American Society of for Dermatologic Surgery, Blackwell Publishing; 2006. Located at http://www.chevychasecosmeticcenter.com/Portals/0/docs/botox.pdf.

10. Adler J. Health: Can You Really Botox the Blues Away? Newsweek May 28, 2006.

11. Travell J, Simons D. Myofascial Pain and Dysfunction: The Trigger Point Manual; Vol. 1: The Upper Extremities. Baltimore, MD: Williams and Wilkins; 1983. p. 285.

CHAPTER 8

Special Treatments

Constitutional Psychospiritual Points

"If you are going to walk on thin ice, you may as well dance."
— Unknown

In Chapter 7, we introduced the idea that the face is the most emotive part of the body, and that facial needling can release not only habitual expressions, but even repressed emotions.

In this chapter, we will explore psychospiritual points and provide you with guidelines for their usage. After seeing a patient 2 to 5 times during the course of a Constitutional Facial Acupuncture treatment series, certain emotions may arise that need to be addressed at the constitutional level.

When this transpires, I usually ask for my patient's permission to palpate and treat either one set of the Kidney Spirit points, which lie over the Heart on the Kidney meridian, or the three Shen points on the scalp. I couple these specialized psychospiritual points with specific essential oils, or other body points that address the Shen.

This approach allows for, and facilitates, a natural transformative process within the patient, one which is accentuated and accelerated by the very nature of the facial treatments.

Our English noun, 'transformation,' is derived from a Latin verb, 'transformare,' meaning to go beyond previously existing form. Therefore, the act of being transformed is a process, a mathematical formula that effects change in structure, as well as composition. This process awakens our cellular memory, and the energies released may alter us profoundly, even shifting our appearance and basic character. Furthermore, through an inner and outer alchemy, it serves to align us with our authentic nature, destiny or vocation.

267

Working at the Shen level has always been considered an integral part of the practice of Chinese medicine, and it does not separate spirit from the body/mind.

I often rely upon the use of these and other Shen points in my practice, particularly when patients are depressed, and/or grieving, due to the death of a loved one, a divorce, loss of employment, or suffering any other emotional stress that manifests as fear, fright or rage.

Sun Si Miao named these imbalances in the psyche *gui,* and treated them with the Thirteen Ghost Points. The *gui* can emerge during a series of Constitutional Facial Acupuncture treatments, when the acu-muscle points holding the facial expressions are relaxed in the needling process. Therefore, I have found it beneficial to integrate these constitutional Shen points within the flow of the treatments.

As previously mentioned, the Kidney Spirit points are found over the Heart on the Kidney meridian. They directly connect to Heart Yin and Kidney water for nourishment, and their precise location is 2 cun on either side of the Ren Mai, and under the intercostal spaces of the ribs.

I palpate each bilateral point separately, pressing it toward the Ren Mai, in order to ascertain which one point is the most exquisitely tender. I instruct my patient to interact with me, and to give me feedback as to whether the points are reactive or not.

I only needle one set of points, and do not recommend that you needle all the Kidney Spirit points, because they are very powerful. In my opinion, needling even more than one set would be excessive and could confuse and disrupt the Shen.

I needle the bilateral points transversely toward the Ren Mai to consolidate the essence back to the Ren, the Mother. I do not disperse these points, and use thin 40 gauge, 30 mm needles for this specific purpose.

Other teachers or practitioners may have different recommendations about needling these Spirit points. I have found that this approach is the most effective when they are integrated into Constitutional Facial Acupuncture treatments.

The Kidney Spirit Points

Kid-26, *Yu Zhong Amidst Elegance*

Location: 2 cun on either side of the Ren Mai in the 1st intercostal space.

When balanced, the Heart fire flourishes and flows gracefully at this point, allowing the spirit to rise and blossom. If there is an imbalance, the patient feels stuck, depressed and caught in the web of old emotional patterns. Their life may look fantastic to an impartial observer, but they are unhappy, miserable, unable to acknowledge the blessings, sweetness or beauty in life – hence, the name; Amidst Elegance. These people appear to have everything – beautiful children, a wonderful spouse, health, wealth, and fabulous successful career. However, they can't appreciate the treasures given to them.

Kid-25, Shen Cang Spirit Storehouse

Location: 2 cun on either side of the Ren Mai in the 2nd intercostal space.

This point houses original Qi or Shen, and represents the patient's spiritual bank account. They have money and other reserves in this Shen bank. However, when imbalanced, these individuals tend to burn the candle at both ends. They are exhausted, feel disconnected from Spirit, and temporarily have lost sight of their path in life.

Needling Shen Cang adds oxygen to dying embers, and helps them remember who they really are, so that they can continue their journey.

Kid-24, Ling Xu, Spirit Ruins/Spirit Burial Ground/Spirit Resurrection

Location: 2 cun on either side of the Ren Mai in the 3rd intercostal space.

This point represents the Ling, or the mysterious, disembodied feminine aspect of Spirit. These patients have difficulty relinquishing their attachment to a deceased loved one, and obsess about them in the middle, Yin hours of the night. They cannot sleep, and are submerged in the most profound grief. The *Su Wen* describes them as having picked up sad entities, with the subjective feeling of a ghost pressing on their chest at night. Life has buried their spirit, and they are 'Shen-less,' and have very little light in their eyes.

They may also be obsessing about the death of a beloved pet, children who may have 'left the nest,' the loss of some cherished vocation, any kind of ego death, or a karmic transformation of past life patterns.

While Yu Zhong manifests as depression related to old dysfunctional emotional expression, Ling Xu patients have been hollowed out by an unbearable sadness; they are a shell of a person, who is unable to let go and move on.

Occasionally, the grief and depression is so severe, that they no longer wish to continue living, but long to join their loved one, and succeed in crossing over to be reunited with them.

Kid-23, Shen Feng Spirit Seal

Location: 2 cun on either side of the Ren Mai in the 4th intercostal space, at the level of Ren-17 Dazhong Chest Center.

This point represents the Yang, masculine aspect of Spirit, and passion. It realigns the soul with the true nature of its life path. When imbalanced, the patient will seek a seal of approval from everyone around them because they have a low sense of self-esteem, and have not yet been able to identify their own authentic passion or voice.

It is crucial for these individuals to give themselves a pat on the back, acknowledging a job well done, and not rely so heavily on others' opinions of them.

Kid-22, Bu Lang On the Veranda

Location: 2 cun on either side of the Ren Mai in the 5th intercostal space.

This beautiful point represents a safe place for convalescence. The patient has been ill, sustained a physical or emotional shock or trauma, and is not yet ready to resume their place in the world. However, from their sick bed, through the open doors of the veranda, they can catch a glimpse of the sun radiantly shining, and view the outside from a distance, knowing that they are still protected. Needling Bu Lang supports their recognition of the fact that they are healing and will soon be able to resume their normal lives.

The Kidney Spirit points are a valuable and recommended adjunct to the constitutional component of this facial acupuncture protocol. I want to stress the importance of palpation in your diagnostics; do not permit yourself to impose your own perception of the patient's situation on the process. It is better to have their body tell you what they need. In my experience, this is a more accurate, effective and respectful strategy.

After you have needled the points, you can then delicately inquire about the patient's personal situation. For example, with Kid-24 Ling Xu Spirit Burial Grounds, you might ask whether they have recently lost a loved one, and are suffering from insomnia, because they are thinking about them constantly.

If the patient is reticent about revealing anything of a personal nature, do not subject them to unnecessary probing. They may be unwilling to show their vulnerability in this fashion and will not be curious as to the nature of your treatment. Nevertheless, they will be affected by it.

The Kidney Spirit points are integrated into the constitutional treatment, and are customarily left in place for the entire duration. However, be sensitive to their effects, and remove them, if you need to do so.

Guidelines for Using the Spirit Points

These points are highly recommended when a patient has manifested all or some of the following conditions:

- An unrealistic perception of themselves in the world.
- They seem out of touch with their core being, or their natural self.
- An inability to form intimate relationships.
- A lack of spontaneity or intuitive insights.
- A loss of connection with their true destiny.
- No heart or Spirit connection.
- An over-reaction to life events, or conversely, they are emotionally dead.

Treatment of the Three Shen Points with Essential Oils

The Three Shen Points located in the scalp are especially effective in transforming Spirit. Their names all contain the word 'Shen,' and they are used to treat psychospiritual issues, ranging from anxiety to manic depression.

I customarily apply these essential oils to the points after needling to augment the potency and efficacy of the treatment, although this is optional.

Essential Oils

Essential oils are similar to the energetic landscape of acupuncture, because they are vibrational in nature, and are also governed by Qi flow. They operate electromagnetically like the meridian system, and can affect the neuroendocrine system that governs both physiological and psychospiritual functions, such as mood, mental states, and behavioral and physical patterns.

Plants and human beings are both examples of organic life and thus they share a similar molecular structure, one based upon molecules of carbon, hydrogen and oxygen; however, their 'blood' contains slightly different constituents. Humans have an iron molecule in their hemoglobin, whereas the active component in the circulatory system of plants is chlorophyll, which is based upon a magnesium molecule.

This molecular affinity illustrates a profound rapport between plants and human beings, a kind of sympathetic resonance that permits the usage of essential oils on acupuncture points, and can produce a powerful Shen effect, or psychospiritual healing potential.

Guidelines for the Application of Essential Oils

1. Apply essential oils directly to the points after you have needled them. Use 3–4 drops on a Q-tip (cotton bud) to ensure that the tip is wet before applying. Some essential oils can be applied 'neat,' while others are too strong, and must be grounded in a carrier oil.

2. For cold and deficient conditions, a Tiger warmer or pole moxa can be used to enhance oil absorption.

3. Choose oils or an oil that resonates with the point, meridian, or body area.

4. Check the patient's pulse to see if there is a clear change, and, most importantly, observe the complexion and the eyes to determine whether their Shen brightens with the application (of the essential oil).

5. Make sure that your patient isn't allergic to the oils by testing them on their inner arm for 12 hours prior to application.

The Three Shen scalp points are excellent for the treatment of any disorders of the Spirit, such as irrational fears, schizophrenia, anxiety, stress or trauma, epilepsy, Bell's palsy and wind stroke. I have also used them effectively to calm hypervigilant, sensitive patients.

Du-24 Shenting Spirit Palace or Spirit Court

The face and scalp are considered to be the court of spirit, and are located near the brain, the storage area for original Qi. Du-24 is located 0.5 cun directly above the midpoint of the anterior hairline, and is a point of intersection with the Bladder and Stomach meridians.

TCM indications	Treats disorders of the spirit and calms the Shen
	Severe anxiety, irrational fears and palpitations
	Schizophrenia
	Insomnia and headaches; vertigo
	Clears the head and sinus
	Brightens the eyes; blurred vision
Psychospiritual indications and qualities	Use for overbearing, impatient and arrogant people
	Calms fear and anxiety, quiets the mind
	Extreme psychosis; Yang mental states with screaming, madness and schizophrenia, as well as Yin mental states, with despair and extreme depression
	Use for a patient who wants to move on, and to further cultivate their Shen

Suggested Essential Oil Pairing: Ou Xie Cao (*Valeriana Officialis*), Valerian

Valerian subdues the Heart and Liver fire, plus Liver wind:

- It treats insomnia, palpitations, anxiety, hysteria, epilepsy, and any other mental disorders.
- Calms the Shen.

Properties	Sedative, venous decongestant, antispasmodic, carminative; valerian can be applied neat to the acu-point
Contraindications	Cooling in nature; do not use with deficient Qi or Yang; overuse can cause fatigue
Psychospiritual	This essential oil is famous for its sedative effects, not only for sleep issues, but also mental problems, from despair and depression to schizophrenia

GB-13 Benshen Root of Spirit

GB-13 Benshen is located 0.5 cun within the hairline of the forehead, 3 cun lateral to Du-24 Shenting, and is a point of intersection with the Yin Wei Mai, Heart, Pericardium and Lung tendino-muscular meridians.

TCM indications	Calms spirit; schizophrenia, jealousy and suspicion
	Expels wind; windstroke, epilepsy, Bell's palsy
	Clears the brain and gathers essence back to the head
	Treats headache, insomnia, epilepsy, stroke, convulsions, split personality, jealousy, lack of will power, confusion
	Calms mood swings, psychic attacks, eases tension
Psychospiritual indications and qualities	Gall Bladder point; aids in courage and decision making
	Roots mind/body connection and balances emotions in the organ systems
	Balances extremes of emotion
	Represents the emotional response to one's worldly challenges
	Supports, grounds and balances life processes

Suggested Essential Oil Pairing: Ai Wei (*Ferula Galbaniflua*), Galbanum

Galbanum smooths Liver Qi flow, Liver overacting on Spleen, expels damp phlegm and wind damp, as well as mucus in the lungs. It is also a cellular regenerator.

Properties	Nervine, expectorant, analgesic, antispasmodic, carminative, emmenagogue, resolvent, vulnerary, stimulant; galbanum can be applied directly to the point without a carrier oil
Contraindications	Galbanum is an emmenagogue, which encourages menstruation, hence it is contraindicated for pregnancy
Psychospiritual	Galbanum balances body/mind and spirit, eases tension and is used to address erratic mood swings, as well as psychic blockages. It facilitates meditation and was used by the ancient Egyptians in embalming, because of its preservative properties

Sishencong Alert Spirit EX-HN-1

Sishencong is a group of four points located at the vertex of the head, 1 cun anterior, posterior and bilateral to Du-20 Baihui Hundred Convergences.

TCM indications	Aids memory
	Headache
	Insomnia
	Dispels wind; epilepsy
	Vertigo and dizziness
	Calms the Shen
Psychospiritual indications and qualities	Treats manic depression
	Self-esteem issues
	Protects patient from negativity and overthinking
	Supports the Ming or true path in life

Suggested Essential Oil Pairing: Ru Xiang (*Boswellia Carterii*), Frankincense

Frankincense aids Lung Qi circulation and is effective in the treatment of asthma, sinusitis and bronchitis, as well as Lung heat issues with coughing and wheezing. It invigorates the blood, and calms the Heart; anxiety, depression. It also reduces swelling and is an strong anti-oxidant.

Properties	Expectorant, vulnerary, sedative; frankincense can be applied 'neat' to the point, without a carrier oil.
Contraindications	Frankincense is slightly cooling in nature, and could further cool the uterus in conditions of Kidney Yang or Qi deficiency
Psychospiritual	Frankincense lifts the spirit, thus it is good for meditation, and treating mental distraction or the feeling of being overwhelmed. It strengthens the immune system, addresses insomnia, irritability, restlessness and supports spiritual freedom and expressiveness. It connects us to our higher selves.

Needling Instruction and Techniques

Use a 36 or 34 gauge, 30 to 40 mm needle to puncture Du-24 Shenting Spirit Palace and GB-13 Benshen Root of Spirit transversely from the point toward the back of the head. Do not use a shorter or thinner needle. You do not need to tonify or sedate these points; unless treating the scalp for windstroke, Bell's palsy and/or neuropathies, I customarily needle them neutrally, without manipulation.

Sishencong Alert Spirit EX-HN-1 can be needled neutrally, tonified or sedated. In my experience, patients with emotional or psychospiritual imbalances often have the vertex area of the head either too open or too closed. If Baihui or the crown of the head is too open energetically, the patient may be ungrounded and won't be able to root their Shen. They can also be vulnerable to invasion by unwanted Qi or *gui,* which can disturb their spirit. If the crown is shut down, they may be too earthbound, and unable to connect with their own Shen to uplift their spirit, or to transcend imbalances, such as depression, anxiety or obsessions. In treating this point, the needle gauge and length is the same, but the technique is different.

Needling Instructions and Techniques for Sishencong

For patients with a closed vertex, tonify by needling clockwise to open the crown. Transversely thread a needle from each one of the four Sishencong points toward the other points. For example:

- Transversely thread the anterior Sishencong point clockwise toward one of the bilateral points.

275

- The bilateral point is then transversely threaded clockwise toward the posterior Sishencong point.

- The posterior Sishencong point is transversely thread clockwise toward the other bilateral point.

- This bilateral point is then transversely threaded clockwise toward the anterior point.

Four needles have been used to open and tonify the crown of the head and also to treat Sishencong.

For patients with an overly open vertex, sedate by needling counterclockwise to close the crown:

- To close the crown, sedate the four points by needling counterclockwise in the same manner.

Neutral needling, to neither open nor close the crown:

- To needle Sishencong neutrally, I insert the needles 90 degrees into each of the four points, and angle them slightly inward in the direction of Baihui.

Different metals can be employed for the various operations described above. The properties of the metals augment the nature of the needling process. Gold needles can further tonify, silver needles have a sedating action, and stainless steel needles can be used for neutral needling.

Of course, the method of needling, and metals used, will vary from patient to patient.

It should be mentioned that, in the *Su Wen*, only Ht-7 Shenmen Spirit Gate was described as a Shen point. But, by 1601, the *Great Compendium of Acupuncture* (*Zhen Jiu da Cheng*) cited twelve or more spirit points.

In my experience, spirit points are essential to the success of a Constitutional Facial Acupuncture treatment series. Facial muscles are referred to as the expressive muscles for a very specific reason.

When the face is needled, tension is relaxed, and emotions trapped in the facial musculature can be appropriately processed. Threading needles through facial lines and wrinkles in the skin triggers the release of cellular memory.

We also needle Windows of the Sky points, *gui* points and other psychospiritual points during the process of a treatment. I strongly suggest that you familiarize yourself with the suggested Shen points in this chapter, and use them, when appropriate. The addition of these powerful treatment strategies will allow you to offer your patients treatments of a truly transformational nature.

CHAPTER 9

Chinese Topical Herbal Treatments and Essential Oil Protocols

"A good dyet is a perfect way of curing,
and worth much regard assuring.
A king that cannot rule him in his dyet
will hardly rule his realme in peace and quiet."
— Regimen Sanitis Salernitanum, 11th century

This chapter presents additional strategies for achieving optimum results in your Constitutional Facial Acupuncture treatments.

These strategies include the use of a variety of topical adjuncts to the facial needling. In addition to internal consumption, Chinese herbs serve as ingredients in masks and poultices that treat dermatological issues, and can be custom-blended for each patient.

Information will also be provided regarding the properties and application of essential oils, which may be blended with Chinese herbs in natural creams, cleansers, or employed as a standalone treatment. After the treatment, hydrosols infused with organic essential oils are sprayed onto the patient's face, to cool, hydrate or balance the skin.

I am also recommending a number of tools that will improve your treatment results, including gem discs, which are placed on the patient's eyes during the treatment, jade rollers, and resonance in the form of tuning forks.

A step-by-step facial protocol integrating topical herbal masks, poultices, creams, natural cleansers and essential oils will enhance your results threefold. Cleansing and hydrating the face is paramount for effective treatments, and the addition of the jade rollers, gem discs, hydrosols and tuning forks, makes this approach more effective. It also creates a safe and nurturing atmosphere in which your patients can relax, allowing them to experience a transformative ritual.

These protocols can be successfully incorporated within a spa environment, or used as a treatment in your existing acupuncture practice. As these protocols employ the strengths of our medicine, are strongly constitutionally based, and use Chinese herbal masks and poultices, there will be no confusion with those offered by estheticians in spas.

I recommend creating a non-sterile, elegant and beautiful environment in your clinic, with the possible addition of a small waterfall, a bonsai plant, a Chinese/Japanese hanging scroll or other tasteful artwork. Remember that the ancient Taoists, in particular, cultivated protocols and specific herbal remedies to promote longevity and enhance beauty.

Topical Chinese Herbs

The herbal preparations discussed below are formulated synergistically to restore the acid/alkaline balance of the skin, tighten pores, and help maintain the suppleness and moisture levels of the skin. As previously mentioned, they can also be tailor-made to clear heat, fire toxins and damp heat from the face.

Integrating Chinese topical herbs into a Constitutional Facial Acupuncture treatment series provides the following additional dimensions:

• Additional nourishment and Lung Qi is brought directly to the skin.

• The acupuncture points are supported and stimulated.

• Specific herbal formulas re-hydrate and bring the Yin to the face.

• Other formulas calm and cool heat in the face, and treat syndromes such as rosacea and acne.

• If the herbal formulas are ingested, and an herbal mask placed on the face externally, there can be a quasi-homeopathic reaction of 'like attracting like,' with the internal substances rising to the skin of the face, augmenting the effects of the treatment.

CAUTION

When using Chinese herbs internally, it is important to be familiar with the contraindications, benefits and properties of the herbs, both singly and in combinations. We are exploring the application of topical herbal formulas only in this chapter.

278

These herbal formulations can be embellished with essential oils, flower essences, gem elixirs, sesame or flax seeds to reinforce the penetration of the herbs into the skin.

Step-by-Step Chinese Topical Herbal Protocol

In Chapter 6, Practical Specifics, I outlined guidelines and presented necessary technical information for Constitutional Facial Acupuncture treatments, including a step-by-step treatment that included the use of topical Chinese herbs.

This chapter focuses on recommendations for the integration of topical Chinese herbs, essential oils, natural creams, cleansers and masks, and other useful tools that will add to the effectiveness of your Constitutional Facial Acupuncture treatments.

Review the detailed facial acupuncture protocol in Chapter 6, and specifically refer to the beginning of the treatment section, which begins with Step 6.

The natural cleansers, face creams, essential oils and Chinese topical herbs and hydrosols illustrated in Figures 9.1–9.4 of this chapter, have been created by the author, and the precise blending and exact proportions of the ingredients in these *Muse L' Herbal* natural foods for the skin are proprietary information.

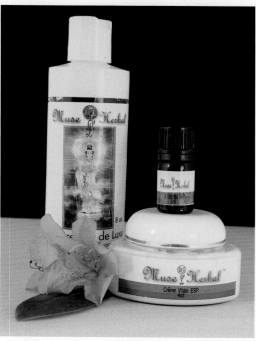

Figure 9.1 Cleanser, cream and essential oil with flower.

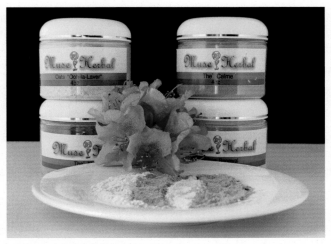

Figure 9.2 Herbal jars with flower.

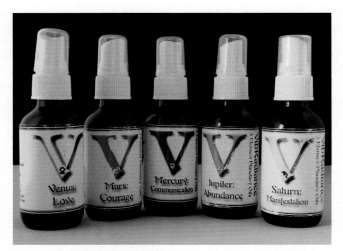

Figure 9.3 Five VibRadiance essential oil bottles.

Some of the ingredients are listed, along with suggestions for additional herbs, essential oils and natural foods, so that you may create a modular mixture for each individual patient.

Step 6: Cleansing

The treatment begins when the patient has entered the bathroom, changed into a robe and put on a headband that holds their hair in place, then washed their face with a natural facial cleanser, *Chevre Lait de Luxe* goat's milk cleanser, combined with a natural exfoliating facial scrub, *Oats 'Ooh-la-Laver.'*

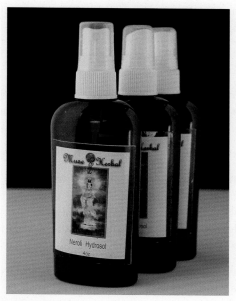

Figure 9.4 Three hydrosol spray bottles.

A Natural Exfoliating Facial Scrub; Oats 'Ooh-la-Laver'

This combination of organic oats, rose flowers, lavender flowers, almonds and French white clay exfoliates and cleanses the skin. Using this natural version of microdermabrasion gently sloughs off dead skin cells, improves the appearance of lines and wrinkles, and can prevent the effect of cross-linking of the collagen elastin fibers.

Organic Oats, *Avena Sativa*

Organic oats used topically are hydrating and when coarsely ground, can gently exfoliate the skin. They contain a high concentration of siliac acid, which reduces the inflammation and itchiness of eczema, psoriasis, and calms the redness and toxicity of facial blemishes, such as acne, blackheads and pimples. It is equally effective for sensitive, normal and oily skin. The skin is considered the third lung in Chinese medicine, and it is literally 'fed' by the ingredients of the topical herbal scrubs, masks, poultices, cleansers, creams and essential oils; it is important to select 'skin foods' that are free of toxic heavy metals and impurities.

Adding oats, with their anti-oxidant properties, to your patients' dietary regimen, combined with their use in topical masks and scrubs, can only enhance their well-being, both internally and externally.

Listed below are some important properties of the vitamins, minerals, amino acids and anti-oxidants contained in oats:

- Calcium: builds healthy bones and teeth, and speeds up wound healing and the body's healing process in general.

- Phosphorus: works in tandem with calcium, but also promotes healthy nerve and brain functions.

- Magnesium: is an important catalyst in enzyme reactions involved in energy production and helps in the utilization of vitamins, minerals and fats. It is essential for a healthy heart muscle, and is also a natural sedative.

- Manganese: nourishes the nerves, brain and the muscles.

- Cysteine: is an amino acid found in the keratin layer of the skin, and supports its structural integrity and resiliency. Keratinocyte cells waterproof and protect the skin, and undergo regular cell death. An imbalance causes the build-up of dead cells, dry skin, pigmentation, inflammation and wrinkles in the dermal layer of the skin.

- Glutatothione: is an anti-oxidant that protects the skin from free radical damage and inflammation.

- Vitamin B1 thiamine: helps prevent premature aging. It is essential for protein metabolism, protects the heart muscle, stimulates the brain, supports the immune system, aids in digestion and metabolism of carbohydrates, maintains the red blood cell count, protects the body from lead poisoning, edema, and congestive heart failure, and also improves blood circulation, prevents fatigue and increases stamina.

- Silicon: renews the bones and connective tissue in the skin, nails, hair and body. Collagen is the principal protein in connective tissue, therefore, silicon can play an important role in strengthening and maintaining the elasticity of the skin, and in preventing wrinkles.

CAUTION

Make sure that your patients do not have an allergy to oats. However, an internal sensitivity to oats may not be a problem in the case of topical application. If there is an oat allergy, prepare an oat paste by mixing oats with a little water, and have the patient spread the mixture on the inside of their arm for 24 hours to check for any negative reaction.

Remember that the Wood element patient has an allergic landscape and may be more prone to topical sensitivities (Chapter 4, under Wood element). If you are concerned about other possible reactions, test each ingredient individually in the same manner.

Rose Flowers, *Rosa Centifolia*

Rose flowers hydrate, rejuvenate and moisturize the skin, and contain a high percentage of the powerful anti-oxidant vitamin C. Vitamin C works synergistically with bioflavonoids to prevent inflammation and premature aging, and has other beneficial, protective qualities:

- Essential for healthy collagen production.

- Strengthens connective tissue.

- Supports the capillary walls and prevents capillary fragility, called thread veins, or cuperose skin.

- Prevents skin and capillary hemorrhages by acting as an anti-coagulant.

- Heals sores, wounds and treats scars, and skin conditions, such as dry skin, eczema and psoriasis.

- Treats sun-damaged skin.

- Firms and tones the skin's tissues.

- Protects the body and skin from environmental toxins and pollutants.

- Supports the function of the Lungs, and encourages a healthy immune system.

Lavender Flowers, *Lavendula Officialis*

Lavender calms anxiety, soothes the nerves, relaxes the Shen and relieves a wind heat headache, with a red face and eyes. It also regenerates cells and balances the skin's sebaceous glands. Some of its properties include the following:

- Regenerates cells, treats burns, sun-damaged skin and scars.

- Treats dermatological issues, such as acne, eczema, and psoriasis.

- Antiseptic and antibacterial: serious wounds, boils, carbuncles.

- Anti-fungal: fungal growths.

- Analgesic: muscular spasms, sprains and rheumatic pains.

- Lowers blood pressure, calms palpitations and relieves insomnia.

- Calms the central nervous system and alleviates depression.

- Treats colds, flu, bronchitis.

Almond, *Amygdalus Communis* Linn. Var. *Dulcis*

According to Chinese medicine, almonds moisturize the Lung, calm coughing, transform phlegm, and balance Qi. They also address facial puffiness, and when ingested, alkalize the blood. Linoleic acid, an omega-3 essential fatty acid, maintains the healthy cell membranes, protects the skin's defensive barrier, and prevents inflammation that can lead to dry and wrinkled skin.

Almonds also contain the potent anti-oxidant, vitamin E, which oxygenates the tissues, and retards aging.

Additional properties of vitamin E include:

- Speeds up the healing process, and prevents scar tissue formation in wounds, burns and pitting acne.

- Improves capillary circulation and addresses spider veins.

- Protects the Lung from environmental pollution, cigarette smoke and other toxins.

- Prevents rancidity when added to essential oils, creams or cleansers.

- Prevents heart disease, asthma, angina pectoris.

- Improves glycogen storage in the muscles.

- Treats reproductive disorders such as impotence and infertility.

French White Clay

French white clay absorbs toxins from the skin, is non-comedogenic, improves lymph flow, stimulates circulation, and delivers trace minerals absorbed through the skin into the blood stream. It is high in silica, which is essential for all healing processes in the body, treats dermatological issues such as eczema and psoriasis, and improves the quality and tone of the complexion. French white clay is gentle and absorbs impurities from the skin without drying out the epidermis.

Different colors of clay contain other minerals and elements, and target various skin imbalances:

- Pink rose clay: is tissue firming and rejuvenates mature skin on a cellular level. It contains iron oxide, which lends it the characteristic color, and silica, which is necessary for skin elasticity and healthy bones, nails and hair. Pink rose clay is gentle, and addresses both broken capillaries around the nose and cheeks and puffiness in the eye area due to Kidney deficiency.

- Red clay: has a higher content of iron oxide, and firms sun-damaged skin, reduces broken capillaries, and heals bruises and burns.

- Yellow clay: is gentle and can be used on sensitive to normal skin for dermatological issues, such as psoriasis, eczema and acne. It contains magnesium, iron oxide and silica.

- Green clay: is high in magnesium and it repairs tissue, draws toxins from the skin, stimulates circulation, eliminates acne, blemishes and cellulite. It also heals sprains and wounds.

Personalize your Constitutional Facial Acupuncture treatments for your patients by blending other natural ingredients with this exfoliating facial scrub. The ingredients can be found in powdered form, ground into fine powder, or slightly ground, to impart the necessary exfoliating properties.

Green tea is effective both in liquid and powdered form, and may be substituted for water when mixing the ingredients. This scrub can be used with the natural liquid facial cleanser, as a standalone cleanser, or as a facial mask when mixed with water, green tea, honey or other natural additives.

Gouqizi, *Fructus Lycii*, Chinese Wolfberry Fruit

Historically, the consumption of goji berries has been considered to promote longevity, enhance beauty and support healthy aging. In ancient China, women who drank goji berry tea, and ate the seeds, were reported to look at least 15–20 years younger than their chronological age.

Chinese medicine recommends Gouqizi in the treatment of deficiency issues, which is a contributing factor in the aging process. It nourishes and tonifies the Liver and Kidney Yin and blood, benefits Jing essence, and moistens the Lung.

Symptoms such as impotence, infertility, nocturnal emissions, diabetes, tuberculosis, blurred vision, dizziness and vertigo, and low-grade abdominal, back and knee pain, are targeted in a treatment.

Gouqizi is contraindicated when excess heat and external pathogens are present, and in cases of Spleen Damp with diarrhea.

Gouqizi has the following attributes:

- Lowers blood sugar associated with diabetes.

- Lowers blood cholesterol and prevents atherosclerosis.

- Enhances immunity.

- Promotes regeneration of Liver cells.

It also contains trace minerals, amino acids, vitamins, polysaccharides, essential fatty acids, phytosterols, carotenoids, such as beta carotene and zeaxanthin, and phenols, which have anti-oxidant properties.

Goji berries can be ingested, as well as added to topical cleansers, masks and poultices, to improve the results of your treatments.

Listed below are some of the more noteworthy constituents of goji berries, and their functions:

Zinc (Zn): is essential for collagen/elastin production; it is also a significant factor in both DNA/RNA repair and cell division. Zinc is involved in the processes of reproduction, tissue respiration, the construction of the insulin molecule, and energy metabolism. It is necessary for the metabolism of vitamin A, which is crucial in bone formation. Other benefits include:

- Healing of wounds and skin diseases.

- Amelioration of lethargy and fatigue.

- Elimination of toxic carbon dioxide from the body.

- Treatment of atherosclerosis, epilepsy and osteoporosis.

- Treatment of white spots on finger and toe nails, which can be a sign of zinc deficiency and/or Liver blood deficiency.

- Aids the normal functioning of the prostate gland.

Iron (Fe): is important for the formation of hemoglobin, which transports oxygen from the lung to every cell in the body. Iron increases general resistance to stress and disease, and also treats conditions such as anemia, fatigue, shortness of breath (SOB), a pale complexion and headaches. It is important to have sufficient hydrochloric acid in the stomach to be able to assimilate iron. Vitamin C aids in the absorption of iron. Wolfberries contain vitamin C, and synergistically contribute to more efficient digestion.

Selenium (Se): is an important anti-oxidant closely related to vitamin E, that protects the hemoglobin in red blood cells from oxidative stress. It also supports healthy aging by inhibiting the activity of free radicals in the body. It also:

- Regenerates the Liver.

- Prevents toxicity from mercury poisoning.

- Is essential for the enzyme function of glutathione peroxidase.

- Prevents muscular degeneration and premature aging.

Vitamin B$_2$, Riboflavin: is important for healthy eyes, skin, hair and nails. It prevents cataracts, itchy, bloodshot, light-sensitive eyes, inflammation, premature facial wrinkles on the face and arms and eczema. It also helps with a wrinkled thin upper lip, which can relate to menopause, a deficiency in the Spleen/Stomach, and the functioning of Chong Mai, which increases blood circulation in the area around the mouth.

Linoleic and Linolenic Acids: are important essential fatty acids (vitamin F), which lower blood cholesterol levels associated with atherosclerosis, prevent heart disease, support the adrenal glands, and make calcium and phosphorus available to the cells. They are necessary for healthy skin and mucus membranes. They also:

- Treat eczema, acne, and dry skin issues.

- Address hair loss.

- Treat retarded growth and impaired reproductive functioning.

- Help with menstrual imbalances.

- Treat Kidney disorders.

- Protect the body from overexposure to radiation.

Zeaxanthin and Lutein: are both anti-oxidant carotenoids located in the macula and lens of the eye, as well as in the skin. They protect both the macula and the skin from oxidative stress and aging.

Beta Carotene: is a well-known source of vitamin A which nourishes the body's mucous membranes, preventing eye diseases. It also:

* Nourishes the skin and hair.

* Prevents premature aging and senility.

* Increases life expectancy.

* Addresses rough, scaly, dry skin, acne, psoriasis, pimples and boils.

* Protects the body from the effects of air pollution.

* Oxygenates the tissues.

* Aids in the digestion of proteins.

Chaye, *Camellia Sinensis*, Green Tea Leaves

According to Chinese medicine, green tea is cold in temperature, and subsequently, treats imbalances that are hot in nature. As an example, green tea can help cool Stomach heat, which causes acid reflux, belching, nausea, vomiting and headaches. It also enters the Heart, Liver Spleen and Kidney, in addition to the Stomach.

The bitter taste functionally detoxifes, drains and dries. Therefore, green tea is a natural diuretic, effective in addressing issues of overweight and obesity, and dampness in the gastrointestinal system that impairs digestion.

Indications:
* Cools heat.

* Drains damp and damp heat.

* Descends rebellious Stomach Qi.

Pharmacological Effects:
* Contains caffeine, stimulates the central nervous system.

* Elevates the mood, clears the mind.

* Increases diuresis of the Kidney.

* Stimulates the secretion of gastric juices.

* Anti-inflammatory.

Contraindications:
Spleen deficiency and cold.

Green tea has many anti-oxidant benefits, if taken both internally and applied topically to prevent damage to the skin resulting from free radicals. Other beneficial constituents of green tea are:

Vitamin C: improves capillary circulation, oxygenates the tissues, and prevents oxidative stress in both face and body. It also contributes to collagen production and improves skin tone, structure and elasticity.

Epigallocatechin-3-Gallante (EGCG): is a powerful anti-oxidant that guards the body from inflammation and protects the skin from ultraviolet light (UV) exposure and radiation-induced DNA damage.

Other Ingredients

Acerola, Malpighia Emarginata Powder: is an anti-oxidant rich in vitamin C, A, B_2 and B_3. It moisturizes, tones, firms and protects the skin from capillary fragility and sun damage.

Horsetail, *Equisetum* Powder or Tea: is rich in silica, which tightens the skin to prevent wrinkles, strengthens brittle nails, and reinforces thinning hair.

Organic Ground Coffee: contains an anti-oxidant that exfoliates, astringes and closes the pores, protects and increases circulation to draw impurities from the skin. Use organic coffee grounds as a substitute for coarsely ground almonds or goji berries when treating oily, blemished skin. Do not use it on dry or aged, parchment skin, which is itchy due to blood deficiency.

Dark Organic Chocolate Shavings: release toxins and have a diuretic, firming action. In particular, they treat the 'orange peel' look on the chin, which I refer to as chin 'cellulite.'

Brown Sugar: moisturizes and exfoliates when added as an ingredient in this scrub.

There are many other herbs, teas and foods you can choose to us as potential additives to this exfoliating scrub. Do some research, look into other ingredients, and customize a treatment for each patient.

A Natural Goat's Milk Facial Cleanser, Chevre Lait de Luxe (Figure 9.1)

This unusual combination of goat's milk, natural fruit and alphahydroxy acids, not only cleanses the face but nurtures and feeds the skin with vitamins and a blend of essential oils. It is gentle, and beneficial for sensitive skin, with issues of eczema, psoriasis and rosacea, and also effective for oily skin. It is recommended for men as a cleanser and shaving cream, because it can heal ingrown hairs and prevent razor burns. This cleanser complements the facial scrub and they may be used in tandem for exfoliating and cleansing the face.

If the patient has any allergies to the ingredients, or has inflamed, dry, sensitive skin, simply eliminate the facial scrub; the cleanser will be sufficient.

Recommended ingredients for a natural facial cleanser:

Organic Aloe Vera Juice or Gel; *Aloe Vera*

Aloe vera contains phytochemicals, and is frequently added to cleansers and creams as an emollient to soothe, soften and moisturize the skin. Topically, it can heal wounds, burns and skin issues, such as psoriasis. Some sources report that it prevents sunburn, however, it has also been known to cause phototoxicity.

In addition to amino acids, it has both antibacterial and antifungal properties, and can address skin infections, boils, cysts, and inhibit fungal growths, as in tinea versicolor, or white spots on the skin. It is also ingested to treat ulcerative colitis and other digestive issues.

The properties of aloe vera in Chinese medicine include the following:

• Eases constipation.

• Reduces internal heat and inflammation.

• Suppresses menstruation.

• Treats children suffering from convulsions.

• Addresses atopic rhinitis, scrofula and boils.

CAUTION

Some patients are allergic to aloe vera, and when it is applied topically, they can react adversely, manifesting inflammation, erythema, skin irritation and dermatitis. Please check for sensitivity if you feel that it is warranted.

Extra Virgin Coconut Oil; *Cocos Nucifera*
Coconut oil is extracted from the meat of the coconut palm tree; it is a heat stable source of fat in the diet, and extremely useful when cooking at high temperatures.

It resists oxidation and rancidity, and is often added as an emollient in facial cleansers and creams, to prevent dry skin by acting as a protective barrier against external pathogens. According to Chinese medicine, coconut meat and milk, when consumed together, eliminate intestinal worms.

Usnea, *Usnea Barbata*
Usnea is a generic name for several lichen species, which grow and hang from trees. Due to its antibiotic properties, it has been used medicinally for thousands of years. Chinese medicine regards it as effective in the treatment of surface infections and skin ulcers.

The active component is usnic acid, which possesses anti-tumor properties that make it effective in treating staphylococcus and streptococcus infections manifesting on the skin. It treats Lung, upper respiratory and urinary tract infections, and its anti-bacterial and antifungal properties make it effective in addressing *Candida albicans*.

Research has found evidence to support the claims of antibacterial properties for usnea. Due to these qualities, usnea is a natural preservative for the facial cleanser.

CAUTION

When ingested, usnea may contribute to potential hepatotoxicity.

St. John's Wort, *Hypericum Perforatum*

St. John's wort is well-known as a natural anti-depressant, and is especially valued as an internal remedy for this syndrome in Germany, Austria and Switzerland.

Its chemical constituent hyperforin, which has anti-viral and anti-inflammatory properties, makes it topically effective in the treatment of infected surface wounds, burns, scars, hereditary atopic dermatitis and other inflammatory skin conditions.

It can be added to the cleanser as an emollient or a skin softener to soothe dry, irritated, inflamed and wrinkled skin.

Grape Seed Extract; *Vitis Vinifera*

Grape seed extract is derived from the whole grape seed and contains vitamin E, vitamin P (bioflavonoids), linoleic acid, and a polyphenol called reservatrol, acknowledged for both its anti-aging properties and its use in the treatment of cancer.

Its powerful anti-oxidants protect the skin cells, and also have excellent cleansing properties when blended into a natural facial cleanser. Other properties and applications include:

- Wound healing, treatment of eczema, acne, dry skin, and spider veins.

- Promotes improved circulation, which prevents the formation of scar tissue.

- Retards the aging process.

- Treats skin cancer: proanthocyanidins prevent malignancy and also protect the skin from ultraviolet (UV) rays.

- Prevents osteoporosis by building bone density.

CAUTION

According to clinical trials, if taken internally for more than 8–10 weeks, grape seed extract can cause headaches, nausea, dizziness and a dry, itchy scalp.

Step 7: Diagnostics

After they have come out of the bathroom, take their pulse, observe their tongue or perform other diagnostics that are relevant to the treatment.

Step 8: Herbal Poultice and Gem Discs (see Chapter 6)

Dip the cotton masks into the warm Nourishing or Calming Tea, and then place the mask on your patient's face. At the same time, immerse 2 cotton eye rounds into the Nourishing Tea only. This tea hydrates the delicate tissues around the eye, and prevents the formation of fine lines and wrinkles in this area. Gem discs are then laid on top of the cotton eye rounds to calm and ground the patient (see Figure 7.1).

Covering the eyes in this manner has a twofold purpose: it prevents the patient from watching you while you are needling their face, which can be disconcerting; and, on a more practical level, it prevents the small intradermal needles from falling in the eyes during the course of the treatment. It also encourages the patient to relax and be more receptive rather than focusing on the mechanics of the facial needling and other aspects of the treatment.

Intradermals

In Figure 7.16, small intradermal needles are threaded through the forehead line, just above the eyebrow. It is important to discern precisely where a line begins and ends; once having done so, angle a needle transversely from one end of the wrinkle toward the middle. Follow the same procedure with the other end. Then, place 1 or 2 intradermals, evenly spaced, in the center of the wrinkle.

Your intention is to shrink the line by terminating it simultaneously at both ends, preventing it from spreading further outward across the face. These small needles induce a microtrauma, which triggers the body's wound healing response, sending blood and fibroblasts to the site of the insertion. It is theorized that fibroblasts are the precursor to collagen/elastin production, and their action may diminish the size of the wrinkle over the course of several treatments, although, as yet, there is no scientific evidence to support this claim for facial acupuncture. Studies have been done that support the validity of this theory for other syndromes.[1] Intradermals are used when lines are present in the skin, but not particularly deep.

Tweezers

These playful tweezers (Figure 9.5) are used to insert and remove intradermal needles. A tweezer allows you to have more control in needling, and keeps

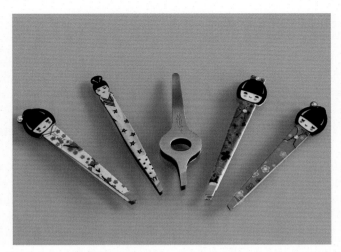

Figure 9.5 Five tweezers. © 2014 Janneke Vermeulen. Published by Elsevier Ltd. All rights reserved.

your fingers from accidentally coming in contact with any blood. When the needles are removed, place them in a cotton ball, and later deposit the needles in a sharps container.

Green Gel Mask (see Figure 7.2)

Heat a gel mask in a microwave for 20 seconds, or in a towel caddy, crock pot, or under hot running water until it is warm; adjust the temperature according to the patient's signs and symptoms. Lay the gel mask over the Chinese herbal poultice for additional penetration of the herbs into the skin. Leave it on the patient's face for 5 minutes while you needle the body points.

When the mask is removed, your patient's complexion should appear balanced; dry skin will look hydrated and glowing after an application of the Nourishing Tea. If you have chosen the Calming Tea, the skin will be less red and blotchy.

CAUTION

Some patients are claustrophobic, and will not want you to cover their faces with a gel mask, or have their eyes covered. Please honor their request to remove these items.

To remedy this situation, I cut a mylar 'space' blanket into a facial mask with holes in the appropriate places, and place it, instead, over the cotton poultice. The lightness of this mylar mask is less oppressive, weight-wise, and helps these patients tolerate the poultice without causing them anxiety. It is rare that they do not want the gem discs on their eyes, because they have holes in the center, and they can see through them. The smoothness of the discs is comforting, and they feel elegant. They also possess wonderful healing properties, which are a product of the unique mineral composition, the physical and psychospiritual indications, and the lore and traditions associated with the gem.

I have chosen 3 different gemstones – green jade, orange aventurine and rose pink rhodonite – based on their different mineral properties, particular color, and the availability of each. Green jade is a stone with a venerable history in Chinese medicine; the green color mirrors nature, is calming, and the stone can be used on all patients. Orange aventurine is warming and promotes blood circulation, and rose pink rhodonite heals both physical and emotional wounds.

Green Jade, Jadeite (Figure 9.6)

Since time immemorial, the Chinese have cherished jade as the most sacred of stones. Bridegrooms presented jade butterflies to their brides to symbolize love, newlyweds toasted each other with jade cups as they affirmed their vows. Chinese royalty drank a ceremonial libation of powdered jade, dissolved in water, immediately prior to death to preserve the physical body; jade and gold were then placed in the Nine Orifices to prevent decomposition and also to affirm the soul's purity on its journey into the afterlife.

In Taoist mysticism, jade represents the Five Virtues – wisdom, justice, modesty, courage and purity – as well as good fortune, prosperity and long life. An elixir of jade was believed to promote longevity, enhance Qi, delay the process of aging, and prevent infections and the formation of pus in the body. Jade worn on the body or applied to the face is cooling and is said to promote clear, unlined skin with bright Shen.

To this day in China, jade is still purported to heal asthma, anemia, leukemia, sepsis and other blood diseases.

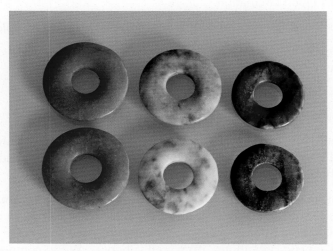

Figure 9.6   Three pairs of gem discs. © 2014 Janneke Vermeulen. Published by Elsevier Ltd. All rights reserved.

Qualities of Green Jade

Jade is composed of aluminum and sodium silicate, and:

- Aids meditation and alleviates stress.

- Instills compassion, virtue and tolerance.

- Regulates the Kidney, adrenals and urinary system.

- Supports awareness and self-realization.

To cleanse a jade stone, immerse it in sea salt and water, and, to clear the Qi, place the gem on top of an amethyst cluster, or leave it in sunlight.

Green jade opens the chest area, CV-17 Tan Zhong Chest Center, and Yintang M-HN-3 Hall of Seal. When placed on your patient's eyes during a treatment, jade can evoke a sense of peace, tranquility and rest.

Orange Aventurine

Aventurine is usually green in color, and therefore it is often confused with jade, as they are both relatively hard stones, 7 on the Mohs scale, and exhibit a similar shade of green. It also occurs in red or peach-orange colors, which arise from the specific mineral content. Orange aventurine is a glittering quartz containing silicon dioxide sprinkled with flakes of hematite. The color of the stone defines its particular properties and applications.

Qualities of Orange Aventurine

- Strengthens self-esteem.

- Promotes the ability to realize goals in a practical way.

- Stimulates blood circulation.

- Enhances blood flow to the skin, warms and enlivens the complexion.

- Supports the immune system and the connective tissue (see Chapter 4, Metal Element: The Immune Treatment).

- Prevents skin issues caused by nervous tension.

- Protects the individual from electromagnetic pollution.

The procedure for cleansing the stone is the same as with jade: immerse it in sea salt and water, place the gem on top of an amethyst cluster, and/or leave it in sunlight to clear the energies.

Use aventurine gem water topically as a wash to ameliorate eczema, rosacea and psoriasis. You can also drink it to treat skin issues related to emotional stress. It will help more sensitive patients who have adverse reactions to electromagnetic vibrations from cell phones, WiFi, computers, and microwaves.

Orange aventurine treats the physical body and its imbalances. It also warms and calms a patient who is cold and blood deficient, with a pale, dry complexion.

Rose Pink Rhodonite

Rose pink rhodonite contains calcium manganese isosilicate, interspersed with black veins of manganese oxide. Its name is derived from the Greek word, *rhodon,* which means rose. Due to its medium hardness of 6.5 on the Mohs scale, it has been carved or faceted into jewelry, vases, goblets and other beautiful objects.

Qualities of Pink Rhodonite

It has other indications and properties relating to its color, mineral content, and historical applications:

- Wound healing, including emotional scars.
- Treats injuries, bleeding sores, and itchy insect bites.
- Strengthens the Heart, and encourages blood circulation.
- Calms the nervous system.
- Has anti-inflammatory properties.
- For trauma and shock, immerse a piece of rhodonite in a pitcher of water to produce a gem elixir. Drinking it will calm the Heart.
- Most significantly, the rose pink color warms the Heart, and encourages compassion, forgiveness, self-acceptance, meditation and quiet.

Chinese Topical Herbal Poultices and Masks (Figure 9.2)

After the patient has exfoliated and cleansed the face, and you have taken the patient's pulse, examined the tongue and palpated the hara, or employed other diagnostic skills, you will ascertain whether the nutritive, nourishing, or cooling, calming facial poultices are needed.

The nutritive tea, *The Nutritif,* nourishes, replenishes and moves blood circulation to the face. It brings a rosy glow to the complexion, counteracting the presence of dry, thirsty, parched, withered skin. The poultice feeds and hydrates the skin of the face, neck and décolletage. It lifts the Yang Qi, to address sagging tendencies, invigorates and tonifies the blood, and fills in lines and wrinkles, while nourishing Kidney Yin, which brings moisture to the skin and supports the tone of the facial muscles.

This formula is based upon the Chinese herbal soup *Si Wu Tang,* Four Substance Decoction. It nourishes the cells of the facial tissue while moistening and tonifying the layers of the skin. The formula is combined with other topical Chinese herbs, essential oils, flower essences and seeds in a modular fashion to address each patient's personal needs.

CAUTION

Please note that in this chapter, I am advocating only the topical application of Chinese herbs. Do not recommend them to your patients for internal consumption, unless you have studied and possess the requisite understanding of the herbs, their indications, contraindications, possible toxicity and side effects, and compatibility and incompatibility with other herbs and pharmaceuticals.

Recipes: If you are using raw herbs, combine about 1 gram of each in a glass or ceramic pot with water, and adjust the formula accordingly, based on the individual patient's needs. Bring the mixture to a boil, and then simmer it for 20–25 minutes.

Strain the herbs and store the remaining liquid in the refrigerator in glass jars. The herbal mixture should last for a week, and can be used for multiple patients, provided that a sterile, disposable cotton mask is immersed in the reheated mixture, and applied to the face.

I prefer to mix Chinese herbal powders, rather than cook the raw herbs. When water is added to the herbal powder, it makes a tea, which also can be refrigerated for up to a week.

Si Wu Tang is a classical formula from the Sung Dynasty (AD 1107–1110) that is noted for treating blood deficiency imbalances. It targets gynecological issues, such as menstrual irregularities, uterine, anal, intestinal and postpartum bleeding, and mild anemia, with associated dry skin, pale complexion and lethargy, among other symptoms.

Si Wu Tang, Four Substance Decoction

The *Si Wu Tang* formula contains:

- Dang gui wei, *Radix angelicae Sinensis*, Chinese angelica root.
- Shu di Huang, *Radix Rehmanniae glutinosae conquitae*, Chinese foxglove root.
- Bai Shao, *Radix Paeoniae lactiflorae*, white peony root.
- Chuang Xiong, *Radix ligustici Chuangxiong*, Szechuan lovage root.

Dang Gui Wei, *Extremitas Radicis Angelicae* Sinensis
Uses the tail of the herb, instead of the head or body of the plant. The tails are the most effective part of the plant for moving blood; therefore, it also promotes circulation to the face.[2] It does tonify Qi, but not as much as the head or body of the herb. The tail relates to Wei Qi, and mirrors the Lung, therefore it invigorates circulation and carries nutrients to the skin.

Dang gui is warm in temperature, has a nourishing sweet taste, and also a pungent flavor, which disperses and moves Qi. It opens to the Heart, Liver and Spleen, has an ascending energetic effect, and its actions target the area of the lower Jiao and the meridians involved.

Indications:
- Tonifies and invigorates blood: Dang Gui Wei brings fresh blood and Qi to the skin, moisturizes and enlivens a pale complexion resulting from blood deficiency, addresses bruises and hematomas from blood stasis, and ameliorates dark circles under the eyes that relate to the Liver, Wood element and blood stagnation (See Chapter 7, under Eye Bags).

- Reduces swelling, pain and generates flesh: it alleviates pain and treats skin sores and abscesses due to wind damp.

- Moistens dryness: it addresses both intestinal and skin dryness.

Pharmacological Effects:
- Stimulates the immune system and has an antibiotic effect.

- Protects the Liver.

- Lessens arteriosclerosis.

- Sedative, analgesic action.

- Lowers blood pressure.

- Contracts the uterus.

- Treats painful neuralgias, and arthritis, when injected into acupuncture points.

Contraindications and Cautions: If taken internally, be cautious with patients who have diarrhea, or abdominal fullness due to dampness. It is contraindicated for Yin deficiency with heat symptoms. Use caution with pregnant women, because it invigorates blood and contracts the uterus, which can result in miscarriage. Take care with patients who are on blood thinners like Coumadin and warfarin.

I have not seen any negative symptoms arise when the poultice is used topically; however, as the skin reflects the Lung, and herbs are absorbed by the body through the skin, use your good judgment.

Shu di Huang, *Radix Rehmanniae Glutinosae Conquitae*, Chinese Foxglove Root

This blood and Heart tonic is cooked in wine to strengthen the Yin, nourish the skin and benefit the face, decrease blood sugar, support vital essence, clear blood heat, and produce fluids. It is a natural diuretic. The herb is slightly warm in temperature, and has a sweet taste. It opens to the Liver, Heart and Kidneys, affects the organs on a deep level, and addresses imbalances in the lower Jiao.

Indications:

- Tonifies and nourishes blood: pale complexion, dyspnea, palpitations, uterine and postpartum bleeding caused by blood deficiency.

- Nourishes Kidney Yin: night sweats and menopause.

- Tonifies Jing essence: premature aging, graying hair, wrinkles, memory loss, weak knees and lower back, exhausted blood and essence.

Pharmacological Effects:
- Treats hypertension.

- Decreases blood pressure.

- Lowers serum cholesterol levels.

Contraindications and Cautions: Be careful with patients who have Spleen/Stomach deficiency, stagnant Qi or phlegm issues; overuse can cause diarrhea, loss of appetite, fatigue and palpitations, if the herb is ingested.

Bai Shao, *Radix Paeoniae Lactiflorae*, White Peony Root

Bai Shao balances the Liver and the emotions, nourishes blood and consolidates Yin essence and vital fluids, soothes Liver Qi and relieves pain. It treats hypertensive headaches, tinnitus, spontaneous sweats and night sweats, chest and abdominal pain, and spasms in the calf muscles. It has a tightening, nourishing effect on the skin. Bai Shao calms the nervous system, and it prevents stress and premature aging.

Its temperature is slightly cold, which consolidates the Yin, and the bitter and sour tastes detoxify and astringe to prevent leakage of vital fluids. The herb opens to the Liver and Spleen, and directs Qi downward to calm and ground the Yang Qi. In treatment, it targets the area of the lower Jiao.

Indications:

- Nourishes blood: regulates menstruation, uterine bleeding and blood deficiency with a pale, ashen, dry face.

- Calms Liver Yang Rising and alleviates pain: the herb quiets and softens the Liver, and aids in the treatment of emotional issues, such as stress, and symptoms of Liver Yang Rising, such as headaches, dizziness and hypertension.

- Preserves Yin and balances Ying and Wei Qi levels: it addresses exterior wind cold with continuous sweating and Yin deficiency, with night sweats and vaginal discharges. It also treats spermatorrhea.

- Moves and regulates Qi: depression, premenstrual syndrome (PMS), cramps in the abdomen, muscles and tendons.

Pharmacological Effects:
- Anti-inflammatory.

- Sedative.

- Initiates platelet aggregation, helps with blood clotting and wound healing.

- Lowers serum glucose levels.

Contraindications and Cautions: Be careful with patients who have diarrhea due to deficiency cold, and also weak Yang Qi and deficiency cold.

Chuan Xiong, *Radix Ligustici Chuanxiong*, Szechuan Lovage Root

Chuang Xiong is a powerful herb for treating menstrual imbalances and hematomas due to blood stagnation. It also has antibiotic properties and addresses chemical burns, and fungal infections such as tinea versicolor, and protects the skin and body from radiation. Chinese lovage root is known for alleviating pathogenic wind-related issues like dizziness, headaches and itchy skin due to urticaria.

It moves Qi upward to the head and eyes to alleviate headache pain in the forehead and temples, as well as aching, painful joints. The temperature of the herb is warm, and it has a pungent taste. It opens to the Liver, Gall Bladder and Pericardium.

Indications:
- Invigorates blood, promotes movement of Qi: for menstrual imbalances like dysmenorrhea, amenorrhea, difficult labor or retained lochia after child-birth. It also moves Qi and blood to treat pain in the chest, limbs and hypochondria.

- Expels wind, alleviates pain: treats external pathogenic wind disorders such as dizziness, headache, wind-related skin issues like urticaria and painful Bi syndrome that affects the joints.

- Ascends Qi: alleviates headache pain due to wind, heat, cold or blood deficiency.

Pharmacological Effects:
- Antibiotic.

- Sedative.

- Inhibits platelet aggregation.

- Protects skin and body from radiation.

- Inhibits dermatomycosis (fungal skin infections).

- Contracts the uterus.

- Lowers blood pressure.

Contraindications: It is contraindicated for pregnancy and also for patients with Yin defiency heat signs, Qi deficiency, excessive menstrual bleeding or Liver Yang Rising headaches; an overdose of this herb can cause vomiting and dizziness when ingested.

Possible herbal additions to your Nourishing Tea:

Tao Ren, *Semen Persicae*, Peach Kernel

Tao Ren invigorates the blood, and enters the meridians and organs of the Heart, Large Intestine, Liver and Lung. Its neutral temperature allows it to replenish fluids while simultaneously enhancing Qi. The sweet taste moisturizes, nourishes, promotes Qi and soothes any wounds or sores on the face and body.

The bitter taste relates to the Heart, and it dries fluids, clears and drains congestion. The therapeutic direction of the herb moves Qi deeply within the body, downward and inward.

Externally:
Tao Ren moves blood and moisturizes dry, parched, thirsty skin. It also addresses swelling and inflammation; dermatologically, it treats dry skin issues, like eczema, and burns, wounds, abscesses and boils.

Internal Indications:
- Invigorates blood and treats blood stagnation: menstrual imbalances, uterine fibroids, traumatic injuries and hematomas, tumors, abscesses and ulcers in the lungs and intestines.
- Moistens intestines: treats dry constipation.
- Drains damp heat: cough, asthma, excess sputum.

Pharmacological Effects:
- Promotes menstruation.
- Treats tuberculosis.
- Anticoagulant effect.
- Anti-inflammatory.

Toxicity and Contraindications: One of the ingredients, amygdalin, is mildly toxic when ingested. It does not normally have the same effect when applied topically. Peach kernel is contraindicated for pregnancy, because it moves blood and could cause a miscarriage. Due to its anticoagulant effect, be careful when treating patients who are taking blood-thinning medications.

Hong Hua, *Flos Carthami Tinctorii*, Safflower Flower

Hong Hua invigorates the blood like Tao Ren, and enters the Liver and Heart. Its warm temperature accelerates Qi movement in the body, and the pungent taste disperses, moves and breaks up stagnation. This herb targets the lower Jiao and the meridians involved.

Externally: Hong Hua moves the blood, promotes facial circulation and encourages a rosy, glowing complexion in a patient who is blood deficient with dull, pale skin. It also addresses blood stagnation and treats skin issues such as eczema, burns, skin ulcers, painful wounds, injuries, hematomas, carbuncles and erythema, often associated with rosacea.

Internal Indications:

- Invigorates blood and treats blood stagnation: menstrual imbalances; amenorrhea, dysmenorrhea, painful abdominal masses, tumors, and tension and pain in the limbs.

- Alleviates pain: edema, swelling and pain from injuries, musculo-skeletal traumas.

Pharmacological Effects:

- Lowers high blood pressure.

- Improves coronary artery disease and arterial thrombosis.

- Stimulates uterine contractions.

- Lowers serum cholesterol.

- Musculoskeletal trauma: a tincture of Hong Hua heals swelling and subcutaneous hematomas due to acute sprains.

Contraindications: Pregnancy and severe bleeding following delivery.

He Shou Wu, *Radix Polygoni Multiflori*, Fleeceflower Root

Hou Shou Wu is a Yin and blood tonic and a longevity herb that enhances Jing essence. It has an astringent quality, stops leakage of vital body fluids, preserves the Qi and essence, and is neither cold, dry, nor oppressive.

The temperature is slightly warm and the sweet taste nourishes fluids and harmonizes Qi. The bitter taste condenses and binds fluids, and the area affected by this herb is the lower Jiao.

Externally: Hou Shu Wu tonifies blood, smooths out and moistens dry wrinkles due to blood deficiency, brightens the complexion, and treats wind rashes such as urticaria, with itchy dermal lesions, as well as eczema, burns, and toxic boils on the neck and body.

Internal Indications:

- Tonifies blood: dizziness, insomnia, blurred vision, sore, tingly extremities.

- Supports Jing and essence: nocturnal emissions, spermatorrhea, vaginal discharge, infertility, impotence, graying hair, weak knees and lower back.

- Moistens the intestines: dry constipation due to blood deficiency.

- Malaria: chronic blood deficient malaria.

Pharmacological Effects:

- Lowers cholesterol.

- Antibiotic properties.

- Treats malaria.

Cautions: Spleen deficient patients with phlegm and/or issues of diarrhea. The raw herb is bitter and cool, and can stimulate intestinal movement. This prepared herb has no side effects. Traditionally, patients should not eat onion, garlic or chives when using this herb internally.

Fu Ling, Sclerotium Poriae Cocos, China Root

Fu Ling has a neutral temperature, and nourishes fluids; its sweet taste regulates and generates fluids and balances Spleen Qi, while the blandness of the herb leaches out dampness in the body. Poriae enters the Heart, Spleen and Lung, has a calming, sinking effect, and addresses issues in the middle and lower Jiaos. Some sources indicate that it enters the Kidney and Bladder, due to its ability to promote urination.

This important herb operates on the physical and psychoemotional levels by leaching out dampness and preventing facial and body edema, promoting urination, transforming phlegm, which can cause palpitations, dizziness, and headache. It also calms the Shen to prevent insomnia, memory loss, nervous tension and stress.

Externally: Fu Ling brightens the complexion and addresses acute facial edema and Spleen-related puffiness under the eyes due to an imbalance in the Earth element, and poor transformation and transportation of Qi, blood and fluids in the Spleen. When phlegm rises to the head, due to Spleen Qi deficiency, there can be facial puffiness; when fluid remains in the body, it tends to collect around the ankles and feet. Often, there is water retention and weight gain with a tendency toward obesity.

Internal Indications:

- Drains and leaches out damp: edema, urinary problems, abdominal distention and heaviness in the body.

- Harmonizes and strengthens the Spleen and middle Jiao: decreased appetite, diarrhea and epigastric distention.

- Transforms phlegm: phlegm rises to the head and causes headaches, dizziness, and palpitations.

- Calms the Shen and anchors the spirit: palpitations, insomnia, forgetfulness.

Pharmacological Effects:

- Diuretic.

- Sedative.

- Antibiotic.

- Used in chemotherapy to support the immune system, improve the Kidney and Liver function, and to stimulate the appetite.

- Lowers blood sugar.

Contraindications: Cold deficiency syndromes and excess urination. Do not take in large doses for an extended period.

Calming Tea, *The Calme*

This herbal mixture cools the blood, addresses heat, fire toxins and wind issues, and quiets redness, damp and stagnant heat associated with skin conditions such as acne, rosacea, eczema, atopic dermatitis, psoriasis, hyperpigmentation and urticaria.

The herbs in this mixture also calm the Shen, reduce anxiety and stress due to excess heat and damp in the body. The calming tea can be combined with the nourishing tea to address combination skin.

Zhi Zi; *Fructus Gardiniae Jasminoidis*, Gardenia, Jasmine Fruit

Zhi Zi drains damp heat, cools the blood, reduces swelling and enters the Heart, Liver, Lung, Stomach and Triple Heater. Its cold temperature replenishes the Yin and the bitter taste purges toxic heat and inflammation from the body. This herb has a therapeutic sinking action, which prevents Yang Qi from rising, and allows it to work internally at a deep level to calm and balance the body.

Externally: Zhi Zi drains fire and damp heat and addresses boils, red, swollen painful eyes and lesions or sores in the mouth and on the face. It also moves blood stagnation, swelling and hematomas from traumatic injuries. The herbal powder is blended into whipped egg whites and applied topically to the area. This is a traditional way to deliver the herbs into the skin and to treat not only traumas, but also dermatological issues such as rosacea, pimples and blemishes.

Internal Indications:
- Clears heat and constrained emotions: anxiety, irritability, restlessness, insomnia, fever.
- Drains damp heat: urinary dysfunction, jaundice.

Pharmacological Effects:
- Increases bile secretion.
- Sedative, analgesic.
- Lowers blood pressure.
- Antibacterial, antifungal.
- Anti-parasitic.
- Increases soft tissue healing.

Contraindications and Cautions: The herb is contraindicated for diarrhea and loss of appetite due to deficiency cold. When ingested, due to its cold nature, nausea and vomiting may ensue, unless the herb is dry fried until it turns yellow prior to consumption.

Mu Dan Pi, *Cortex Moutan Radicis*, Moutan

Mu Dan Pi cools and moves the blood, treats Yin deficiency, disinfects and drains pus from sores, and reduces swelling both externally and internally. It does not induce nausea and vomiting when ingested. It enters the Heart, Liver and Kidney, and its temperature is slightly cold but not as cold as Zhi Zi. The pungent and bitter tastes disperse Qi and treat inflammation. The action of the Qi moves deeply into the lower Jiao.

Externally: Mu Dan pi moves blood, cools red purpura on the skin, treats blood stasis causing bruises and swelling from traumatic injuries; it has an antibacterial effect and drains pus from hard sores, abscesses and wounds.

Internal Indications:
- Clears heat, cools blood: nose bleeds, bloody sputum and stools, and excessive menstrual bleeding.
- Treats Yin deficient heat: low-grade fever, Steaming Bone syndrome without sweat, heat in the Five Palms – menopause.
- Clears Liver Fire: headaches, eye pain, flushing.
- Invigorates blood: menstrual issues due to blood stagnation, amenorrhea, fibroids.

Pharmacological Effects:
- Antimicrobial.
- Antibiotic.
- Lowers blood pressure.
- Lowers high fever.
- Sedative and analgesic properties.
- Anti-inflammatory.
- Treats allergic rhinitis.

Contraindications: Pregnancy, cold disorders, profuse menstrual bleeding and Yin deficiency with excessive sweating.

Ku Shen, *Radix Sophorae Flavescentis*, Sophora Root

Ku Shen addresses skin issues characterized by purulent damp oozing sores, chicken pox, scabies, itchy skin diseases like urticaria, as well as genital rashes, yellow, viscous leucorrhea, and fungal infections. It treats damp heat skin lesions, ulcerative sores and eczema, and clears dysentery, jaundice and cystitis.

The temperature of the herb is cold and the bitter taste clears heat and damp issues. Ku Shen opens to the Heart, Liver, Small Intestine, Large Intestine, and Bladder meridians.

The direction of the herb is sinking, which prevents empty Yang Qi from floating upward; it acts on the skin like Ju Hua, but its energy moves toward the lower Jiao.

Externally: Sophora root benefits the complexion and treats eczema, psoriasis, acne and rosacea due to damp heat, and wind issues, which add itchy skin into the equation. Boils, fungal infections, scabies caused by skin parasites (mites), skin lesions, oozing sores and genital itching can be treated effectively with a topical poultice of Ku Shen.

Internal Indications:
- Clears heat and drains damp: amoebic dysentery, jaundice, leukorrhea, vaginal itching.
- Clears heat and promotes urination: cystitis, hot edema, damp heat in the Small Intestine, scanty urination.

Pharmacological Effects:
- Antibiotic.
- Anti-parasitic.
- Anti-mycotic (fungal skin infections).
- Treats arrhythmia.
- Dysentery.
- Dermatological diseases.
- Anti-asthmatic.
- Antibacterial.
- Used in treatment of cervical, stomach and liver cancer.

Contraindications: Do not use with deficiency cold patterns in the Spleen/ Stomach.

Huang Bai, *Cortex Phellodendri*, Phellodendron
Huang Bai addresses damp heat issues related to fire toxins seen in sores, damp skin lesions, burns, ulcerations, eczema, fungal nail infections, herpes zoster, pruritis, boils and abscesses.

The temperature is cold, and the taste is bitter, as is the case with most of the heat clearing herbs. Huang Bai opens to the Kidney and Bladder, and some sources also add the Small Intestine and Large Intestine meridians. Its direction is sinking, and it travels to the lower Jiao.

Externally: Phellodendron treats sores, damp skin lesions, eczema, particularly visible around the ears, boils, infections, abscesses, and herpes zoster.

Internal Indications:

- Drains damp heat in the lower Jiao: yellow, thick leucorrhea, foul smelling diarrhea, dysentery, red, swollen, painful knees, legs and feet, damp heat-related jaundice.

- Yin deficiency: night sweats, malar flush, afternoon and nocturnal sweats, Steaming Bone syndrome, due to deep internal heat from Yin deficiency.

Pharmacological Effects:
- Meningitis.

- Dysentery.

- Conjunctivitis.

- Lowers blood pressure.

- Increases intestinal peristalsis.

- Increases pancreatic secretions.

- Fungal skin infections.

Contraindications: Spleen deficiency with or without diarrhea.

Ju Hua, *Flos Chrysanthemi Morifolii*, Chrysanthemum Flower

Ju Hua is a harmonizing herb that is effective both by itself, and in combination with other herbs. It is recognized for its ability to treat eye disorders due to wind heat in the Liver meridian. It also detoxifies and clears blood heat that manifests as infected, painful skin ulcerations and sores. It vents allergic skin rashes and treats headache, dizziness, vertigo, and deafness due to Liver Yang Rising.

The herb has a sweet taste that generates fluids, combined with a bitterness that drains heat from the body. It is slightly cold and cools heat, but not fire toxins like cold herbs, such as Zhi Zi and Ku Shen.

The herb sinks Qi downward to anchor the Yang, and addresses the area of the head, eyes and skin.

Externally: The chrysanthemum flower clears wind heat and treats inflamed, dry, bloodshot eyes. It is also employed effectively in topical eye compresses to dispel these symptoms. A tea can be brewed from the powdered herb for internal consumption, and the remainder of the tea used as a compress or poultice over a patient's eyes during a Constitutional Facial Acupuncture treatment. Tea bags can also be used.

I recommend placing the dried chrysanthemum flowers, slightly warmed in water on a tissue over the patient's eyes. The tissue protects their eyes from stray pieces of the flower, and also allows the herbal essence to penetrate the eyes.

Ju Hua also addresses dermatological conditions such as eczema, infected purulent sores, skin ulcerations and boils, and it vents skin rashes arising from heat and wind.

Internal Indications:
- Releases the exterior and addresses wind heat: treats fever by inducing perspiration, eases red, inflamed eyes and blurred vision, dizziness and vertigo.

- Harmonizes the Liver: treats Liver Yang Rising, with symptoms including tinnitus, hypertension and deafness.

Pharmacological Effects:
- Antibacterial, anti-viral.

- Antifungal.

- Treats hypertension and atherosclerosis.

- Anti-inflammatory.

- Reduces fever.

Contraindications and Cautions: Be careful with patients who have Qi deficiency, with poor appetite and/or diarrhea.

Step 9: Needle the Body (see Chapter 7)

When you have placed the gel mask on the patient's face, over the herb-infused poultice, needle the body, completing your constitutional treatment.

Step 10: Remove Gel Mask and Poultice

Remove the gel mask and cotton poultice, and give your patient arnica 6C to prevent bruising.

Step 11: Jade Rollers

Prior to needling the face, cool it down and prevent hematomas by gently rolling it with two jade rollers. Jade rollers are utilized twice during this

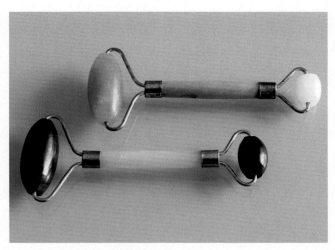

Figure 9.7 Two double-headed jade rollers. © 2014 Janneke Vermeulen. Published by Elsevier Ltd. All rights reserved.

protocol, prior to facial needling, and again at the end of the treatment, to even out the complexion, calm redness and enhance the penetration of the natural cream into the skin (Figure 9.7).

Jade has been prized in China for centuries for both its mystical and practical attributes; its natural cooling properties preserve and protect the skin. It was an intrinsic part of the beauty regimens of the Chinese Empresses, and it is believed that the stone nurtures beauty and fosters longevity.

Instead of applying cold sponges, a cold cloth or ice to your patient's face, it is more elegant, comfortable, effective, and consistent with the traditions of Oriental medicine to incorporate jade rollers. You only need to roll over the patient's face and neck 3 times to cool the facial tissues sufficiently to minimize the risk of bruising.

Be sure that you use the smaller head of the roller gently around the eyes to avoid harming the delicate skin in this area of the face. If your patient wears contact lenses, be cautious with this step of the protocol.

You are now ready to begin the facial needling component of your Constitutional Facial Acupuncture treatment.

CAUTION

Please note – Do not apply alcohol directly to the face prior to needling; the Chinese herbal formulas previously introduced have a myriad of antibacterial and anti-viral properties, and protect the face naturally. Alcohol is unnecessary, and it will dry and irritate the skin.

Step 12: Remove Facial Needles

When the appropriate amount of time has passed, gently remove the facial needles, and some of the body needles. I usually leave a few body needles in place to keep the patient grounded and anchored while I paint on the Renewal Facial Mask.

Step 13: Mask with Brush

At this point in the treatment, the Renewal Mask is applied to the face, décolletage and the neck with a fan brush (see Figure 7.17). If there are any herbs left on the skin from the herbal poultice, do not wash them off. Simply paint the Renewal Mask directly over them, to close the pores, and drive the nourishment of the poultice and mask directly into the epidermis.

Renewing Facial Mask; Masque Renewal

This Chinese herbal powdered tea becomes a lifting mask when mixed with egg whites. The cool frothed egg whites allow the herbs to penetrate the skin more effectively, while toning, astringing and stimulating the flow of fresh blood to the facial tissues.

Masque Renewal can be blended with a variety of other ingredients to address the specific needs and constitutional imbalances of a given patient. Just as a reminder, all of these herbs are to be applied topically; consult a Chinese herbalist about their internal use if you do not have the requisite knowledge and experience.

Mu Li, *Concha Ostreae*, Oyster Shell

Mu li grounds and calms the spirit; it benefits Kidney Yin and treats insomnia, irritability, palpitations, a red,flushed face, and leakage of vital fluids which debilitates the body. It also relieves epigastric pain and peptic ulcers.

It has a tendency to manifest a cool temperature with a salty taste which astringes fluids, softens and loosens nodules and lumps in the neck and body. It opens to the Liver and the Kidneys, and its direction is sinking, and therefore calming and anchoring. It works deep in the body by targeting the lower Jiao.

Externally: As an ingredient in the Renewal Mask, Mu li functions as an anchoring, binding agent to calm Yin deficiency imbalances, such an excessively flushed, red face or restlessness that occur after the facial needling. Mixed in the frothed egg whites, Mu li tends to astringe, close the pores, cool and calm irritability and anxiety, and alleviate any headache or hot flashes that may arise during the treatment.

309

It helps to prevent menopausal sweating, and softens nodules, goiters, fatty tumors or an enlarged thyroid gland.

Internal Indications:
- Calms and anchors the spirit, benefits the Yin: palpitations, anxiety, insomnia, dizziness, tinnitus, bad temper.

- Prevents leakage of vital essence: spontaneous and continuous perspiration, night sweats, Steaming Bone syndrome, nocturnal emissions, spermatorrhea, leukorrhea, uterine bleeding.

- Softens nodules and masses: scrofula, goiters, enlarged thyroid, tumors, cysts.

- Relieves pain and absorbs acidity: epigastric pain and gastric or duodenal ulcers.

Pharmacological Effects:
- Neutralizes gastric acid and treats ulcers.

- Prevents night sweats arising from tuberculosis.

Contraindications and Cautions: Contraindicated for high fever with an absence of perspiration arising from an excess condition. Overdosing can lead to indigestion or constipation.

Zhen Zhu, *Margarita*, Pearl
Pearl powder has been used as a beauty treatment in China for centuries to brighten the complexion, sharpen vision, reduce redness, even out blotchy or discolored skin, and to encourage the healing of burns, wounds and mouth ulcers.

It is a cold herb that supports the Yin and calms internal heat. It has a sweet taste to nourish fluids, and also salty, so that it collects fluids and softens any nodules or masses within the body. Like Mu li, it sinks down deeply into the interior, enters the Liver, and, in the case of Zhen Zhu, also the Heart.

Externally: Pearl powder contains a high amount of calcium, which is essential to the vital functioning the body; it accelerates the healing process, and addresses palpitations, insomnia and irritability. Another mineral, silica, is similarly important for healing and the maintenance of healthy hair, nails and teeth. It prevents skin aging through minimizing the formation of wrinkles by supporting the skin's resiliency and flexibility.

Topically, it can treat rashes, pimples, blemishes, blotches, hyperpigmentation, and eczema caused by heat. Silica has a beneficial impact on facial wrinkles because of its smoothing, softening and clearing actions; it is an important ingredient in creams and masks. Internally, it can be taken in capsules for insomnia, or as a powder dissolved in water. (See Chapter 4: Seasonal Allergies, Wood Element treatment).

Internal Indications:

- Grounds the heart and anchors the Yang: convulsions (children), seizures, epilepsy, vertigo, tinnitus, insomnia, palpitations, easily frightened or angered.

- Clears the Liver and sharpens vision: clears vision, blurred vision and red eyes.

- Promotes healing and generates flesh: used topically for chronic, non-healing wounds or ulcers, mouth ulcers, burns and skin issues such as eczema.

Pharmacological Effects:

- A daily intake of pearl powder has been found to improve memory, energy levels, concentration, and boost the immune system in elderly patients.

- Treats gastric acid and painful peptic ulcers.

Contraindications and Cautions: Be cautious with patients who have a cold abdomen, otherwise there are no contraindications.

Ren Shen, *Radix Ginseng*, Ginseng Root

Chinese medicine practitioners value Ren Shen for its ability to promote longevity; and it is said to have 'superpowers' because of its many important functions. It is an adaptogen, allowing the body to absorb what it requires from the herb, and it is a Qi tonic and augments vital energy. It hydrates and protects fluids in the body and face, calms the spirit and emotions, benefits the brain and stimulates memory. Ren Shen also prevents prolapses of the uterus, anus and platysma muscle of the neck, which alleviates sagging. It is a Heart tonic, lowers blood pressure and enhances the immune system. Chinese ginseng is slightly warm and slightly bitter, which dries and detoxifies the body; it also has a sweet taste, which tonifies Qi. It opens to the Spleen and Lung, and targets the area of the middle Jiao to lift and direct Qi upward.

Externally: Chinese ginseng is a Qi tonic; it especially tonifies Lung Qi, which promotes the flow of fluids throughout the body. The skin is the third Lung in Chinese medicine and has rulership over Qi; therefore, Ren Shen augments Qi, and assists the Lung in conveying fluids and nutrients to the skin, to hydrate and enliven a tired, pale complexion. Ren Shen also raises Spleen Qi, and it can treat prolapses, sagging skin and muscles in the face.

Internal Indications:

- Tonifies Lung Qi: augments Qi and treats wheezing, shortness of breath (SOB), Lung Qi deficiency and the pattern of Kidney not Grasping Lung Qi.

- Raises the Qi: prolapses of the uterus, stomach, and rectum. Also effective for diarrhea and severe blood loss.

- Generates fluids: diabetes, injury to fluids by high fever, profuse perspiration.

- Calms Shen: tonifies Heart Qi; palpitations, anxiety, insomnia, poor memory, restlessness due to Qi and blood deficiency.

Pharmacological Effects:
- Increases endurance.
- Stimulates memory.
- Supports the immune system.
- Cardiac tonic.
- Lowers blood sugar and cholesterol.
- Treats peptic ulcers.
- Increases wound healing.
- Reduces toxicity of certain chemicals.

Contraindications and Cautions: Yin deficiency with heat, heat excess or an absence of significant Qi deficiency, hypertensive patients with Liver Yang Rising, and very high blood pressure.

Hua Shi, Talcum

Hua Shi is a diuretic herb that drains damp heat from the Bladder and Stomach. It is a cold herb that eliminates summer heat with signs of fever, thirst, and irritability and absorbs the damp from skin lesions and the heat from prickly rashes.

The bland taste eliminates excess fluids from the body, and acts as an emollient; the sweet taste of the herb tonifies, nourishes and harmonizes Qi. The herb moves Qi downward and targets the lower Jiao, opening to the Bladder and Stomach.

Externally: Talcum powder applied topically has been known to demonstrate antibacterial properties; it treats skin lesions and wounds, and protects the mucus membranes by absorbing toxins. It promotes the formation of scar tissue, and addresses both eczema and prickly heat rashes. Talcum has moistening properties, and nourishes the skin; it also releases the heat and toxicity from blemishes and pimples.

Internal Indications:
- Promotes urination and drains heat: hot, painful urination, cystitis, damp heat-related diarrhea.
- Clears summer heat: fever, vomiting, thirst, irritability, scanty urine.
- Absorbs damp: skin lesions, eczema, edema.

Pharmacological Effects:
- Protects skin mucosa from toxic chemicals.
- Protects the stomach from gastritis, vomiting and diarrhea.
- Inhibits the absorption of poisons in the gastrointestinal tract.
- Antibacterial.
- Diuretic action.

Contraindications and Cautions: Contraindicated for absence of damp in the body. Long-term use may injure the Yin fluids.

Sang Ji Sheng, *Romulus Sangjisheng,* **Mulberry Parasite, Loranthus**
Sang Ji Sheng is a parasite found on the white mulberry plant that tonifies deficient Liver and Kidney Yin, and also dispels wind damp, which can cause arthritic pain. It can prevent miscarriages, addresses blood deficient dry skin and calms hypertension.

The temperature of Loranthus is neutral and regulates fluid metabolism and the bitter taste dries, detoxifies and drains fluids. Some sources also report that it has a tonifying, sweet, taste.

The targeted organs are the Liver and Kidney and the treatment direction is deep within the lower Jiao.

Externally: It treats blood deficiency that manifests as dry, scaly skin, and a pale, withered complexion with wrinkles. Sang Ji contains vitamin P, and important bioflavonoid called quercetin, which not only prevents spider and varicose veins, but also addresses hypertension, eczema and psoriasis.

Traditionally, chicken eggs mixed with brown sugar are applied topically to hydrate and ameliorate the appearance of dry, scaly skin.

Internal Indications:
• Tonifies Kidney and Liver Yin and expels wind damp: arthritic pain in the back, knees and joints, and atrophy of the tendons and bones.

• Nourishes the blood: prevents miscarriage and calms a restless fetus.

• Alleviates hypertension: lowers blood pressure.

Pharmacological Effects:
• Diuretic.

• Sedative.

• Lowers blood cholesterol.

• Treats hypertension.

• Treats capillary fragility.

• Anti-viral.

• Cardiac tonic.

Contraindications and Toxicity: Large doses taken internally can cause diarrhea and vomiting.

Other Ingredients

Chicken Eggs
Whole chicken eggs are considered a complete source of protein, and can be integrated into your diet and ingested and/or employed topically

313

for dermatological imbalances. A whole egg is veritable treasure trove of vitamins, minerals, amino acids, essential fatty acids and CoQ10, among other important nutrients. The yolk of the egg contains the majority of these nutrients, like choline, a significant member of the family of B complex vitamins.

Choline: teams up with inositol, a constituent of lecithin, for proper fat metabolism. It is also necessary for the synthesis of DNA and RNA nucleic acids, which are the building blocks of our physical structure. Choline also addresses the following conditions:

- Glaucoma.

- High blood pressure.

- Atherosclerosis.

- Gall stones and cirrhosis of the Liver.

- Kidney damage.

Retinol (Vitamin A): strengthens the immune system, and maintains the health of the mucus membranes. It also addresses:

- Poor vision and night blindness.

- Unhealthy teeth and gums.

- Rough, scaly, dry skin.

- Acne, pimples, psoriasis, eczema, boils and wrinkles.

- Hair loss and brittle nails.

Riboflavin (Vitamin B_2): is important for physical growth and a healthy constitution. It also addresses:

- Photosensitivity.

- Itchy, burning eyes.

- Cracks in the lips and mouth.

- Dull, oily hair.

- Premature wrinkling of the face and skin.

- Eczema.

- Thinning upper lip, due to aging.

Folic Acid (vitamin B_9): works in tandem with B_{12} to support the formation of red blood cells, and it protects the DNA and RNA, nucleic acids that carry our genetic patterns. It also addresses:

- Immune system support and prevents infection.

- Protein metabolism.

- Healthy hair and skin.

- Encourages normal growth.

- Prevents premature hair graying.

- Anemia.

- Atherosclerosis.

- Radiation injuries and burns.

- Acute diarrhea and stomach ulcers.

- Depression.

- Anemia during pregnancy and other reproductive disorders.

Pyridoxine (Vitamin B_6): **aids in the assimilation of food and protein and fat metabolism. It supports the functioning of DNA and RNA, fortifies the brain and nervous system, and regulates the body's balance between sodium and potassium. It also addresses:**

- Anemia.

- Edema.

- Depression.

- Acne, eczema.

- Nervous tension and irritability.

- Insomnia.

- Migraine headaches.

- Premature senility.

- Parkinson's disease.

- High cholesterol.

- Diabetes.

- Heart disease.

- Lessens the severity of seizures.

Vitamin B_{12}: is important for the production of red blood cells. It also addresses:

- Anemia.

- Growth in children.

- Chronic fatigue syndrome.

- Difficulty concentrating.

- Poor appetite.

- Neuropathies in the body.

Vitamins A, D and E are found in the egg yolk only:

Vitamin D: assimilates calcium, phosphorus and other minerals in the intestine and stomach, and supports the functioning of the parathyroid gland, which regulates blood calcium levels. Vitamin D is absorbed by the body through the skin. It also addresses:

• Tooth decay and poor gums.

• Osteoporosis.

• Retarded growth and poor bone formation in children.

• Fatigue.

• Deficient assimilation of minerals.

• Rickets.

• Weak muscles.

• Premature aging.

Vitamin E: oxygenates the tissues, prevents rancidity when added to other substances, improves blood circulation, and prevents the formation of scar tissue. It also addresses:

• Heart disease.

• Reproductive diseases.

• Capillary fragility and varicose veins.

• Aging tendencies.

• Asthma, arthritis.

• Hypoglycemia.

Traditional Chinese medicine has historically recognized the value of chicken eggs both as a source of dietary nourishment and in the treatment of constitutional imbalances. Eggs are also valued as an additive in poultices, masks and plasters, which are then applied to the body and face.

In Constitutional Facial Acupuncture, frothed organic egg whites, blended with various powdered Chinese herbs, are used to address specific dermatological conditions. The part of the egg that is selected depends on the patient's individual skin type, signs and symptoms.

Organic eggs benefit Lung Qi, and ameliorate symptoms such as dry cough, sore throat and hoarseness; they also treat conjunctivitis, diarrhea, and are topically effective in treating burns.

The temperature is neutral, and the taste is sweet, which nourishes and lubricates the skin. The egg yolk by itself tonifies the blood and treats issues of blood deficiency that manifest as dry skin and pale complexion. Whole organic eggs are effective topically in addressing the following:

- Neurodermatitis.

- Psoriasis.

- Severe skin itching.

- Blotchy, hyperpigmented skin.

- Lines and wrinkles.

Organic egg whites also ease conditions such as sore throat, cough, diarrhea, conjunctivitis, burns and laryngitis. However, the temperature is cool, not neutral, and therefore, they can alleviate issues of Lung heat. The taste is sweet, which lubricates and moistens the Lung and skin.

Organic egg whites also possess anti-inflammatory properties, and are especially good for treating first, second and third degree burns. They are used in treatment in various ways:

- Inflamed skin infections and wounds.

- Otitis media (when mixed with sesame oil).

- Vaginitis after childbirth.

- Firming, toning and tightening the skin.

- Hyperpigmentation and red blotches on the face.

- Astringing and tightening the pores.

Egg whites contain more protein than the yolks; frothing them aerates and activates the proteins, which creates a powerful synergy with Chinese herbs. After the mask is painted on the face with a fan brush, the herbal mixture is readily absorbed by the skin, and the protein feeds the facial muscles.

Organic egg whites are more beneficial for normal and oily skin, because of their heat clearing properties. Conversely, egg yolks tonify the blood, and improve dry, blood deficient skin.

Whole eggs may be used to treat combination skin. The neutral temperature and coolness of the egg white can both nourish and cool heat. The sweetness hydrates and moisturizes the skin.

CAUTION

Please note that some patients have an allergy to eggs, especially to the whites. I do not recommend using eggs topically on a person with this allergy.

You may substitute other ingredients for chicken eggs in the Renewing Mask:

Champagne

Champagne is a lively, festive substitute for eggs. It contains potent anti-oxidants that stimulate the metabolism of the skin, and promote cellular growth. Champagne leaves the skin looking vibrant and glowing. The tartaric acid component, which gently exfoliates dead skin cells, is an anti-oxidant that is found in all wines.

Just combine the powdered herbs with the champagne, and froth them together. The natural effervescence of the champagne will transport the Chinese herbs directly to the epidermis. Champagne can be used for all skin types.

Feng Mi, Mel, *Apis Melifera*, Honey

Honey is a sweet natural food manufactured by bees with the nectar that they collect from flowering plants. Bees transform the nectar into honey by a process of regurgitation and evaporation, and it is stored in the hive for the benefit of the colony.

Honey contains anti-oxidants, monosaccharides, fructose, glucose, flavonoids, and amino acids such as gluconic acid, proline and malic acid, which provides honey with its characteristic taste and aroma. Other natural ingredients include vitamins A, B_2, C and D.

The ancient Chinese cultivated honey for centuries, consumed it as food, and used it topically on skin rashes, burns, wounds, and dry, cracked skin to prevent wrinkles and nourish the skin.

Honey

Honey is considered a general tonic for the body, like ginseng. It is neutral in temperature, and sweet, which strengthens, tonifies, lubricates and harmonizes the body. It affects the Stomach, Spleen and Lung, and also the Large Intestine, according to some sources. It has the following properties and effects:

* Tonifies the body.
* Protects the mucus membranes from inflammation. demulcent.
* Moisturizes and nourishes the skin and body.
* Works as a laxative.
* Expectorant. removes phlegm from the Lungs.
* Antibiotic effects.
* Astringent. protects the body from leakage.
* Relieves pain; analgesic.

Indications (External and Internal):
* Dry cough.
* Dry constipation.
* Stomach aches.

- Dry eyes.

- Sinusitis.

- Hypertension.

- Tuberculosis.

- Heart and Liver disease.

- Calms anxiety and hysteria.

- Gastric and duodenal ulcers.

- Bacillary dysentery.

- Heals dry, cracked skin, burns.

Clinically, honey is reported to heal the pain of gastric and duodenal ulcers, treat acute bacillary dysentery, plus chronic and temporary constipation in elderly patients and pregnant women. It relieves insomnia due to anxiety, headache and anemia.

Honey can be substituted for both chicken eggs and champagne, and is a good medium for powdered Chinese herbs. This resulting facial mask is more sticky and messy, but it produces wonderful results with all skin types, especially dry and mature skin.

Step 14: Remove Needles

Remove the remaining needles from the body while the Renewal Mask dries on the patient's face. It dries and sets rather quickly when blended with frothed egg whites or champagne. A honey-based mask will not dry, and it will be necessary for you to wash it off at the appropriate time. I usually leave the mask in place for 5 minutes.

Step 15: Towel

When the mask is sufficiently dry, use a bar towel, which is thinner and longer than an ordinary hand towel, to remove it (see Figure 7.18). See Chapter 6 for more detailed instructions.

Step 16: Vitalizing Face Cream and Essential Oils

Vitalizing Face Cream; Crème Vitale ESP (Figure 9.1)

Take a small amount of the Vitalizing Face Cream (Crème Vitale ESP) and massage it into the patient's face (see Figure 7.19A, which demonstrates facial massage: hands on temples; and Figure 7.19B, facial massage: hands on forehead).

Crème Vitale ESP is a lush, non-greasy cream containing the anti-oxidant, penetrative qualities of organic camellia seed oil. It is an emollient rich in fatty acids, in particular oleic acid, which mirrors the sebum of the skin.

Crème Vitale ESP also contains organic neroli essential oil, which treats skin conditions such as scars, stretch marks and thread veins. Psychoemotionally, neroli also relieves anxiety and instills inner peace. This vitalizing cream is easily absorbed by the skin, and it is recommend for both men and women and all skin types.

To create a custom blended facial cream, begin with a natural cream base, and then add essential oils, Chinese herbs and other ingredients to the formula. A natural cream base can be found in health food stores, online stores that carry cosmetic products, and from companies that carry spa supplies. Make sure that you purchase a natural or organic cream bases free of heavy metals or toxic chemicals.

A number of possible additions to a vitalizing cream appear in the sections on the goat's milk cleanser (Chevre Lait de Luxe) and the Renewing Mask (Masque Renewal), earlier in this chapter. For example:

• Organic usnea.

• Virgin coconut oil.

• Organic aloe vera juice or gel.

• St. John's wort.

• Grape seed extract.

• Pearl powder.

• Green tea.

Ge Hua, *Citrus Aurantium/Vulgaris*, Organic Neroli Oil

Organic neroli, orange blossom essential oil, is a distillate of the white flowers of the bitter Seville orange tree; it has a floral smell and a sweet, spicy taste. Its nature is neutral according to Chinese medicine, being neither hot nor cold. Therefore, it can treat both temperatures, and signs and symptoms such as a dry, pale complexion and an inflamed, sunburned face. The oil is considered to be a middle note, which means that it evaporates at a moderate rate. The petals were, and still are, used in China in creams, cosmetics and perfumes.

Neroli essential oil is very precious and expensive, because it takes a large amount of flowers to produce a thimbleful of oil. It was named after an Italian princess, Anne-Marie, Countess of Neroli, who was famous for using neroli oil to scent her gloves and bath water.

Properties:

- Sedative, anti-depressant, antiseptic, digestive, anti-spasmodic, aphrodisiac, emollient, tonic, carminative, euphoric, bacteriacide, anti-fungal, cytophylactic.

Benefits:

- Relieves anxiety, depression, stress, highly charged emotional states.

- Very hypnotic and euphoric, instills peace.

- Treats insomnia related to depression.

- Addresses nerve pain, headaches, vertigo and bouts of yawning.

- Aphrodisiac qualities, treats sexual dysfunction.

- Relieves emotional depression and irritability associated with premenstrual (PMS) and menopausal symptoms.

- Anti-spasmodic effect, calms the intestines, and treats colitis and diarrhea.

- Tonifies Spleen Qi: promotes digestion, transforms damp and ascends Qi.

- Clears Heart Fire: palpitations, fibrillations, angina, hysteria and shock. It also improves circulation and cleanses the blood.

Skin Benefits:

- The cytophylactic effect regenerates skin cells and improves elasticity.

- Good for all skin conditions, especially dry, sensitive and mature skin.

- Decreases scars, stretch marks and thread veins (cuperose skin).

- Protects the skin from X-ray treatments.

Camellia Oleifera, Organic Camellia Seed Oil

Organic *Camellia oleifera* seed oil has been used in Asia for centuries as an exceptional multi-purpose, soothing moisturizer. It is extracted from the seeds of the flowering *Camellia oleifera* tree. The seeds are then cold-pressed into a scentless, clear yellow oil.

Because of its amazing anti-oxidant properties, it not only prevents damage from free radicals to the skin, but also has a long shelf life. In Japan, the samurai used it to protect their swords from rust and corrosion. It is considered to be the most penetrative of all the plant oils.

Properties:

- Softens and deeply penetrates skin, an emollient rich in fatty acids, omega 3s, 6s, 9s and linoleic acid.

- Anti-oxidant: contains vitamins A, B, C, E and polyphenols protects skin from ultraviolet B rays.

- Anti-inflammatory and analgesic: heals wounds and lessens pain.

- Mirrors the sebum of the skin: contains 82% oleic acid. It is similar to the fatty acid produced by the skin's sebaceous glands, and is easily absorbed into the cellular membrane.

- Improves immune function and enhances anti-viral and anti-bacterial properties.

Benefits:
- Hydrates and softens skin, and addresses fine lines and wrinkles.

- Treats both acne and dry skin.

- Heals cracked, sunburned, damaged and sensitive skin.

- Prevents stretch marks and scars, including acne scars.

- Treats eczema, psoriasis, rosacea and hyperpigmentation.

- Protects skin from UV-B rays and skin cancer.

- Prevents razor burns.

- Aids chemotherapy and radiation patients.

- Good for dry and brittle hair.

Sea-buckthorn, *Hippophae Rhamnoides*
Sea-buckthorn is a shrub that grows in dry, sandy areas. The berries contain both saturated and unsaturated fats that are often included as ingredients in cosmetic face creams and body moisturizers. The fruit is rich in vitamin C, which is the precursor to collagen/elastin production, and tones and firms the skin. It also contains anti-oxidants, carotenoids, vitamin E, amino acids, polyphenols and flavonoids. The seeds and the oils pressed from the pulp both nourish and hydrate the skin. The berries can be ingested or applied topically as an emollient or skin softener.

Sea-buckthorn is an additive in herbal formulas that address metabolic imbalances, like obesity, and gastrointestinal, cardiac and blood imbalances.

Kukui Nut/Candlenut Tree Oil, *Aleurites Moluccana*
When I was teaching in Hawaii some years ago, one of my colleagues educated me about the benefits of Kukui nut seed oil, especially as a treatment for very dry skin, and other difficult skin conditions, such as psoriasis.

Kukui seed oil has no known toxicity; it is non-irritating and very gentle in effect. Its high oil content makes it a natural emollient, which moisturizes and protects the skin. It may also be substituted for castor oil.

The aroma of the oil is sweet, and it is hydrating and healing for the skin. Kukui nut seed oil is a valuable addition to the vitalizing cream.

VibRadiance Five Element Planetary Essential Oils
(Figure 9.3)

Acknowledgment

I would like to acknowledge and express my appreciation to two of my colleagues for the fine work that they are doing on the application of essential oils within the field of Chinese medicine. Dr. Jeffrey Yuen has catalogued essential oils according to the meridian functions, and outlined contraindications, actions, properties, and other qualities. Peter Holmes, L.Ac., M.H., has created essential oil blends according to Five Element principles.

Organic essential oil blends, based upon the Five Elements, are an interesting addition to your facial cream, and can be added just before you apply it to the patient's face. These oils address specific skin conditions, constitutional issues, and psychoemotional imbalances.

The Five Elements

In Oriental medicine, the Five Elements, or Five Phases, are a system of relationships that describe humanity's connection to the environment. In primordial times, our early ancestors lived in a respectful and mutually supportive balance with nature, and not only observed, but also honored, the perennial changes of the seasons.

They understood that their interaction with the cycles of the natural world was mirrored in the internal workings of the human organism, and manifested outwardly in its most harmonious state as abundant health and well-being.

As did all ancient peoples, the ancient Chinese sought to harmonize the structures and rituals of their culture with the manifold and mysterious symmetries that they observed in the heavens. They viewed the five planets of their cosmography as being related to the Five Elements, and subsequently documented these associations in the *Nei Jing*, assigning the elements to the planets as follows:

Venus: Metal

Mars: Fire

Mercury: Water

Jupiter: Wood

Saturn: Earth

The VibRadiance Five Element Planetary Essential Oils are blended with organic grapeseed and apricot seed carrier oils, and the anti-oxidant vitamin E, to prevent premature rancidity. These essential oil blends are formulated using planetary correspondences, Chinese Five Element and Traditional Chinese Medicine (TCM) theory. This section of the chapter presents the specific meridian involvement, contraindications, dermatological applications, associated constitutional imbalances, and psychospiritual indications for the specific oil. The taste, aroma, the part of the plant from which the oil is distilled, and the temperature of the oil are also included in this petite Materia Medica.

Metal Element: Venus

This organic essential oil blend represents the feminine principle and embodies the qualities of the goddess Venus and the bodhisattva Kuan Yin. The constituent oils have aphrodisiac, phytoestrogenic, cellular regenerating, antidepressant and spiritually uplifting qualities.

The principal oil in this blend is organic Bulgarian rose, which is synergized with geranium to enliven the complexion, ylang-ylang to balance oily and dry skin and calm the Shen, lemongrass, which tones the skin promotes mindfulness, and other oils which have Metal element characteristics.

Rose Otto, *Rosa Damascena;* Mi Gui Hua

Aroma	Floral, sweet
Parts distilled	Blossoms
Taste	Sweet
Nature	Neutral
Meridians	Heart, Liver, Kidney
Contraindications	Pregnancy
Actions	Anti-depressant, hemostatic, nervine, hepatobiliary, stimulant, hormone balancer, emmenagogue, aphrodisiac
Skin	Regenerates skin; particularly good for mature, dry or sensitive skin, eczema, broken capillaries, can address all skin types
Properties	Promotes circulation, soothes asthma, calms coughs, clears Liver; is phytoestrogenic, therefore treats premenstrual syndrome (PMS) and menopause. It also treats depression, exhaustion, stress, and shock, and uplifts emotions. It aids memory, promotes self-acceptance; historically, it was used as a hangover remedy
Other	Rose otto essential oil is a nervine, and it supports the parasympathetic nervous system. It also enters the Heart meridian and organ to transform passion into compassion, fostering unconditional love

Geranium, *Pelarganium Graveolens*, Shi La Hong

This essential oil is neutral in temperature, and addresses the Liver and Kidney meridians. It is phyto-estrogenic, and regulates the hormonal system, and therefore caution should be taken with pregnant women. Geranium increases blood flow, enlivens the complexion, and treats sagging flesh on both face and body.

It moisturizes mature, sensitive skin, balances the sebum, and treats stretch marks, eczema and broken capillaries on the face. It also calms the Shen and lightens the mood. Geranium speeds recovery after an illness or operation, and harmonizes mind and emotions.

Ylang-ylang, *Unona Adorantissimum*

Ylang-ylang is cooling, and enters the Liver, Heart and Kidney meridians. Consequently, it is contraindicated for empty Yang syndromes because of its cool nature. It clears blood heat, and addresses anxiety, palpitations and calms anger. It supports Kidney essence, and is a famous aphrodisiac, which helps with frigidity, impotence and infertility. It balances oily and dry skin. The aroma is both haunting and lingering.

Lemongrass, *Cymbopogon Citratus*, Xiang Mao Cao

This warming oil is not recommended for use with patients who have Yin deficiency or heat issues; it opens to the Liver and Spleen meridians, and has anti-bacterial, antifungal and diuretic properties. It tones the skin and astringes the pores, clears acne, balances oily skin, promotes digestion, treats fatigue and loss of concentration. It also moves Qi, lifts the spirit and promotes increased awareness.

Fire Element: Mars

This organic essential oil blend represents the masculine principle and the explosive, dynamic energy of the god Mars. Its oils have stimulating, aphrodisiac, analgesic and anti-inflammatory qualities; they are also cellular regenerators, balance phytohormones, and support the adrenal glands.

The main oil is organic ginger, blended with basil to treat sinus congestion and hysteria, myrrh for powerful skin preservation, and pine, which supports the adrenals, plus other Fire element essential oils.

Ginger, *Zingiber Officialis*, Jiang

Aroma	Spicy, sharp
Parts distilled	Rhizome
Taste	Spicy
Nature	Hot
Meridians	Lung, Spleen, Stomach, Kidney
Contraindications	Can irritate sensitive skin; full and empty heat conditions

Continued

Actions	Stomachic, carminative, expectorant, analgesic, aphrodisiac, laxative, stimulant, antiseptic
Skin	Helpful with bruising, sores and carbuncles
Properties	Treats nausea, poor appetite, indigestion, flatulence, motion sickness, diarrhea, and stimulates circulation. It helps with cold phlegm and influenza. Ginger also warms the emotions, sharpens the senses, aids memory, uplifts, stimulates and grounds a tired person

Basil, *Ocimum Basilicum*, Jiu Zeng, Lo Le

Basil is warming, and addresses the Liver, Stomach and Kidney meridians. As an emmenagogue, it is contraindicated during pregnancy, because it encourages menstruation. Basil is a tonic for sluggish, congested skin, and is beneficial for treating acne. It improves protein digestion, alleviates headaches, sinus congestion and muscle tightness. Its aphrodisiac qualities are beneficial in the treatment of frigidity and infertility. It lessens depression, calms hysteria, and engenders confidence.

Myrrh, *Cammifora Myrrha*, Mo Yao

This essential oil is cooling in nature, and opens to the Liver, Spleen and Stomach meridians. Myrrh is contraindicated for treatments during pregnancy, and if there is excessive uterine bleeding, because it promotes menstruation.

Myrrh was one of the precious oils employed by ancient Egyptian embalmers, as it possesses powerful skin preservation attributes. It checks the progress of tissue degeneration, and encourages the regeneration of the skin.

Its anti-viral and regenerative properties promote wound healing, cool inflammation in sores, skin ulcers, and eczema. Myrrh also treats bruises, varicose veins, and clears Lung and Stomach heat with coughing, gum swelling and hyperthyroidism. It fortifies the Spleen and has a carminative effect, eliminating gas from the digestive system, and strengthening digestion.

Pine, *Pinus Sylvestris*, Song Jie

Pine is warming, and addresses the Lung and Kidney meridians; it should be used with caution on patients with deficient Yin and blood symptoms.

It is a powerful antiseptic, transforms phlegm, and is a respiratory tonic; it alleviates conditions such as bronchitis, and clears the sinuses. It also supports the Kidney, stimulates the functioning of the adrenals, and can treat issues of exhaustion and adrenal burnout.

The warming properties relieve arthritis and muscle aches; as it is decongestant, it addresses blemished skin, eczema and psoriasis. Psychoemotionally, it restores a fatigued and tired mind to alertness.

Water Element: Mercury

This essential oil is a multifaceted blend, representing the adaptable energy of Mercury, the messenger of the gods. The constituent oils have sedative, analgesic, digestive, and anti-inflammatory properties, and are excellent cardiac tonics. The principal oil is the euphoric Clary sage, which is combined with lavender to calm the spirit, carrot seed to treat hyperpigmentation and fennel, which lessens the appearance of wrinkles, and is purported to enhance longevity, plus other oils with Mercurian qualities.

Clary sage, *Salvia Sclarea*

Aroma	Sweet
Parts distilled	Flowering tops and leaves
Taste	Spicy; sweet
Nature	Cooling
Meridians	Liver, Heart, Kidney
Contraindications	Phytoestrogenic; be careful if the patient is pregnant or has cancer. Sedative: do not drink and drive wearing Clary sage
Actions	Sedative, hypotensive, anticonvulsant, antifungal, euphoric, emmenagogue, aphrodisiac, carminative, antiseptic
Skin	Dry, mature or inflamed skin, cellular regenerating properties; also good for rosacea, blemishes and acne
Properties	Uterine hormone balancer, eases menstrual tension, menopause, insomnia, hemorrhoids, varicose veins, panic attacks, fright and hysteria. The euphoric effect encourages well-being

Lavender, *Lavendula Augustifolia*

Lavender has a cool temperature, and opens to the Lung, Liver and Pericardium meridians. It is also an emmenagogue, and therefore contraindicated for pregnant women, and those with uterine or other bleeding, because it is an anti-coagulant.

Lavender calms the Shen, and treats palpitation, insomnia and irritability. It releases wind heat with accompanying headache and sore throat, and encourages the smooth flow of Liver Qi, opens the chest and diffuses the Lung. Lavender is perhaps the premier cellular regenerator among all essential oils, and therefore it reduces scarring, and treats dry, sun-damaged skin and burns.

Lavender should be included in a first aid kit that you have on hand in your clinic, at home, or when you travel.

Carrot seed, *Daucus Corota*, Hong Lo Bai Zi

Carrot seed oil is sweet in nature, and addresses the Liver and Kidney meridians. Another emmenagogue, it should not be used to treat pregnant women. It nourishes blood, and treats blurring vision, dry skin, pale complexion, age spots and wrinkles, eczema and psoriasis. Kidney Yin deficiency, menopausal symptoms and blemished skin due to hormonal imbalances can also be addressed.

Fennel, *Foeniculum Vulgaris*, Xiao Hui Xiang

This oil is warming, and opens to the Liver, Spleen, Stomach and Kidney. It is phytoestrogenic, and contraindicated during pregnancy and for patients with cancer. Fennel has a cleansing and tonic effect on the skin, and prevents the formation of wrinkles. It bestows the gift of longevity, as well as strength and courage.

It also fortifies the physical kidneys, and the Zhi, the spirit of the Kidneys. It supports digestion, treats cellulite because of its diuretic properties, and is purported to be a good tonic for hangover and snakebite. Its phytoestrogens alleviate the symptoms of menopause, menstrual tension and low libido.

Wood Element: Jupiter

This expansive organic essential blend represents the optimistic and powerful energy of the god Jupiter. All the constituent oils have aphrodisiac, anti-inflammatory, sedative, diuretic and anti-spasmodic qualities. The principal component is sensual, organic jasmine, which is blended with grapefruit for weight loss, Roman chamomile to soothe burns and wounds, balsam fir for respiratory issues, and other Jupiterian organic oils.

Jasmine, *Jasminum Officinale*, Mi Li Hua

Aroma	Floral
Parts distilled	Flowers
Taste	Sweet
Nature	Cooling
Meridians	Liver/kidney
Contraindications	Pregnancy until just prior to giving birth; eases labor
Actions	Anti-depressant, uterine tonic/stimulant, emmenagogue, galactagogue, aphrodisiac, sedative and anti-spasmodic
Skin	All skin types, especially dry and sensitive skin
Properties	Treats severe depression, calms nerves and emotions; gives confidence. Promotes childbirth, balances hormones, treats sexual problems, impotence, infertility, and helps the respiratory system. Softens stretch marks and scarring

Grapefruit, *Citrus Paradisi*, Da Guo Pi

Grapefruit is slightly warming, and treats the Lung, Stomach and Gall Bladder meridians; as a citrus oil, it can cause photosensitivity, and it is contraindicated for heat issues. Grapefruit is a well-recognized remedy for weight loss, and helps with water retention and lymphatic congestion. It increases fat metabolism, treats cellulite and can dissolve gallstones.

As a Liver tonic, it can relieve migraine pain and premenstrual syndrome (PMS). It has an anti-depressant effect, and lifts the mood. When including grapefruit in an essential oil blend, vitamin E should be added to prevent rancidity, because it has a short shelf life.

Roman Chamomile, *Athemis Nobilis*

This essential oil is cooling, and opens to the Liver and Spleen meridians. It should be avoided when treating patients who are in the early months of pregnancy, because it is an emmenagogue. Roman chamomile is contraindicated for patients with a sensitivity to ragweed. It calms the Shen, alleviating symptoms of anxiety, restlessness, insomnia and anger, soothes the Stomach, and relieves gastritis and colitis.

As an anti-inflammatory, it treats burns, wounds, acne, and other issues, including psoriasis, hypersensitive skin, broken capillaries, itching, and symptoms associated with Liver Blood deficiency.

Balsam Fir, *Abies Alba*

Fir is another cooling essential oil, and enters the Lung and Kidney. It has no significant contraindications. It has a grounding effect, and, because it expels phlegm from the Lung, is beneficial for a wide range of respiratory issues, including asthma. It relieves fatigue and aching limbs, and addresses urinary tract infections.

Earth Element: Saturn

This astringent essential oil blend represents the Sage and Keeper of Time, Saturn. It contains oils that have sedative, expectorant, digestive and analgesic properties. The principal oil is cooling organic cypress, synergized with cumin, which increases fertility and libido; Atlas cedar treats memory loss; and frankincense, a cellular regenerator, is included, among other Saturnian organic oils.

Cypress, *Cupressus Sempervivens*

Aroma	Spicy
Parts distilled	Needles, twigs
Taste	Bitter

Continued   329

Nature	Slightly cooling
Meridians	Lung, Spleen, kidney
Contraindications	Pregnant women or patients with breast or prostate cancer, or hypertension
Actions	Astringent, sedative, anti-spasmodic, diuretic, hepatic, insecticide, vasoconstrictor
Skin	Mature skin, sweaty, oily skin
Qualities	Soothes anger and calms the Shen. Treats hemorrhages, edema, nosebleeds, heavy menses, sweaty feet, incontinence, and cellulite. Cypress is especially good for addressing prolapses of the bladder and uterus. Helps with bronchitis, asthma, hemorrhoids and varicose veins

Cumin, *Cuminum Cyminum*

Cumin is slightly warming, and enters the Liver, Spleen and Heart meridians. It is contraindicated during pregnancy, and can cause a slight level of photo-sensitivity. Cumin dispels lethargy and fatigue. It also stimulates digestion, increases fertility and libido, and normalizes the menstrual cycle. It invigorates the blood, and as a Heart tonic, treats palpitations, hypotension and poor circulation.

Atlas cedar, *Cedrus Atlantica*

Like cypress, cedar is also cooling, and affects the Lung, Heart and Liver meridians. It is contraindicated for both pregnancy and when treating pre-pubescent children. Cedar has pronounced mucolytic qualities, and addresses Phlegm Misting the Mind, with symptoms of depression and memory loss. It also treats Liver Qi Stagnation, associated with irritability, abdominal pain, and heat issues, including insomnia, and cystitis. Atlas cedar has the ability to break up cellulite; it promotes the healing of scar tissue and skin issues like dermatitis and psoriasis.

Frankincense, *Boswellia Carterii*, Ru Xiang

This essential oil is slightly cooling, and opens to the Liver, Heart and Lung meridians. Some sources report that it is contraindicated during pregnancy. It is another resinous oil, like myrrh, and is a cellular regenerator; it preserves the skin, smooths out wrinkles and gives new life to aging skin. Frankincense reduces swelling and treats scars, wounds, ulcerated skin and carbuncles.

Frankincense addresses the Lung, aids with breathing, and associated issues of asthma and bronchitis. It alleviates symptoms of anxiety and depression, calms the Shen and quiets the mind, and treats digestive complaints like gas, belching and indigestion. It also benefits urogenital issues, such as cystitis.

Insure that your Five Element essential oil blend achieves a significant result by custom blending it according to your patient's specific needs. If he or she has skin that requires more hydration, cooling, calming or balancing, add it to the vitalizing cream.

CAUTION

Please note that some patients are allergic to both the aroma and the topical application of certain essential oils. Please inquire about these allergies prior to any application, or even opening the bottles in your treatment room.

If there is a question of a possible allergic reaction, test your patient by applying some of the oil on the inside of the arm, and checking the site after a 24-hour period. Patients who are allergic will report their experience with certain oils to you, and ask you not to use them in your treatment.

Jade Rollers

After you massage the patient's face, neck and décolletage with the Vitalizing Cream and essential oils, jade rollers are gently used on the face and neck to call forth the Yin moisture, cool and even out the complexion, and facilitate deeper absorption of the cream by the skin (see Figure 7.20).

As previously noted, since the time of the Tang dynasty (AD 618–906), jade was featured prominently in the daily regimens of the Chinese Imperial family, to protect beauty and promote increased longevity. It is cool by nature, enhances blood circulation, decreases hyperpigmentation and regenerates the skin. It also firms and tightens the skin and muscles.

Sun Si Miao, a famous doctor of that era, authored two important books that included prescriptions for beauty and longevity, *Important Formulas with a Thousand Gold Pieces for Emergencies,* and its sequel, *Important Formulas with a Thousand Gold Pieces.* He also ground jade stones into powder for topical application and medicinal purposes.[3]

Other functions of jade include:

- Closes the pores.
- Reduces fine lines, wrinkles and puffiness.
- Opens the sinuses.
- Reduces inflammation and redness after facial needling.
- Increases lymphatic drainage.

The Chinese honor jade as a sacred stone both for its beneficial impact on outer beauty and its ability to support the inner glow of the Shen.

Step 17: Hydrosol Spritz

The last stage of the Constitutional Facial Acupuncture treatment protocol features the choice of one of three essential oil hydrosols, organic Bulgarian rose, organic lavender, or organic neroli. The hydrosol is sprayed upon the face to seal in the vitalizing cream and activate the healing properties of the essential oil (see Figure 7.21).

A hydrosol is the aromatic water that remains after the distillation of an essential oil, either by steam or water (Figure 9.4). We refer to them by a variety of names – hydrosols, hydrolats, distillates, or floral waters. However, you may come across certain mixtures marketed as floral waters that are not the end product of a distillation process; rather, the essential oils contained in them have simply been added to water. Consequently, these floral waters possess neither the therapeutic properties of the plant, nor the exquisite aroma.

The indications and usages for hydrosols are different, and should be selected carefully for each individual patient. The sense of smell is the first to develop in the womb, and the olfactory sensory receptors link directly with the limbic system of the brain. It is oldest part of the brain's structure from an evolutionary perspective, and thought to be the seat of emotion. Some patients react strongly to the scent of certain essential oils, because they have unpleasant memories attached to them, arising either from personal experience, or excessive contact with individuals who may have favored these fragrances. Bear in mind that some patients are simply allergic to certain essential oils.

The organic Bulgarian rose hydrosol is especially beneficial for dry or mature skin. It nourishes the Yin, and hydrates and regenerates flesh. It also calms the symptoms of Yin Deficiency heat, such as hot flashes and irritability. Rose is a hormonal balancer, an anti-depressant, and regulates the free flow of Liver Qi and calms the Shen. It communicates with the Heart on both a physical and an emotional level.

The organic lavender hydrosol is cooling and releases heat from the head. It treats Wind heat symptoms, with blocked sinuses, and Liver Qi stagnation, causing headaches, tight shoulders and neck, hypertension and stiffness in the chest. It is also effective for sun-damaged skin, sunburn, burns and insect bites.

The organic neroli hydrosol increases blood circulation and regenerates skin cells, improves the elasticity of the skin and heals scar tissue. Its emollient action promotes hydration of dry, sensitive and mature skin, as well as couperose skin with thread veins, and it can alleviate stretch marks from pregnancy or weight loss. It is also known to protect the skin from exposure to X-rays.

Neroli has euphoric properties, clears Heart fire, and relieves anxiety, depression, stress, insomnia and palpitations. It is also good for treating severe shock and hysteria, calms intestinal spasms, and ameliorates the symptoms of colitis and diarrhea.

Spray the hydrosol of your choice gently on the patient's face; avoid spraying it directly into their eyes. This direct spray may startle them, and it will not be in keeping with the relaxation and quiet they experienced during the treatment.

Tuning Forks

An optional step, that you may wish to incorporate into the flow of your treatments, involves the use of calibrated tuning forks; these are extremely versatile tools, which can be used in a variety of different ways. Customarily, I begin and end a treatment by grounding my patient with two Ohm[4] tuning forks, which engender an Earth tone. Prior to this step, however, I have them listen to the specific tonal combination, and then I apply the forks to the soles of the feet at Kid-1 Yongquan Gushing Spring, to quiet, calm and connect them to their Earth Qi.

In my experience, these tuning forks increase the effectiveness of Constitutional Facial Acupuncture treatments. They can ameliorate symptoms of Yang Qi rising, facial redness, headache, and irritability caused by facial needling, simply by bringing the energy down to the feet.

There is an entire range of planetary frequencies associated with this system, and these forks can be employed upon acupuncture points and meridians at your discretion.

To ground the patient and to bring the Constitutional Facial Acupuncture treatment to a conclusion, two Ohm tuning forks, referred to as an Ohm Unison, are vibrated on Du-20 Baihui and Ren-17 Tanzhong, and then bilaterally on Kid-1 Yongquan (see Figure 7.22).

Once having completed all the stages of your treatment, offer your patient the mirror while they are still lying on the table, so that they may observe the renewed brightness of their Shen. Then have them sit up, and look again to ascertain the effect of gravity on the newly enlivened facial landscape. After they have changed back into their street clothes, you can then consult with them about how many treatments they will need to become more healthy, vibrant, youthful and balanced, both in body and spirit.

REFERENCES

1. Langevin HM, Sheaman KJ. Pathophysiological model for chronic low back pain integrating connective tissue and vous system mechanisms, Elsevier; 2007, p. 77;

also Department of Neurology, University of Vermont, Burlington, VT, Center for Health Studies, Group Health Cooperative, Seattle, WA ... "a microtrauma or ... tissue injury and histamine release is a powerful driver of fibroblast collagen synthesis ..."

2. Dan B, Andrew G, Ted K. Chinese Herbal Materia Medica. revised ed. Seattle, WA: Eastland Press; 1993. p. 330.

3. Huang F-L, Cui H (Rebecca Parker, translator). Cosmetology in Chinese Medicine. Beijing, China: People's Medical Publishing House; 2011. p. 10–11.

4. Ohm is the central tone of a system of tuning forks referred to as Acutonics®; its frequency is 136.1 Hz, which is approximately a C# in standard tunings. This value is calculated using the orbital velocity of the Earth around the Sun, hence I have referred to it as an Earth tone. Acutonics® tuning forks are used instead of needles in my vibrational facial treatment protocol, Facial Soundscapes: Harmonic Renewal™, which can be a very effective adjunct to Constitutional Facial Acupuncture treatments. For more information: www.chiakra.com/soundscapes.htm.

CHAPTER 10

A Personal Note from the Author

"Time spent laughing is time spent with the gods."
— Japanese Proverb

Even though I have treated many patients with Constitutional Facial Acupuncture in my clinic, and taught these protocols to students worldwide, I am still amazed and pleased by the efficacy and profound impact that these treatments have on both student and patient alike.

A Constitutional Treatment Approach and Philosophy

Facial acupuncture seemingly targets only the visible signs of aging, and consequently is often labeled as cosmetic by the general public and many of my fellow acupuncturists.

However, without a strong constitutional component, this modality effects neither long-term change in the patient's general health, nor does it ameliorate any significant dermatological issues. The face is the mirror of our health and well-being, and the most emotive part of the anatomy. These attributes make the face a perfect indicator of physical and psychoemotional imbalances.

As I stated in Chapter 7, "The Shen leads the Qi," and the truth of this old Chinese axiom is even more apparent when we consider the facial terrain. For example, a deep crease between the eyebrows may herald your diagnosis of Liver Qi Stagnation, originally caused by long-term frustration that has disturbed the Shen. The persistent suppression of anger can cause the appearance of this Liver line, referred to as a suspended sword in Oriental physiognomy.

335

Chinese medicine views the patient as a unified whole, and does not separate the physical from the mental or spiritual. Neither can the face, head and trunk be separated from the body in treatment. It is such an elegantly simple and organic relationship, and yet the constitutional treatment approach that follows from this connection is omitted from some facial acupuncture protocols; or in a teaching situation, only the face is needled, or the body is treated after the facial needling.

A failure to needle the body prior to the face in a treatment, may cause the patient to become ungrounded. It can also trigger headaches, or exacerbate pre-existing hypertension, hot flashes, acid reflux, or other conditions. I recommend that you focus on the constitutional treatment, and your patients will rarely experience any side effects from facial needling.

Other Facial Syndromes

I also treat other more serious facial syndromes such as Bell's palsy, windstroke, post-operative neuropathies, facial paralysis, trigeminal neuralgia, and temporomandibular joint dysfunction (TMJ). I believe that the specialized knowledge required to treat non-cosmetic issues should be an essential part of the training offered by any facial acupuncture program; they are a natural adjunct to an approach that focuses solely on beauty. As a facial acupuncturist, it is important to have the skills to address both these facial syndromes and cosmetic concerns, but not simultaneously.

A Definition of Aging

"What is Aging?" was a question that one of my students asked in a facial acupuncture seminar in Australia a few years ago. The question took me by surprise, and I really wasn't sure as to how I should answer it. However, I like challenges and appreciate questions that are thought provoking. After a pause, the answer popped out, without further reflection: "Aging is not hardening of the arteries; it is hardening of the attitudes."

To further clarify this response, aging may be described as an inability to adapt to the changing circumstances of one's life. A person who is vibrant, and learns new skills, like painting, singing, a new language, sport, dance or Qi-gong, remains youthful. They also choose to live with courage and a sense of adventure, and are willing to reach out to new friends of every age.

In Chinese medicine, aging is described as chronic blood stasis; when this vital essence does not move, circulation to the brain, muscles, tissues, extremities, and vital organs becomes stagnant and we ossify, become rigid and die.

It is therefore important to recommend lifestyle changes to your patients, in addition to encouraging them to adopt a balanced diet and exercise regimen. I often like to assign them 'homework,' suggestions like dancing, singing and painting. These creative expressions feed the soul, as well as the body, and foster 'ageless aging.'

The Patient's Age

In my seminars, practitioners and students usually inquire about the significance of the patient's age, and want to know how old or young they should be to achieve optimum results. I do not set an age limit for my patients; the efficacy of the treatments depends on a combination of factors – individual genetics, lifestyle, diet, exercise, water intake, and their psychospiritual health and well-being.

I have treated teenagers for acne and other dermatological concerns with facial acupuncture, combined with the topical Chinese herbal poultices presented in Chapter 9, with good results. My oldest patient to date, was 90 years young, possessed remarkably good genes, pursued a healthy, active lifestyle, and exhibited a rare combination of youthful exuberance and wisdom. She responded very well to the Constitutional Facial Acupuncture treatments, and her inner beauty radiated forth from a clear, open and characterful face.

Most of my patients are women, from age 49–66. They are Baby Boomers, and upwardly mobile, professional people, working or retired. Their lifestyle choices include the consumption of organic food, with supplemental vitamins and minerals, exercise, meditation and yoga. They do not take Western medications unless it is necessary, and they prefer using complementary medicine modalities to stay healthy. Most have not had any kind of cosmetic surgery, but a few have had Botox injections. The majority of them have authentic creative passions, which they pursue with zeal.

Some of them contact me about the possibility of treating a sagging neck prior to undergoing plastic surgery. After experiencing facial acupuncture treatments, which not only improve the appearance of the droopy neck, but also help them with constitutional issues, such as Spleen Qi deficiency, about 65% of them choose not to pursue the surgical option.

Recently, I have treated more artists, actors and singers of all ages. Performers, in particular, are under pressure to look their best; accordingly, they are compelled to safeguard their health and get enough sleep to maintain a youthful, vibrant appearance.

Professional men, including lawyers and doctors, are very discreet about their facial acupuncture treatments. Usually, after a few treatments, they receive compliments at the office on how they look, and people ask whether they have had a vacation – a question to which they answer "Yes." Despite their successful and observable results, they tend not to refer patients to you, because they simply don't want their circle of family, friends and colleagues to know about their facial acupuncture treatments.

In New York City, facial acupuncture continues to increase in popularity, and I see more patients of both sexes, and all ages and nationalities. Please be aware that your target audience for your facial acupuncture treatments will vary, depending on where your clinic is located.

I have outlined some basic guidelines for Constitutional Facial Acupuncture treatments in Chapter 6, Practical Specifics. Let me offer some additional insights that I have gleaned from my many years of experience in this field:

Prescreen Patients: Make sure that patients are not contraindicated for facial acupuncture treatments. For example, a person who is not migraine-free for at least 3 months prior to their first appointment should not receive facial needling until that period of time has passed. Focus on treating the constitutional source of the migraines, and later you can choose to embark on the facial acupuncture treatment series. Remember that facial acupuncture is not for everyone.

I always interview each prospective patient personally on the telephone before I see them at my clinic. I want to educate them about the treatments, make sure that they don't have any contraindicated conditions, and clarify the exact nature of the process, especially if they have had no previous exposure to facial acupuncture, or acupuncture in general.

I also listen carefully to the quality and timbre of their voice and pay attention to the sound as it relates to the Five Element correspondences. This helps me to ascertain whether they will benefit from facial acupuncture treatments. Some prospective patients have issues of depression and certain psychological imbalances that cannot be resolved with facial acupuncture.

My previous experience with these patients has taught me that, despite their enthusiasm for facial acupuncture, they will be difficult, and their needs would be best served elsewhere. Honor the wisdom of your own intuition when you encounter these individuals and make an informed decision. Do not hesitate to say "no" to a difficult situation, and refer them out to other professionals if that is warranted.

Realistic Expectations: It is crucial that, prior to a first treatment, you inform a prospective patient about the results that they may expect from Constitutional Facial Acupuncture. Do not misrepresent the outcome of the treatments.

Do not Advertise your Services as an Acupuncture 'Face Lift': This makes new patients think that they will experience instantaneous results, and they will be disappointed. Facial acupuncture is an organic process that treats both face and body in a series of treatments that are cumulative in effect.

Do not Guarantee Results: Every patient is unique in their response to these treatments, and the results will vary. Patients may pressure you for some kind of guarantee; do not give into this demand. Remind them of the benefits, and that their results will depend on their genetics, lifestyle choices, and outlook on life.

Educate Patients about Possible Bruising during Treatment: Do not treat patients with facial acupuncture less than 1 week prior to a special event. Use other non-needle modalities instead – Tui-na, microcurrent or the *Facial Soundscapes*™ tuning fork facial. I have learned that even patients who have never previously bruised may bruise unexpectedly (see Chapter 6 for how to prevent bruises).

Patients can bruise because the acupuncturist is not sufficiently skillful or knowledgeable about the techniques. However, this is not always the case; sometimes, bruising cannot be avoided with patients who have systemic blood stagnation, or have puffiness under the eyes in the area of St-2 Sibai Four Whites.

Other factors may contribute to the formation of hematomas. I work with a television anchor person, who, because her employment is more than a bit contingent upon remaining slim and attractive, and is, ordinarily, extremely careful about her lifestyle, diet and exercise regimens. Unfortunately, I discovered the hard way, after months of successful results, that she was a closet 'sugar-holic.'

Apparently, the night before one of our appointments, she binged on every dessert on the menu in a well-known restaurant. Not surprisingly, she bruised, and it took some acupuncture detective work to determine what had happened. As the Spleen holds in the blood in the vessels, the Earth element was severely compromised that particular morning.

I managed to lessen the hematoma on her neck, but not completely. Thanks to professional make-up, no one was any the wiser. However, she became wary of facial needles after this transpired, and took little responsibility for her binge. Nevertheless, I honored her wishes and continued to treat her with a combination of modalities.

Please be aware that the process of facial acupuncture treatments is a learning experience for not only for the patient, but also the practitioner.

Smokers, Saggers, and Patients with Poor Dietary Habits: I always inform smokers that they will not achieve the results they desire if they continue to smoke. I do accept smokers as patients, and offer them the necessary assistance to stop smoking when they are ready. I have encountered those individuals, who motivated by 'healthy vanity,' have quit smoking with my help. However, the majority of smokers do not quit. I recommend that you make an informed decision whether or not to work with these patients.

Patients who sag excessively will require more sessions. It is important to notify them of this fact at the outset of their first treatment series, bearing in mind that more than one series may be necessary. If there are no visible results after the first treatment series, I customarily recommend that they discontinue treatment, and they usually agree.

Patients who have poor dietary habits, and who resist recommendations regarding lifestyle and dietary changes, will not experience the best results. I emphasize that this is a collaborative effort, in which both practitioner and patient have their particular responsibilities. If an individual expects to achieve a miraculous transformation of their appearance without an investment of energy and a commitment to the process, they are not a good prospect for a treatment series. The patients who want 'me' to fix 'them' are usually more difficult, and I often refer them to another practitioner or health care professional.

Cosmetic Surgery, Botox, Cosmetic Fillers: Patients are not always entirely forthcoming regarding their cosmetic surgery and other procedures, even in a detailed intake form and subsequent interview. It is crucial to tell them that needling the face at the insertion sites of Botox and cosmetic fillers will undo the Botox and/or fillers in that area. For example, the corrugator muscle, which is responsible for the glabellar crease that forms between the brows, is needled in close proximity to Botox injection sites; needling the corrugator will increase circulation in the area, and unfreeze the muscle. They will not be pleased if you eliminate the effects of their Botox injections with facial needling.

Advise them to wait 3–6 weeks for effects of their procedures to wear off, before you needle that area of their face. Make sure that they agree not to have additional injections during your treatment series.

Wait 3 weeks to begin facial acupuncture treatments after laser resurfacing, and 2 weeks after microdermabrasion and chemical peels. Patients who have had cosmetic surgery require at least 6 months prior to facial needling, although it is unusual that they will want to experience facial acupuncture. However, you can treat the scars and adhesions from the surgery after a period of 6 months.

Addiction to Facial Acupuncture: It should be noted that some patients become addicted to facial acupuncture, because the needling stimulates production of the body's natural endorphins, particularly facial needling.

Be firm and do not give into a patient's request for more sessions simply because you want to please them or because you see this as an opportunity to make more money. Remain grounded in the face of these demands, in a place of integrity and professionalism. The body needs time to integrate the results of facial acupuncture treatments, and effects of the treatments will continue after each session.

Other patients who have pathologically addictive personalities will try to persuade you to see them more often to feed their compulsion. Refer these individuals out to other professionals, and be realistic about whether you feel that it is appropriate for you to have them as patients.

As I said earlier, facial acupuncture is not therapy, and it is important to be conscious of your own limitations. Each treatment session involves the meeting of two psyches, and patients can 'push our buttons,' so to speak, and cause us to react inappropriately to their behavior and emotions. Once again, stay grounded, do not react, and later take some time to reflect on what it was about their behavior that provoked your response.

Often, this is a gift, because it brings to light certain unconscious attitudes and feelings. I recommend that you honor and respect your patients, and be grateful for the gifts that they bear you, either consciously or unconsciously. They are our best teachers.

Cancellation Policy: If a patient fails to provide me with 24 hours' notice prior to canceling an appointment, I charge them in full for the session, unless there has been an emergency or a situation of *force majeure*. Usually, they will have paid in advance for their entire treatment series of 12–15 sessions, and they will have an assigned time slot every week.

I also offer new patients the option to pay for half of a treatment series in advance, and half later, with the stipulation that they will complete all their treatments so as to achieve optimum results.

If there are no discernible results by the 5th treatment, I will have a candid discussion with them about whether we should continue their series, or terminate. This rarely occurs, but in this instance, I refund any payments made in advance for treatments they will not receive. Please note: saggers and smokers will require more than one course of treatments.

It is important to be thoroughly acquainted with the guidelines regarding treatment series as outlined in your malpractice insurance. Some insurers do not recognize the validity of treatment series options and will not permit you to accept payment in advance, except under certain conditions.

I have terminated a treatment series when I felt that I was not helping the patient, or they had psychological issues that could not be addressed with acupuncture. They have usually agreed with me.

Maintenance Treatments: Following the completion of an entire treatment series, the patient moves on to a period of maintenance. During this time, I customarily recommend one treatment per month for basically healthy patients, and twice monthly for saggers or people who need more care. If patients travel, or cannot adhere to the schedule you have established for them, they will usually call to remind you that they need a treatment.

Final Insights

I would like to share some final insights: the patient/practitioner dynamic is a relationship that depends upon respect and clear communication. Honor your patient's wishes, but remain true to yourself, anchored in your integrity, wisdom and good judgment.

My entire philosophy of facial acupuncture, as presented in the Introduction to this book, focuses on the idea of renewal. The patient who embarks upon a Constitutional Facial Acupuncture treatment series has made a commitment to a profound transformational journey; you are their Sherpa,[1] their psycho-pomp,[2] their native guide, accompanying them every step of the way. Each of you shares in the responsibility for the continued well-being and personal evolution of the other.

I recommend that you savor each unique relationship with a patient, while acknowledging the reality of *your* own personal transformation. This process is a blessing, and the voyage is a mutual one, filled with important lessons and the potential for joyful collaboration – during which you will share their triumphs and setbacks, tears and laughter. Do take time to laugh a bit along the way, and, if the Japanese proverb I have quoted at the beginning of this chapter is correct, you will indeed spend time "with the gods."

REFERENCES

1. The Sherpas are an indigenous enthic group in eastern Nepal, who often guide travelers during their journeys in the Himalayas; perhaps the most famous Sherpa was Tenzing Norgay, who accompanied Sir Edmund Hillary on his epic climb to the summit of Mt. Everest on May 29, 1953.

2. Our word 'psychopomp' is derived from the Greek *psychopompos,* which translates as 'guide of souls.' The most famous psychopomp in Greco–Roman mythology is the god Hermes (Mercury), the Winged Messenger, who can travel from the heights of Mt. Olympos to the depths of Hades, and was often entrusted by Zeus with crucial communications; there are many other noteworthy examples, including the Roman poet Virgil who guides Dante throughout the *Divine Comedy*. From my perspective, a psychopomp can be seen to traverse the three realms, the three Treasures of Heaven, Earth and Humanity.

Bibliography

Bensky D, Gamble A, Kaptchuk T. Chinese Herbal Medicine: Materia Medica. Revised ed. Seattle, WA: Eastland Press; 1993.

Bridges L. Face Reading in Chinese Medicine. 2nd ed. London, UK: Churchill Livingstone; 2012.

Cain S. Quiet: The Power of Introverts in a World That Can't Stop Talking. New York, NY: Crown Publishers; 2012.

Callison M. Motor Point Index: An Acupuncturist's Guide to Locating and Treating Motor Points. San Diego, CA: Acu-Sport Seminar Series, LLC; 2007.

Carey D, Franklin E, MichelAngelo, Ponton J, Ponton P. Acutonics: From Galaxies to Cells, Planetary Science, Harmony and Medicine. Llano, NM: Devachan Press; 2010.

Chase C, Shima M. An Exposition on the Eight Extraordinary Vessels: Acupuncture, Alchemy and Herbal Medicine. Seattle, WA: Eastland Press; 2010.

Clemente CD. Anatomy: A Regional Atlas of the Human Body. 4th ed. Baltimore, MD: Lippincott, Williams, Wilkins; 1997.

Connelly D. Traditional Acupuncture: The Law of the Five Elements. 2nd ed. Washington, DC: Wisdomwell Press; 1994.

Deadman P, Al-Khafaji M. A Manual of Acupuncture. 2nd ed. East Sussex, UK: Journal of Chinese Medicine Publications; 2007.

Deng LY, Gan YJ, He SH, Ji XP, Li Y, Wang R. Chinese Acupuncture and Moxibustion. Beijing, China: Foreign Languages Press; 1987.

Denmei S. Introduction to Meridian Therapy. Seattle, WA: Eastland Press; 1990.

Eco U. History of Beauty. New York, NY: Rizzoli International Publications; 2004.

Ellis A, Wiseman N, Boss K. Fundamentals of Chinese Acupuncture. Revised ed. Brookline, MA: Paradigm Publications; 1991.

Ellis A, Wiseman N, Boss K. Grasping the Wind: An Exploration into the Meaning of Chinese Acupuncture Point Names. Brookline, MA: Paradigm Publications; 1989.

Huang F-L, Parker R, Cui H. Cosmetology in Chinese Medicine. Beijing, China: People's Medical Publishing House; 2011.

Gienger M. Crystal Power, Crystal Healing: The Complete Handbook. London, UK: Cassell Illustrated; 2005.

Gladwell M. Blink: The Power of Thinking Without Thinking. New York, NY: Little, Brown & Co.; 2005.

Gladwell M. The Tipping Point: How Little Things Can Make a Big Difference. New York, NY: Little, Brown and Co.; 2002.

Hall J. 101 Power Crystals: The Ultimate Guide to Magical Crystals, Gems and Stones for Healing and Transformation. Beverly, MA: Fair Winds Press; 2011.

Helm JM. Acupuncture Energetics: A Clinical Approach for Physicians. Berkeley, CA: Medical Acupuncture Publishers; 1995.

Hempen CH, Fischer T. A Materia Medica for Chinese Medicine: Plants, Minerals and Animal Products. Exeter, UK: Churchill Livingstone; 2009.

Jablonski NG. Skin: A Natural History. Berkeley and Los Angeles, CA: University of California Press; 2006.

Jacob JH. The Acupuncturist's Clinical Handbook. New York, NY: Integrative Wellness; 2003.

Jeffreys S. Beauty and Misogyny: Harmful Cultural Practices in the West. New York, NY: Routledge; 2005.

Wu J-N. Ling Shu or The Spiritual Pivot. Honolulu, HI: University of Hawaii Press; 1993.

Kaptchuk T. The Web That Has No Weaver: Understanding Chinese Medicine. Chicago, IL: Congdon & Weed; 1983.

Chen KJ. Imperial Medicaments: Medical Prescriptions Written for Empress Dowager Cixi and Emperor Guangxu with Commentary. Beijing, China: Foreign Languages Press; 1996.

Kuczynski A. Beauty Junkies: Inside Our $15 Billion Obsession with Cosmetic Surgery. New York, NY: Doubleday Books; 2006.

Langer EJ. Counterclockwise: Mindful Health and the Power of Possibility. New York, NY: Ballantine Books; 2009.

Langer EJ. Mindfulness. Cambridge, MA: Da Capo Press Books; 1989.

Lao-Tzu, Blakney RB. The Way of Life. New York, NY: New American Library, Inc.; 1955.

Larre C, Schatz J, Rochat de la Vallee E. Survey of Traditional Chinese Medicine. Columbia, MD: Institut Ricci (Paris) and Traditional Acupuncture Foundation Institute; 1986.

Low R. The Secondary Vessels of Acupuncture: A Detailed Account of Their Energies, Meridians, and Control Points. New York, NY: Harper Collins; 1984 (out of print).

Maciocia G. The Channels of Acupuncture: Clinical Use of the Secondary Channels and Extraordinary Vessels. London, UK: Churchill Livingstone; 2006.

Maciocia G. The Psyche in Chinese Medicine: Treatment of Emotional and Mental Disharmonies with Acupuncture and Chinese Herbs. London, UK: Churchill Livingstone; 2009.

Matsumoto K, Birch S. Extraordinary Vessels. Brookline, MA: Paradigm Publications; 1986.

Matsumoto K, Birch S. Five Elements and Ten Stems: Nan Ching Theory, Diagnostics and Practice. Brookline, MA: Paradigm Publications; 1983.

Matsumoto K, Birch S. Hara Diagnosis: Reflections on the Sea. Brookline, MA: Paradigm Publications; 1988.

Mojay G. Aromatherapy for Healing the Spirit: Restoring Emotional and Mental Balance with Essential Oils. Rochester, VT: Healing Arts Press; 1997.

Netter F. Atlas of Human Anatomy. Summit, NJ: Ciba-Geigy Corporation; 1989.

Nguyen VN, Dzung TV, Recours-Nguyen C. Huangdi Neijing Lingshu, Vol. 1. Sugar Grove, NC: Jung Tao Productions; 2005.

Ni MS. Yellow Emperor's Classic of Medicine: A New Translation of the Neijing Suwen with Commentary. Boston, MA: Shambhala Publications; 1995.

Ni YT. Navigating Channels of Traditional Chinese Medicine. San Diego, CA: Oriental Medicine Center; 1996.

Nietzsche FW, Geuss R. Speirs R. The Birth of Tragedy and Other Writings. London, UK: Cambridge University Press; 1999. p. 154.

O' Connor J, Bensky D. Acupuncture: A Comprehensive Text. Seattle, WA: Eastland Press; 1981.

Rifkin B, Ackerman MJ. Human Anatomy: From the Renaissance to the Digital Age. New York, NY: Harry N. Abrams; 2006.

Sellar W. The Directory of Essential Oils. Essex, UK: Random House; 1992.

Travell JG, Simons DG. Myofascial Pain and Dysfunction: The Trigger Point Manual Vol. 1. Baltimore, MD: Williams and Wilkins; 1983.

Unschuld PU. Medicine in China: A History of Ideas. Berkeley and Los Angeles, CA: University of California Press; 1985.

Unschuld PU, Nan Ching: The Classic of Difficult Issues. Berkeley and Los Angeles, CA: University of California Press; 1986.

Walker BG. The Book of Sacred Stones: Fact and Fallacy in the Crystal World. San Francisco, CA: HarperCollins Publishers; 1989.

Wallnöfer H, von Rottauscher A. Chinese Folk Medicine and Acupuncture. New York, NY: Bell Publishing Company, Inc.; 1965.

Watson L. Lifetide. New York, NY: Bantam Books; 1980.

Worwood VA. The Complete Book of Essential Oils and Aromatherapy. Novato, CA: New World Library; 1991.

Index

Page numbers followed by 'f' indicate figures and 't' indicate tables.

347

Printed in the United States
By Bookmasters